ON CALL
Psychiatry

ON CALL

Psychiatry

4th Edition

CAROL A. BERNSTEIN, MD

Professor of Psychiatry and Neurology
Vice Chair for Education and Director of
  Residency Training
New York University School of
  Medicine/NYU Langone Health
New York, New York
Past President, American Psychiatric Association

MOLLY POAG, MD

Director of Medical Student Education
  in Psychiatry
Clinical Associate Professor of Psychiatry
New York University School of Medicine
New York, New York

MORT RUBINSTEIN, MD

Clinical Associate Professor of Psychiatry
New York University School of Medicine
Deputy Associate Chief of Staff,
  Mental Health
VA New York Harbor Healthcare System
New York, New York

CHRISTINA AHN, MD

Clinical Assistant Professor Department of
Psychiatry
New York University School
  of Medicine
New York, New York

KATHERINE F. MALOY, MD

Clinical Assistant Professor
Department of Psychiatry
New York University School
  of Medicine
New York, New York

PATRICK YING, MD

Assistant Professor
Department of Psychiatry
Director
Psychiatry Resident FGP Program Director
ECT Program New York University School
  of Medicine
New York, New York

ELSEVIER

ELSEVIER

1600 John F. Kennedy Blvd.
Ste 1800
Philadelphia, PA 19103-2899

ON CALL PSYCHIATRY, FOURTH EDITION ISBN: 978-0-323-53109-2

Previous editions copyrighted 2006, 2001, and 1997.

Library of Congress Cataloging-in-Publication Data

Names: Bernstein, Carol A., editor.
Title: On call psychiatry / editors, Carol A. Bernstein, Molly Poag,
    Mort Rubinstein, Christina Ahn, Katherine F. Maloy,
    Patrick Ying.
Other titles: On call series.
Description: 4th edition. | Philadelphia, PA : Elsevier, [2019] | Series:
On
    call series | Preceded by Psychiatry / [edited by] Carol A. Bernstein ...
    [et al.]. 3rd ed. c2006. | Includes bibliographical references and index.
Identifiers: LCCN 2018001818 | ISBN 9780323531092 (pbk. : alk. paper)
Subjects: | MESH: Crisis Intervention | Emergency Services, Psychiatric |
    Handbooks
Classification: LCC RC480.6 | NLM WM 34 | DDC 616.89/025–dc23
LC record available at https://lccn.loc.gov/2018001818

Executive Content Strategist: James Merritt
Senior Content Development Manager: Kathryn DeFrancesco
Publishing Services Manager: Catherine Jackson
Senior Project Manager: Daniel Fitzgerald
Design Direction: Amy Buxton

Printed in the United States of America
Last digit is the print number: 9 8 7 6 5 4 3

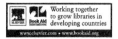

Preface

On Call Psychiatry was first developed by the general psychiatric residency training program at the New York University School of Medicine 20 years ago as a practical guide for clinicians who deal with psychiatric emergencies while on call. We have retained a situational approach to the organization of this book, because psychiatric signs and symptoms are frequently evident long before the patient's diagnosis has become clear. We hope that this book will continue to serve as a useful manual for psychiatrists and other mental health professionals and for physicians from other disciplines. We also look forward to feedback from our readers.

Revisions in this edition include new chapters on "Telepsychiatry" and "Cross-Cultural Issues"; Appendices on the Montreal Cognitive Assessment (MoCA) and on updated detoxification protocols on opiates, benzodiazepines, and alcohol; and an extensive update of all chapters.

Foreword

Since the publication of the first edition of *On Call Psychiatry,* this book has remained faithful to its original mission: to serve as a practical resource for psychiatrists, other physicians, and mental health professionals who deal with psychiatric emergencies while on call. Since its initial printing, knowledge of *Psychiatry's* neuroscience foundation, of psychopharmacology, and of evidence-based practice have all expanded. Our health care delivery system has changed dramatically, with an increased focus on decreasing inpatient length of stay, decreased availability of inpatient psychiatric beds, and increased acuity in psychiatric and other emergency services, intensive care units, and other inpatient services. Physicians providing emergency care now need to provide increasingly complex, cost-effective, and compassionate care for more critically ill patients, many at increased risk of violence, 24 hours per day, 7 days per week. The psychiatric house staff of New York University School of Medicine have risen to these challenges by producing an updated guide to the assessment, management, and treatment of patients in emergency and inpatient settings, which is both practical and grounded in rigorous scientific evidence. Their knowledge and skills have been developed and tested while responding to challenging psychiatric emergencies and crises while on call in the diverse clinical facilities affiliated with New York University. These hospitals serve patients from every ethnic and socioeconomic group, suffering from every diagnosable psychiatric illness, often with co-occurring complex medical and substance abuse disorders, involvement in the criminal justice system, and inadequate access to resources. Under these challenging conditions, carefully supervised by experienced attending psychiatrists, our house staff are expected to diagnose, treat, and manage their patients; to provide consultation to other disciplines; and to give direction to the patient's multidisciplinary team. Drawing on these valuable educational and training experiences, our house staff have written a book that translates what they have learned into concise recommendations, which will enable multidisciplinary clinicians to manage successfully the psychiatric emergencies of their patients. The text provides comprehensive coverage of the most common symptom-based medical and psychiatric emergencies, including psychosis, agitation, substance withdrawal, and delirium. It also addresses common medicolegal concerns, such as capacity assessment, the use of seclusion and restraint, and the initial response to abuse, neglect, and physical and sexual trauma.

We are confident that readers of this edition of *On Call Psychiatry* will find inside its pages the knowledge that they need to provide superb and compassionate emergency care.

We commend the authors for their commitment to medicine's educational mission and for their willingness to transform their challenging clinical experiences into sound and wise guidance for their colleagues.

Charles R. Marmar, MD
Lucius N. Littauer Professor
Chair
Department of Psychiatry
New York University Langone Medical Center
New York, New York

Mary Anne Badaracco, MD
Chief of Psychiatry
NYC Health and Hospitals/Bellevue
Professor and Vice Chair
Department of Psychiatry
New York University Langone Medical Center
New York, New York

Contributors

Elizabeth Allan, MD
Resident Physician
Department of Psychiatry
New York University School
    of Medicine
New York, New York

Bem Atim, MD
Fellow
Department of Child and
    Adolescent Psychiatry
New York University School
    of Medicine
New York, New York

Diya Banerjee, MD
Resident Physician
Department of Psychiatry
New York University School
    of Medicine
New York, New York

Laura Black, MD
Resident Physician
Department of Psychiatry
New York University School
    of Medicine
New York, New York

Janice Chou, MD
Resident Physician
Departments of Psychiatry
    and Neurology
New York University School
    of Medicine
New York, New York

Jillian Copeland, MBA, MD
Clinical Instructor
Department of Psychiatry
New York University School
    of Medicine
New York, New York

Elizabeth Dohrmann, MD
Resident Physician
Department of Psychiatry
New York University School
    of Medicine
New York, New York

Kristin Gill, MD
Resident Physician
Department of Psychiatry
New York University School
    of Medicine
New York, New York

Fayrisa Greenwald, MD
Resident Physician
Department of Psychiatry
New York University School
    of Medicine
New York, New York

Allison Grossman, MD, MPH
Resident Physician
Department of Psychiatry
New York University School
    of Medicine
New York, New York

Amanda Paige Harris, MD
Child and Adolescent Psychiatry
    Fellow
Clinical Instructor
Department of Child and
    Adolescent Psychiatry
Hassenfeld Children's Hospital at
    NYU Langone
New York, New York

Louisa Hong, MD
Clinical Instructor
Department of Psychiatry
New York University
New York, New York

Kathryn Keegan, MD
Resident Physician
Department of Psychiatry
New York University School
    of Medicine
New York, New York

Katherine Kerr, MD
Resident Physician
Division of Child and Adolescent
    Psychiatry
Department of Psychiatry
UCLA-Semel Institute for
    Neuroscience and Human
    Behavior
Los Angeles, California

Omar Khan, MD
Resident Physician
Department of Psychiatry
New York University School
    of Medicine
New York, New York

Maya Koenig-Dzialowski, MD
Resident Physician
Department of Psychiatry
New York University School
    of Medicine
New York, New York

Jesse Koskey, MD
PGY3 Resident
Department of Psychiatry
New York University School
    of Medicine
New York, New York

Danielle La Rocco, MD
Child and Adolescent Psychiatry
    Fellow
New York University School
    of Medicine
Department of Child and
    Adolescent Psychiatry
New York, New York

Samantha J. Leathers, MD
Attending Physician
Department of Psychiatry
Bellevue Hospital
New York, New York

Erin Li, MD
Psychiatry Resident
New York University School
    of Medicine
Department of Psychiatry
New York, New York

Megan Ann V. Mendoza, MD
Resident Physician
Department of Psychiatry
New York University School
    of Medicine
New York, New York

Eugene Mortison, MD
Resident Physician
Department of Psychiatry
New York University School
    of Medicine
New York, New York

Rita Ouseph, MD
Resident Physician
Department of Psychiatry
New York University School
    of Medicine
New York, New York

Acknowledgments

We would like to thank the editors of previous editions of *On Call Psychiatry:* Drs. Waguih IsHak, Brian Ladds, Ze'ev Levin, Ann Maloney, and Elyse Weiner. We are indebted to Charles Marmar, MD, Lucius N. Littauer Professor and Chair of the Department of Psychiatry at the New York University School of Medicine, Mary Anne Badaracco, MD, Vice Chair and Director of Psychiatry at Bellevue Hospital Center, David Ginsberg, MD, Vice-Chair for Clinical Affairs and Director of Psychiatry at NYU Langone Medical Center, Adam Wolkin, MD, Vice Chair and Associate Chief of Staff for Mental Health at the NY VA Harbor Healthcare System, and Donald Goff, MD, Vice Chair for Research and Director of the Nathan Kline Institute, for their ongoing support and commitment to psychiatric education. We would also like to acknowledge the invaluable support of our friends and families as well as our trainees, faculty, and supervisors, who have been a constant resource. Finally, we remain humbled by and deeply grateful to our patients, who are our finest teachers and without whom none of this would be possible.

Palak S. Patel, MBBS
Resident in Combined Psychiatry/
    Neurology Program
Departments of Psychiatry and
    Neurology
New York University Langone
    Medical Center/Bellevue
    Hospital Center/VA NY
    Harbor Health Care System
New York, New York

Yona Silverman, MD
Fellow
Department of Child and
    Adolescent Psychiatry
New York University School
    of Medicine
New York, New York

Rubiahna L. Vaughn, MD, MPH
Clinical Assistant Professor
New York University School
    of Medicine
Director of External Relations
    and Attending, Consultation—
    Liaison Psychiatry
Tisch Hospital, New York
    University Langone
    Medical Center
New York, New York

Jennifer Zhu, MD
PGY-4, Chief Resident
Adult Psychiatry Residency
New York University School
    of Medicine
New York, New York

Structure of the Book

PHONE CALL

Questions

Pertinent questions to assess the urgency of the situation.

Orders

Urgent orders to be carried out before the housestaff arrives at the bedside.

Inform RN

RN to be informed of the time the housestaff anticipates arrival at the bedside.

ELEVATOR THOUGHTS

The possibilities in the differential diagnosis to be considered by the housestaff while on the way to assess the patient (i.e., while in the elevator).

MAJOR THREAT TO LIFE

Identification of the major threat to life is essential in providing focus for the subsequent effective management of the patient.

BEDSIDE

Quick Look Test

The quick look test is a rapid visual assessment to place the patient into one of three categories: well, sick, or critical. This helps determine the necessity for immediate intervention. Other relevant information:

- Vital signs
- Selective history and chart review
- Selective physical examination

MANAGEMENT

The Appendices consist of reference items that we have found useful in managing calls.

Contents

Approach to Emergency Psychiatric Evaluation

The purpose of this book is to provide an organized overview of the knowledge and problem-solving approaches relevant to the most common emergencies that arise in the course of providing psychiatric care. Psychiatric providers inevitably face unexpected emergencies in outpatient offices, inpatient units, emergency department (ED) wards, and consult services. In all environments the management of psychiatric emergencies starts with safety. Triage, formulation, and disposition follow, keeping in mind that the true nature of the emergency may not be plain to see. An informed, systematic approach is a prerequisite to life-saving emergency psychiatric care. This chapter discusses an overall approach to evaluating a psychiatric emergency.

By definition, a psychiatric emergency involves dangerousness on the part of a patient to himself or herself or to others. Acute agitation is the most obvious emergency and can incorporate both danger to self and others—for example, a delirious postoperative patient pulling out his intravenous (IV) lines and swinging them at others. Often less obvious, but no less dangerous, are suicidal ideation, inability to care for self, and homicidal ideation. All of these emergencies are discussed in detail in their respective chapters; here we provide an overview of the general principles and steps involved in psychiatric emergency response.

One principle that is difficult to describe—and probably difficult to accept for scientific-minded physicians—is instinct. Although we often make much of the unconscious verbal clues that patients provide us when formulating their personality structures or drives, clinicians may tend to overlook their own countertransference or instincts in emergency settings. However, if a patient makes you uncomfortable, pay attention! A clinician's "gut" feelings are likely the result of an assimilation of subtle and key unconscious or subconscious information and experiences that do not translate verbally into the language of risk assessment but are no less vital to safety.

Logistically, safety can be maximized by following practices common to emergency or inpatient psychiatric settings. Patients should be searched and interviews conducted in a room free of potential weapons, such as intravenous poles, sharps, or glass. Clinicians should allow the patient to enter the room first, and then sit closest to, but not blocking, the door, so that the clinician can easily escape or be assisted by other providers or security if necessary. If the patient is too agitated or menacing to be seen in a closed room, find a relatively private space within a larger setting where you will not become trapped with the patient. Clinicians should not hesitate to terminate the interview to get security backup if they feel uncomfortable. It may be appropriate to have staff prepare medication and restraints based on your phone triage of the consult. A one-to-one watch may be required until more stable arrangements can be made if there is any chance of immediate self-harm, elopement, or violent behavior. Finally, clinicians should remember that the safest thing to do may be to defer the interview and return for further assessment after the patient's level of acute agitation has subsided.

Triage

The ability to triage quickly and accurately is a "must-have" skill for any busy on-call psychiatrist. Our colleagues in critical care use "Airway, Breathing, Circulation" to prioritize their triage assessments. In psychiatry, we too can follow the ABC model.

AGITATION/ALERTNESS

The first step in evaluating a psychiatric patient is to assess the level of agitation and alertness. How severe is the agitation? Does the patient's level of agitation need to be addressed before evaluation can safely proceed? If there is an acute level of dangerousness, the clinician may need to consider medications to help the patient calm down or restraints/seclusion if less restrictive options fail. Is the patient arousable, alert, and oriented, with stable vital signs? The clinician should recognize signs of delirium or altered mental status and not delay treatment of potential life-threatening illnesses, such as an accidental heroin overdose or an evolving delirium tremens. If any potentially dangerous physical abnormality is suspected, the clinician should consult internal medicine or emergency medicine colleagues promptly.

BEWARE OF MASQUERADING MEDICAL CONDITIONS

After ruling out life-threatening emergencies that would require emergent transfer, the clinician should perform a thorough medical evaluation. Behavioral or emotional difficulties are often the first manifestations of serious illness. The clinician should check medications, vital signs, laboratory data, and radiologic evidence for medical causes of psychiatric morbidity and consider the patient's past medical history. Abnormal vital signs should lead to consideration of infection, cardiovascular abnormalities, neuroleptic malignant syndrome, withdrawal syndromes, poisoning, or toxicities of medication. A thorough history and physical examination may implicate seizures, delirium, dementia, poisonings, adverse drug reactions, neurologic conditions, or even pancreatic or brain tumors as the cause of the presenting psychiatric symptoms. Electrolyte abnormalities may induce mental status changes, as can central nervous system events, autoimmune or endocrine disorders, withdrawals, and infections. Liver pathology invites a consideration of alcohol-related disease and hepatic encephalopathy. Numerous medications can affect the central nervous system, so review the patient's current medication regimen carefully. When available, check beta-human chorionic gonadotropin (beta-HCG), human immunodeficiency virus (HIV), thyroid function, B12/folate levels, rapid plasma reagin, and urine toxicology.

CONSIDER A WIDE DIFFERENTIAL OF PSYCHIATRIC DIAGNOSES

After the patient's immediate safety has been addressed and acute medical conditions ruled out, consider psychiatric disorders. In embarking on any psychiatric assessment, a few key aspects of the case should be kept in mind. First, who is the patient? A quick once-over can reveal signs of disorganization or paranoia, anxiety, medical instability, or intoxication. Second, what is the setting? Did this patient walk into the emergency room on his or her own, or was the patient brought in by an ambulance? If this is an inpatient on a nonpsychiatric floor, what is the reason for the consult and why has the primary team chosen this moment to call for help? Remember that the initial diagnosis/assessment of the patient will greatly affect the patient's treatment and ultimate disposition. It is often impossible to make a certain diagnosis on the first assessment because many disorders can look identical on initial presentation. The clinician should not limit the differential prematurely; including all of the diagnostic possibilities early on can ensure that a patient is not misdiagnosed. Common types of diagnoses encountered include substance-induced psychiatric symptoms, mood disorders with or without psychotic symptoms, primary psychotic disorders, and personality disorders.

Patient Interview

Within the psychiatric interview, the mental status examination is one of the most useful tools for assessment. A competent mental status examination provides not only rationale for treatments implemented but also a snapshot of the patient at a particular point in time, thereby allowing for the establishment of longitudinal benchmarks in the care of the patient. Although the clinician can at times tailor the examination to the demands of the differential diagnosis at hand, it is also important to always assess for safety. A thorough mental status examination will ultimately guide treatment decisions.

Collateral Information

Interventions are primarily informed by effective history taking, and collateral sources of information are essential components of a patient's history. A medical emergency is a valid reason for waking someone up in the middle of the night; family members, former psychiatrists, old medical records/discharge summaries, case managers, and nursing staff on the patient's floor can prove invaluable, particularly when the patient wishes to deny all past psychiatric history to avoid admission to the hospital. Clinicians should remember—and remind collateral if necessary—that in an emergency setting the Health Insurance Portability and Accountability Act (HIPAA) allows for sharing of relevant patient health information (PHI) without a patient waiver.

Documentation

Documenting all interactions with the patient or a collateral informant is a must both for quality patient care and for medical-legal reasons. Statements made about suicidality, homicidality, hallucinations, or delusions must be recorded just as clinicians record vital signs or physical examination findings. Any change in mental status, emergence of new symptoms, or initiation of a new treatment all have significant clinical implications that can only be fully appreciated by a thorough and chronologic record of events. Risk assessments should be documented and include analysis of stable and dynamic risk factors, a treatment plan that addresses modifiable risk factors, and the clinician's reasoning in reaching a disposition. Good documentation reflects "reasonable professional judgment" and demonstrates that the clinician has thoughtfully considered clinical aspects of the case.

Final Thoughts

The full range of psychiatric symptoms and diagnoses makes the job of the psychiatric clinician fascinating; keeping in mind the vastness of potential differential diagnoses of acute behavioral changes makes it possible to provide thorough and safe evaluations. Developing a sound differential helps to ensure the provision of competent care for the psychiatric patient. A thorough understanding of mental illness comes with time and detailed evaluation and study; however, in the emergency setting the focus is on the immediate assessment and provision of a safe channel for management and diagnosis of the situation at hand. Interventions made during psychiatric emergencies can save lives as powerfully as in any other specialty of medicine.

Suggested Readings

Atakan Z, Davies T. ABC of mental health: mental health emergencies. *BMJ.* 1997;314:1740–1742.

Hughes DH. Suicide and violence assessment in psychiatry. *Gen Hosp Psychiatry.* 1996;18:416–421.

The Role of the On-Call Psychiatric Consultant

On-call physicians are often asked by medical or surgical colleagues to evaluate their patients. This chapter addresses some of the major issues involved in such consultations.

Being an Effective Consultant

The job of being a psychiatric consultant can be exciting, intellectually challenging, and unpredictable. These evaluations involve evaluating patients with diverse conditions, including those with a long-standing psychiatric illness, a new complaint, or a sudden change in mental status. At times, such consultations will be requested not because of the patient's distress but because of the distress the patient's behavior has generated among the staff (e.g., experiences of projective identification with a patient who has borderline personality disorder). A wide range of questions may occur to the consultant including: Why is this patient so agitated? Why does this patient have an altered mental status? Does the patient have the capacity to consent to surgery? Is this patient safe to be discharged from the hospital?

The role of the on-call consultant has two main components including:

- The relationship with the patient:
  - Remember that in most cases the consultant provides a one-time evaluation only and that follow-up care will be provided by the regular consultation-liaison team. The relationship between the consulting physician and the patient is established with the goal of answering the consult question.
- The relationship with the primary treatment team (this includes but is not limited to):
  - Generating a differential diagnosis and recommendations that help the consultee.
  - Supporting the team in managing challenging cases (e.g., managing personality disordered patients, recommending restraints for agitated patients, deciding on the need for

involuntary psychiatric treatment, and recommending guardianship for demented patients).
- Functioning in the liaison role, which entails (1) linking medical and psychiatric knowledge and skills to enrich the diagnostic formulation of the patient and help the team to generate a comprehensive treatment plan; (2) facilitating communication between the patient and the consultee; (3) educating the consultee about psychiatric issues impacting the presentation; (4) providing information about determination of decision-making capacity and involuntary psychiatric hospitalization.

Quick suggestions in doing an on-call psychiatric consultation:
1. Clarify the consult question with the consultee
2. Preform a guided evaluation of the patient
3. Create a differential diagnoses
4. Gather pertinent collateral from the chart, outpatient psychiatrist, family, friends, coworkers, etc.
5. Communicate key findings and recommendations to the team
6. Assist the team in implementing the recommendations as necessary
7. Cogent documentation of findings and recommendations

Reasons for Consultation

The most common requests for consultation involve the following categories of psychiatric diagnoses.

PSYCHIATRIC DISORDERS MANIFESTING AS MANAGEMENT PROBLEMS

Suicidal ideation or behavior
Violent threats or behavior
Personality disorders
Assessment of decision-making capacity

PSYCHIATRIC DISORDERS DUE TO MEDICAL CONDITIONS

Delirium, dementia, amnesia, and other cognitive disorders
Psychotic disorder due to a general medical condition
Mood or anxiety disorder due to a general medical condition

SUBSTANCE-RELATED DISORDERS

Intoxication
Withdrawal
Substance-induced psychiatric disorder

PSYCHOPHARMACOLOGIC MANAGEMENT

Drug-drug interactions
Adverse effects
Pharmacokinetic profiles

OTHER PSYCHIATRIC DISORDERS

Any preexisting psychiatric disorder (e.g., schizophrenia)
Neurodevelopmental disorders (e.g., intellectual disabilities, autism spectrum disorders)
Sleep disorders

PSYCHIATRIC DISORDERS RELATED TO ADJUSTMENT TO MEDICAL CONDITIONS

Adjustment disorder with depressed mood, anxious mood, disturbance of emotions and conduct, etc.
Psychological factors affecting other medical conditions

PSYCHIATRIC DISORDERS MANIFESTING AS MEDICAL CONDITIONS

Somatic symptom disorder
Illness anxiety disorder
Conversion disorder (functional neurologic symptom disorder)
Factitious disorder
Malingering

How to Complete a Consult

PHONE CALL

The first contact with the team requesting the consult could be via an electronic order, an in-person request, a page, or a phone call to the consultation service. Independent of the specific hospital system, it is important to speak directly with the consultee via phone or in person. Use the questions below to guide communications with the requesting service.

Questions

1. How urgent is the situation? Is there any immediate danger to the patient, the staff, or others? Is the patient suicidal or homicidal?
2. What questions does the requesting physician want answered?
   For all consults, except emergencies, speak directly to the physician ordering the consult. The requesting physician should be able to provide a brief history of the patient, including the reason

for admission, current medical status, presence or absence of substance abuse or known psychiatric conditions, current medications, and the presenting problem. At times, the requesting physician will need help to define what questions need to be addressed. Make sure to note the physician's name and pager number.

3. Is the patient aware that a psychiatric consultation has been ordered? If not, ask the physician to let the patient know.
4. What is the patient's primary language?

If the patient does not speak English, arrange for an interpreter or for the use of a telephone interpreter.

Orders

Order one-to-one observation if needed. Based on the information obtained in the initial phone call, it may be important to have the patient placed on one-to-one observation until an in-person assessment can be conducted. Potential reasons for immediate institution of a one-to-one may include the following:

Patients who are:

1. suicidal
2. homicidal
3. disorganized
4. agitated
5. at a high risk for elopement
6. delirious and repeatedly pulling at intravenous (IV) lines, nasogastric tubes (NGTs), or wound dressings or trying to get out of bed

Staff may resist initiating a one-to-one for a variety of reasons, including negative countertransferential feelings towards the patient. In these situations, it is useful to remind the treatment team that one-to-one observation is recommended to maintain patient and/or staff safety. After the patient is examined, one-to-one observation may be discontinued if indicated.

Medication orders should be deferred until the examination has been conducted, whenever possible. If consulted for extreme agitation, it may be helpful to ask that intramuscular or intravenous medications be available on the floor and ready for use.

Collecting Data

Collecting data can be difficult, especially in emergency situations. Immediate interventions may need to be taken before a thorough evaluation can be done. When time permits, the following process can be followed.

CHART REVIEW

Review the patient's history systematically, noting the chief complaint; the history of present illness; the medical, surgical, and psychiatric history (including alcohol and substance abuse); the physical examination and laboratory test results; and the mental status at admission, if available. Note the circumstances of the admission (e.g., emergency transport, came in with friend or spouse), and read any social work and nursing evaluations. Review the patient's course in the hospital, and read the events leading up to the request for the current psychiatric consultation. Pay special attention to any recent changes in medications or medical status, notes from other consult services, and the nursing notes. Note whether the patient has "do not resuscitate" (DNR) status and/or any other advance directive information, and the identity of the patient's emergency contact.

INFORMATION FROM THE TREATMENT TEAM

Inquire from the nursing staff about the patient's behavior; attitude toward illness, staff, and visitors; compliance with medication regimen; and sleeping and eating habits. It is also helpful to personally observe the patient's behavior both alone and with the treatment team. This process helps to consolidate the team approach. It is also helpful, if time allows, to personally observe the patient's interactions with the physician and with staff.

OTHER SOURCES OF INFORMATION

Check old charts whenever possible; patients may have had a psychiatric evaluation during a previous admission.
- If the patient also receives outpatient treatment at the same facility, try to obtain those records for review, and check which outpatient medications the patient has been taking. Sometimes this will reveal a psychoactive medication that was discontinued at the time of an admission.
- Contact family or friends, especially when dealing with delirious, intoxicated, demented, or disorganized patients.
- Call the patient's regular psychiatrist or therapist, after obtaining consent if the patient is no longer in the emergency room. Valuable data may be obtained, especially about longitudinal history and current psychotropic medications.
- Be sure to get a release of information before obtaining collateral information in nonemergent settings.
- Reviewing old records is most helpful where patients are unable to provide this information themselves.

MAJOR THREAT TO LIFE

Immediate threats to life include patients who are acutely agitated and potentially harmful to themselves or others, those who are suicidal, or those who are refusing life-saving treatment (a decision-making capacity consult). Separate chapters in this book cover each topic. In addition, remember that any sudden and acute change in mental status may be a sign of an underlying life-threatening medical condition (e.g., cerebrovascular accidents, seizure, hypertensive encephalopathy, endocarditis, arrhythmia). Be alert to the patient's medical history, and do not assume that all medical conditions that might influence the mental status have been ruled out.

BEDSIDE

Quick-Look Test

Does the patient look comfortable, distressed, agitated, or depressed? Is the patient resting in a bed, in a chair, or pacing the floor? Is the staff calm or anxiously awaiting your intervention?

Establishing Rapport

After establishing that the patient is safe in their environment, introduce yourself. Explain that the patient's physician has asked you to perform a psychiatric examination, and explain the reason for it. Try to make the patient as comfortable as possible in the situation before proceeding with the interview.

Some patients may be resistant to the idea of seeing a psychiatrist, particularly if they have not been notified in advance by the requesting physician that a psychiatric consultation was ordered and told the reasons for the consultation.

The Interview

Focus on the presenting problem and on the patient's current mental status and cognitive exam. Consider having a copy of the neurocognitive assessment (e.g., the Montreal Cognitive Assessment [MOCA], the Folstein Mini-Mental State Examination [MMSE], Saint Louis University Mental Status Examination [SLUMS], or Confusion Assessment Method for the intensive care unit [CAM-ICU]) because it may be an important baseline measurement for later consults.

Consult Note

The consultation note should be clear, concise, and goal directed. Begin with a summary statement that is a one- or two-sentence description of the patient and the reason given by the treatment team for the consultation, such as, "This is a 32-year-old male with no known psychiatric history who was admitted for pneumonia 1 week ago. Psychiatric consult was requested because the patient has been eating very little for the past 2 days, appears depressed, and is refusing all medical tests." After this, your note should contain the following sections.

HISTORY OF PRESENT ILLNESS

Summarize the interview with the patient, including the patient's chief complaint and his or her own explanation of the current situation, preferably in the patient's own words. Note the patient's report or denial of relevant subjective symptoms such as hallucinations or suicidal ideation. Include a summary of the hospital course.

Past Psychiatric History
Past Medical History
Medications
Allergies
Pertinent Labs, Imaging and Studies
Mental Status Exam
Cognitive Testing and Neurologic Exam

ASSESSMENT

The assessment should include all data used to reach a preliminary conclusion or differential diagnosis. The assessment is the part of the note that will likely be read first and perhaps the only section read by the treatment team. Avoid abbreviations for psychiatric terms, and clarify the reasons for the assessment in a few sentences so that the medical team understands the conclusions and recommendations. Give only the most relevant information, including positive and negative findings. List the provisional diagnosis or differential diagnoses (in descending order of likelihood) using the *Diagnostic and Statistical Manual of Mental Disorders*, 5th edition (DSM-V) nomenclature.

Avoid drawing premature conclusions or offering an overly simplistic explanation of the patient's behavior (e.g., writing that the patient is somatizing), which may lead to neglect of associated medical problems.

RECOMMENDATIONS

The usefulness of the psychiatric consultation is directly proportional to the clarity of its recommendations. Here are some points to take into account when writing recommendations:

Recommendations for management of acute problems should be given first. Precautionary measures for suicide, such as a one-to-one observation and medications for agitation or insomnia, should be implemented immediately, leaving less pressing decisions to the regular consultation team (e.g., prescribing an antidepressant).

Give specific recommendations for tests or additional consultations that are needed to clarify the diagnosis (e.g., arterial blood gases or neurology consult), and be specific about which psychiatric or medical conditions you are considering.

General recommendations for ongoing psychiatric care while in the hospital should be given, if appropriate. Provide pager information, including the number of the consultation service that will monitor the patient during regular work hours. If the patient does need to be monitored by the consultation service in an ongoing way, this should be clearly documented, along with information about how and by whom follow-up will be arranged. Finally, be very clear about recommendations for follow-up care on stabilization of the patient's medical condition. Is he or she a candidate for admission to the psychiatric unit? Will he or she need a referral to another health care facility at the time of discharge, such as an outpatient psychiatric clinic or drug and alcohol treatment program?

Communicating With the Treatment Team

It is best to communicate conclusions personally to the requesting physician and to the nursing staff whenever possible. This helps to clarify the plan for the treatment team and resolve further questions immediately. Although the primary physician is responsible for following up on recommendations, immediate personal contact will facilitate an integrated team approach to the patient's management.

Whenever possible, use the consultation as an opportunity to inform and educate the requesting physician and staff about the psychiatric issues related to patient care, such as management of difficult patients, identification of patients who are at psychiatric risk, the use of psychotropic medications, therapeutic interventions (supportive or behavioral techniques, such as limit setting), and countertransference issues.

Follow-Up

The consultation process is incomplete without appropriate follow-up. Be sure to inform the regular consultation-liaison team of your consultation. This is especially important for patients seen on weekends or holidays.

Suggested Readings

Leigh H. The function of consultation liaison psychiatry. In: Leigh H, Streltzer J, eds. *Handbook of Consultation-Liaison Psychiatry*. 2nd ed. New York, NY: Springer; 2015:11–14.

Querques J, Stern TA. Approach to consultation psychiatry: assessment strategies. In: Stern TA, Fricchione GL, Cassem NH, Jellineck MS, Rosenbaum JF, eds. *Handbook of General Hospital Psychiatry*. 6th ed. Philadelphia, PA: Elsevier; 2010:7–14.

Psychodynamic Issues

The psychiatrist on call faces a number of emotional challenges in interacting with patients, families, and other medical personnel. This chapter focuses on some of the more difficult emotional reactions that may arise in the psychiatrist and outlines ways to address and manage them.

General Principles

Psychodynamic terms have numerous definitions, and are used in different ways in different contexts. However, some of the basic psychodynamic terms and principles that are useful in understanding the ways that people relate to one another emotionally include:

1. Transference—the feelings the patient has for the psychiatrist. Some of these arise in response to the psychiatrist as he or she truly is in reality, whereas some of these are reactions to characters in the patient's past (parents, teachers, bosses, etc.) being displaced on to the psychiatrist.
2. Countertransference—the feelings aroused in the psychiatrist in reaction to the patient (or the family of the patient, other medical professionals, etc.). Some of these responses may originate from the patient, such as in a psychiatrist's reaction to a patient who has a history of malingering presenting to the emergency room and demanding to be seen immediately. In other cases, countertransference may come from the life of the physician, such as when a patient who has recently lost a family member reminds the on-call psychiatrist of a recent loss in his or her own life.
3. Conscious mind—the part of the "mind" that is experienced as the ongoing thought process during waking hours of the day.
4. Unconscious mind—the part of the "mind" that is not always accessible as conscious thoughts (although there are glimpses of it visible in dreams) but that also influences behavior and decisions people make.
5. Defense mechanisms—patterns of behavior that help people deal with the day-to-day conflict between what they really want

for themselves and the demands of real life (e.g., financial obligations, the needs of other people).

All people use defense mechanisms to cope with the stressors of everyday life, and generally do so at an unconscious level (i.e., the person is usually not aware of the behavior). The kinds of defense mechanisms used (often considered on a scale from "immature" to "mature"), or the rigidity with which they are used, make them adaptive or maladaptive. For instance, many people adaptively use the mature defense of humor as a way to deal with what might otherwise be an overwhelming situation (e.g., a cancer patient who has lost her hair because of chemotherapy joking about how she will not have to spend money on the hairdresser for a while). However, sometimes less adaptive defenses come to the fore, especially in psychiatrically ill patients, or even generally well-functioning patients who are under medical stress. Understanding some of these more immature defenses through the case examples in this chapter may help the on-call psychiatrist deal with patients and other people on call. The defense mechanisms illustrated will include:

1. Denial—refusing to acknowledge the reality of a situation without being consciously aware of this refusal.
2. Projection—attributing one's own ideas or emotions to another person.
3. Projective identification—one person has unconsciously "telescoped" his or her feelings "into" a second person, and the second person has unconsciously taken these feelings as his or her own.
4. Splitting—seeing people as being either all good or all bad; this involves the process of idealizing and/or devaluing another person.
5. Somatization—focusing on the body to avoid focusing on emotions.
6. Help-rejecting complaining—asking for help with a problem and then rejecting the help that is offered.

Recognizing defenses used by a patient on call serves essentially two purposes for the psychiatrist:

1. If the psychiatrist is able to recognize what is happening, he or she can then exercise a choice to not react countertherapeutically. For instance, if the psychiatrist finds himself or herself on the bad side of a split (i.e., devalued), he or she can try to understand why the patient is reacting in this way. Being able to think this through will provide valuable information about the patient and help the psychiatrist develop the short-term alliance that is essential in dealing with patients on call.

2. The goal of the psychiatrist on call is not necessarily to help patients change, but to help them through their current current emergency safely. Therefore recognizing defenses and attempting to encourage the patient to use his or her most adaptive ones in the present is often helpful. Alternatively, if no adaptive defenses seem to be available to the patient in the moment, the psychiatrist can sometimes use awareness of the patient's maladaptive defenses to educate other staff on how to best deal with the patient acutely.

Clinical Examples

These clinical examples will further elucidate some of the principles listed and demonstrate the ways they will be useful on call.

TRANSFERENCE

The psychiatrist on call is paged to the emergency room to perform a suicide risk assessment. The patient is a young woman who took 30 tablets of acetaminophen after her boyfriend threatened to leave their relationship. The psychiatrist attempts to conduct an interview, but the patient is reluctant to answer questions and accuses the psychiatrist of not listening to her, although the consultant believes he or she has been listening quite attentively.

It is important to keep in mind that patients bring their own sets of experiences to every situation and what may seem like an irrational reaction at first glance can have meaning. Perhaps this young woman was sexually abused in her childhood, and no one would listen to her complaints. Although in emergency room evaluations the psychiatrist will not always have time to get to the underlying meaning of the patient's reaction, he or she will do well to keep in mind that a patient may be acting on transference feelings and thus avoid taking the reactions of the patient personally. In addition, with the patient noted previously, one may use the knowledge of transference to realize that with this patient it is especially important to take a little extra time to build an alliance—otherwise the evaluation will be a very poor one because the patient will not really be able to cooperate.

COUNTERTRANSFERENCE

The on-call psychiatrist is called by the inpatient psychiatry unit to evaluate a patient who is complaining to the staff that he has not seen a doctor for hours. The psychiatrist arrives on the floor to speak to him and finds that he wants a stat dose of lorazepam for "anxiety." Chart review and discussions with the staff reveal that over the past several days the patient has made such requests on a frequent basis and the staff suspects that the patient is seeking drugs for pleasure or a "high." Not wanting to assume that this is the case right away, the psychiatrist attempts to speak with the patient about his symptoms but is immediately challenged by the patient: "You look way too young to be caring for me. Are you even a doctor?" The patient continues, "You are obviously too inexperienced to really know how to treat someone with anxiety as severe as mine." The psychiatrist begins to feel angry, a feeling that is obviously justified on some level; however, this patient most likely brings up anger in many people by the ways he interacts with them and thus alienates even those who try to help him.

Without being able to understand what is happening, the psychiatrist is liable to act on his or her anger in any number of ways, such as saying something rude or terminating the interview early, with the associated risk of the patient then acting on his difficult-to-manage feelings by becoming agitated. However, the psychiatrist who is aware that his or her feeling of anger is informative rather than just a random emotion can handle this difficult situation without "losing his or her cool." Self-reflection on one's own vulnerabilities and insight into what kinds of words and actions may be most personally upsetting will prove invaluable in the field of mental health, especially in an on-call setting.

DENIAL

Returning to the patient in the first example: after the on-call psychiatrist forms an alliance with the woman and she begins to answer the clinician's questions, she states she wants to leave the hospital immediately because she now feels completely better. This may be true, but at the same time she may be engaging in denial. Assuming she has never done anything like this previously, she is now faced with the troubling information that she has the capability to become so upset that she considers taking her own life. To avoid dealing with this, she may attempt to push this danger out of her conscious awareness.

It is very important for the psychiatrist to be aware that denial may be at play. A patient's denial may be so powerful that the psychiatrist may also begin to believe that the patient does not need help and miss important information that this woman is at risk for further self-injurious behavior. Despite the patient's assertion, the psychiatrist must proceed through the same risk assessment that he or she would otherwise. Denial is also often used in patients who are actively abusing alcohol or other substances. By walking through the benefits and risks of continued use rather than joining in denial, the on-call psychiatrist may be able to bring some of the conflict out of unconscious denial and into their conscious mind to enable informed decision-making about continued substance use.

PROJECTION AND PROJECTIVE IDENTIFICATION

An intern on the medical floor calls for a consultation on a young patient admitted for a complicated urinary tract infection who is also depressed. The psychiatrist mentions to the intern at the time of the initial consult that she may not be able to see the patient immediately because of an urgent situation in the emergency room. Over the course of the next half hour, the intern pages the psychiatrist twice more, and the psychiatrist hurries to the medical floor somewhat exasperatedly. She goes to the nursing station to speak with the medical intern and review the chart before meeting the patient. While she is there, a middle-aged woman comes twice to speak to the intern and nurses about when the psychiatrist is coming. The psychiatrist realizes that this woman is the mother of the patient she has been called to see. Although the patient's mother seems relatively calm as she speaks with the staff, she mentions to the intern, "I know how anxious you are to have the psychiatrist come."

The patient's mother seems to be unconsciously projecting her anxiety state onto the intern through her behavior, perhaps because she has difficulty dealing with her own anxiety. The intern is internalizing and acting on this anxiety in having trouble giving the psychiatrist a reasonable amount of time to come to the floor before paging the psychiatrist again. Being aware of the intrapsychic mechanisms at play may help the psychiatrist on call avoid internalizing this "infectious" anxiety and so not act on it.

One also often sees a more primitive level of projection in dealing with patients in an acute state of psychosis. Such a patient may state to the psychiatrist, "You want to hurt me." The psychiatrist has no such intent, but the patient is unable to realize this. The patient is actually projecting his or her own aggressive urges onto the psychiatrist because these urges are overwhelming to the patient. It is important to know this is happening—if the patient is unable to respond to reassurance and gentle reality testing, such as the psychiatrist reminding the patient of the intention to be helpful, the patient may act aggressively because he or she feels threatened. It would be important in such a situation to take steps to ensure the safety of both the patient and staff (e.g., giving the patient a quiet place to relax, asking for security help if necessary, or offering medication).

SPLITTING

Continuing the story of the young woman in the first example, she expressed denial about the need for psychiatric treatment but now agrees to stay for the necessary medical observation given that she has made an overdose attempt. The psychiatrist is paged again several hours later after the patient is admitted to the medical floor, where she has been put on one-to-one observation. She demands to speak to the psychiatrist on call; when the consultant arrives, she complains that she does not like having a staff member sitting with her all the time because "it is disrespectful of my privacy." The one-to-one aide taking care of the patient throws her hands up when approached by the psychiatrist for collateral information. She states that the patient has been demanding and hostile ever since arriving on the floor. In contrast, the nurse taking care of the patient has found the patient to be pleasant and appreciative each time she has entered the room and has difficulty understanding why the aide cannot seem to get along with the patient. The patient reveals to the psychiatrist that the nurse is "wonderful" in her opinion, but that the aide is "an undereducated excuse for a nurse."

The nurse and the aide are astutely picking up on the patient's disparate attitudes toward each of them and responding accordingly. The psychiatrist can help by speaking to both the nurse and the aide to validate their experiences of the patient and to provide psychoeducation about splitting processes. In a way, they are both right, and if they can each see both sides of the patient they will be able to see her more realistically and work with her more productively.

SOMATIZATION

Psychiatrists on call often encounter patients who present with physical symptoms that mask emotional issues. For example, an elderly man comes to the emergency room with complaints of stomach pain for the fourth time in a week. On his first three presentations, he received the full medical work-up including physical examination, laboratory tests, and radiologic studies, all of which were unremarkable. On his fourth presentation, the emergency room doctors begin to suspect something "psychological" may be going on. Although the psychiatrist must be watchful that other medical professionals do not automatically assume that physical complaints are emotional in nature (medical problems may be missed when this happens, especially when a patient has a prior history of a psychiatric diagnosis), in this case the work-up has already been obtained. The psychiatrist, in focusing on the patient's recent stressors and possible symptoms of depression, anxiety, or psychosis, may learn that one month ago his daughter who was living with him moved out into her own apartment and since then the patient has been having trouble with sleep and appetite. More recently, he began having stomach pain. When the psychiatrist asks about the stomach pain, the patient reveals that in the months following his wife's death several years ago he developed similar symptoms. Thus, the appropriate treatment, rather than further medical tests, is treatment of his mood symptoms. For this man, stomach pain serves the function of a defense by diverting his and everyone else's attention away from the intolerable feelings associated with his loss.

HELP-REJECTING COMPLAINING

A middle-aged man presents to the emergency room with a chief complaint of depression. He tells the emergency room physician that he has been feeling unwell for a few weeks and the consulting psychiatrist determines that his depression is severe enough to warrant admission because of his suicidal thoughts. The patient voluntarily signs into the inpatient psychiatry unit but expresses the worry that he will not be able to sleep. The psychiatrist suggests the use of a medication to help with sleep, but the patient declines, saying, "It will not help me anyway." At 9 PM the psychiatrist receives a call from the nurses that the patient is complaining of still not being able to sleep. The psychiatrist prescribes diphenhydramine, but when the nurses take it to the patient he refuses because he wants to wait to fall asleep on his own. The nurses call the psychiatrist again at 10:30 PM because the patient still cannot fall asleep. They have offered him diphenhydramine again, but he says that his outpatient psychiatrist prescribes that medication for him and that it does not always work. The psychiatrist offers to prescribe trazodone. When the nurses offer this medication, the patient reports feeling worried about feeling groggy in the morning and refuses. The psychiatrist is called again. In a moment of frustration, the psychiatrist thinks about giving the patient a neuroleptic, in part to punish the patient for his constant complaining and refusal of treatments offered.

In thinking about the situation a little more, this man seems to complain repeatedly and then find a way to reject the help that is offered. Perhaps the experience of being admitted to the psychiatric unit is overwhelming. Although the patient came to the hospital for treatment, he may be frightened, with mixed feelings about being there and may be acting out this internal conflict. One way of dealing with this patient is to return some control he fears he has lost by discussing what he thinks might be helpful rather than simply putting in orders for different sleep aids, all of which he may reject. Taking some time to sit with the patient and listen to his fears may relieve some of his anxiety. In the worst-case scenario, the psychiatrist may have to resign himself or herself to the fact that this patient may continue this way throughout the night. Understanding the explanation behind the behavior makes this situation more tolerable.

Conclusion

Knowledge of basic psychodynamic terms, how they may manifest clinically, and how to incorporate them into one's clinical thinking will make the call smoother for both the clinician and the patient.

Suggested Readings

Cabaniss D, Cherry S, Douglas CJ, Schwartz AR. Transference. In: *Psychodynamic Psychotherapy: A Clinical Manual.* New York, NY: Wiley-Blackwell; 2011a:217–232.

Cabaniss D, Cherry S, Douglas CJ, Schwartz AR. Countertransference. In: *Psychodynamic Psychotherapy: A Clinical Manual.* New York, NY: Wiley-Blackwell; 2011b:233–241.

Telephone Consultations

There are two types of telephone calls you should be familiar with when you are on call. Most calls will come from hospital staff (doctors, nurses) requesting a psychiatric consultation for a hospitalized patient. The other type of call may come from patients or family members outside of the hospital seeking advice. As an on-call psychiatrist with limited time, you need to handle both types of calls efficiently and prioritize consultations so that the more urgent cases are dealt with first.

This chapter does not address calls relating to medical concerns from a psychiatric service because these are discussed elsewhere in the book.

Psychiatric Consultations for Hospitalized Patients

When you get requests for consultations from various staff members in the hospital setting, always obtain the name and discipline of the person calling, as well as a way to reach them to communicate your recommendations. Patients who require a psychiatric consultation (or any specialty consultation) should first be triaged by the primary clinician in charge of their medical care.

The information you obtain upfront will set the tone for the remainder of the consult. You may not have another opportunity to reach the clinician who is calling for the consult or to obtain clarifying information. By developing a system for gathering information—and following it every time—you will ensure that you always get the basic information you need and ask for the information confidently. Your confidence will help to contain the team's anxiety, who may be calling because they are confused, scared, or otherwise uncertain of how to best care for their patient. We recommend obtaining the following information: patient's name, location, medical record number, presenting problem, and reason for consult. A brief summary of the hospital course thus far is also useful (Box 4.1).

BOX 4.1	Information to Obtain for All Consults

- Primary team discipline
- Caller's name and contact number
- Primary team contact information
- Patient's name
- Patient's location
- Patient's medical record number
- Presenting problem
- Reason for consult

Your goal while taking the initial consult information is to obtain enough data from the primary service so that you can be best prepared to arrive in the room. By getting a picture of what the patient's presenting symptoms are and the question the team is asking, you will not only be able to triage across cases, but you will also be able to begin to think of the relevant information you will need from the patient, staff, and collaterals to formulate the case.

The primary team should have a psychiatric question for you to answer so that you can provide a focused evaluation (Box 4.2). In instances when the team cannot formulate a reason for the consult, try to help them with questions regarding the patient's behaviors or symptoms. If they cannot answer your questions because they have not evaluated the patient, you should ask them to medically evaluate the patient and call you afterward so you can help to identify the question. Examples of things you should listen for in a medically ill patient include (1) agitated, violent, or out-of-control behavior, in which case the team may need your help for behavioral management; (2) a change in mental status or new-onset psychotic symptoms that may cause imminent danger to the patient or others and may suggest delirium; (3) acute risk of suicide, such as the presence of suicidal ideation or plans, depression, recent substance use, severe anxiety, or global insomnia; and (4) refusal to accept important medical evaluations or treatments requiring

BOX 4.2	Common Reasons for Emergent Psychiatric Consultation for Medically Ill Patients

- Concerns for agitation or dangerousness
- Change of mental status or new onset psychosis
- Concerns for patient safety (e.g., suicidality)
- Questions regarding patient capacity to refuse or consent to treatment
- Medication recommendations for chronic psychiatric illness in setting of new-onset medical or surgical illness

capacity assessment. If after prompting with questions about the patient, the team still cannot define a specific question for you, use your clinical judgment as to whether or not the patient must be seen emergently. Sometimes, the primary team has a vague sense that something is wrong and cannot verbalize their concerns specifically, in which case there may be danger lurking, and only you as the specialist can clarify the situation.

If you have several emergent consults pending and cannot see the patient immediately, always inform staff callers that you have other more urgent evaluations to perform and let them know the approximate time you will be available. This will alleviate anxiety and decrease resentment from the primary team. If the caller cannot wait for you to arrive in person, you may be able to advise him or her how to handle certain situations over the phone until you are available. For example, in case of an agitated patient who is trying to leave the hospital premises against medical advice, you can recommend that security be called to retain the patient and have the team offer the patient medication to calm the patient down. In case of a suicidal patient, you can have the patient placed on one-to-one observation. When the patient's decisional capacity is the question, you can inform the team that any physician is qualified to do an evaluation for treatment capacity if he or she cannot wait for your consult. If there will be a significant delay, you should communicate to the team that you will come as soon as possible, and have them page you again if the situation escalates, in which case you may need to respond to this request on an urgent basis.

You may get calls for nonacute, routine psychiatric problems at night, such as clearing a patient for discharge to a shelter, providing psychotherapy for a medically ill inpatient, or evaluating a patient with a chronic psychiatric illness who is not acutely ill. Ask the caller if the patient can be seen the next day by the consult-liaison team, because you are only available for urgent psychiatric problems and questions. If the caller agrees that this is clinically sound, you should inform him or her of the procedure to obtain the consultation for the next day. It is also useful for you to communicate all such requests to the daytime psychiatry service, because you may give some advance insight to the team, minimize the chance that the patient will "fall through the cracks," and obtain feedback from the team about what is acceptable to wait until the next day as different hospitals may have different thresholds for deferring consults.

Outside Calls

Occasionally, you may receive telephone calls from patients or family members outside the hospital seeking advice. Before you respond to this type of call, you need to know from the hospital administration whether or not you are responsible for these outside calls. Some hospital systems routinely direct all such calls to the psychiatrist on call and may provide malpractice coverage for these calls. At other facilities, it may be the protocol to direct the caller to a crisis hotline, 911, or the emergency room.

If you are responsible for outside calls, before engaging in any discussion with the caller you must obtain his or her full name, date of birth, telephone number, and current location. It is essential to get the person's contact information. In the event of an emergency, you can direct emergency medical service to the caller's location. If the caller refuses to give you this information, explain that this is routine procedure. If he or she continues to refuse and starts to tell you his or her problem, you should interrupt and say that you cannot take the call unless you have the necessary identification data and that you will otherwise have to direct him or her to call 911 or go to the emergency room.

Above answering the caller's question or responding to his or her concerns, your job is to query for any signs of acute dangerousness that may require a face-to-face evaluation. Try to determine if he or she is a patient at your hospital and if you can view his or her medical records to give you additional information as you take the call. Ask if he or she has a psychiatrist currently and for their doctor's contact information, which will provide more options for a follow-up plan. Remember: you will not know the person well enough to give treatment advice or do any type of psychotherapy on the phone. Never treat a patient or give medication recommendations over the phone. Giving medical advice could be considered establishing a doctor-patient relationship, which has implications for liability for any subsequent bad outcomes.

Try to establish the caller's concerns and the reason for the call at that specific time. Your questions should focus on any signs of imminent danger to self (e.g., suicidality), aggressive ideation or violence to others, and medical complications from psychiatric medications. Be direct with your questions about suicidal or violent ideation. If you suspect any dangerousness or you are not clear if an acute risk is present without a face-to-face interview, you must direct the person to the nearest emergency room. If the person refuses to go to the emergency room, you may need to call the police immediately. Try to keep the person on the phone while you direct someone else to make the 911 call. Remember, when in doubt of the person's safety, always take the conservative route and call the police. If the person agrees to go to the emergency room, when possible, ask permission to speak to a family member or friend who can help to ensure that the person follows up. If the caller is a family member or friend who is concerned about someone else, ask the caller if he or she feels the situation is unsafe or cannot leave the person alone for fear that person may harm himself or herself. In that case, it is best to advise the caller to contact 911 or to convince the person to go to the emergency room for an evaluation and accompany the person if possible.

For nonemergent calls, direct the caller to contact his or her psychiatrist during the day. If he or she is not already in treatment, you can give referrals to outpatient psychiatric clinics at your facility or elsewhere. If there is any concern about a drug reaction, explain your concern about the possible reaction and direct the patient to get evaluated immediately in an emergency room, if appropriate.

Be sure to document your phone calls. Jot down the identification data and summary of your assessment and outcome. You should also encourage the caller to give you permission to contact his or her treating physician to inform the doctor of the encounter for follow-up care.

Seclusion and Restraint

This chapter defines seclusion and restraint; outlines the indications and contraindications for these procedures; and provides step-by-step guidelines for the implementation, documentation, and discontinuation of seclusion and restraint for patients. Medication for the agitated patient, which often accompanies seclusion and restraint, is discussed in the management sections of the Agitated Patient, Violent Patient, and Psychotic Patient chapters.

General Principles

The regulations and procedures concerning the seclusion and physical restraint of patients vary from state to state and among different institutions within the same state. It is important for physicians to know the laws and policies governing seclusion and restraint in the states and the institutions in which they are working. Seclusion and restraint restrict a patient's movement, environment, and rights. These procedures, no matter how necessary, are often frightening for patients and are generally experienced in a negative way and as punishment. Given the increasing effort to provide restraint-free environments, locked seclusion and restraint should be used as a last resort and only to maintain patient and staff safety and/or to facilitate therapeutic intervention.

Literature Review

Fisher (see Suggested Readings) reached the following conclusions concerning the risks and benefits of these interventions:

Seclusion and restraint are efficacious in preventing injury and reducing agitation.

Some form of seclusion or physical restraints is necessary to maximize patient and staff safety in treatment settings for severely symptomatic individuals.

Restraint and seclusion may have deleterious physical and psychological effects on patients and staff.

Local nonclinical factors, such as cultural biases, staff role perceptions, and the attitude of hospital administration, have a substantial influence on rates of restraint and seclusion. Overall, Flammer et al. found that illness severity and violent behavior in the past 24 hours were the strongest predictors of restraint use, whereas voluntary admission status was the strongest protective factor.

In recent years, many hospitals have initiated restraint-reducing programs, with reported success, particularly with behavioral and cognitive-behavioral programs in children; however, systematic data are still lacking to identify the common elements of successful programs.

D'Orio et al. ascertained that a hospital program founded on principles of early identification and management of problematic behaviors was associated with a 39% reduction in the use of seclusion and restraint and an increase in compliance with hospital standards. Specifically, the program used two-way radios, which alerted staff when emergency codes were called, and continuous video monitoring by staff to enhance early identification, communication, and responsiveness. Although these measures may not be available where all residents train, residents should inquire about the particular safety measures in place at each facility. Often, units will have alert buttons that notify additional staff of a behavioral emergency immediately when pressed.

Jonikas et al. have shown that incidents of seclusion and restraint can be reduced by helping patients identify personal stress (or agitation), triggers, and individual calming measures during the initial evaluation. This worked in conjunction with staff education, focusing on factors that precipitate agitation and nonviolent means for its management.

Hellerstein et al. found that decreasing the initial time spent in restraint/seclusion before a new order for restraint/seclusion was placed, educating staff about patients at risk of restraint/seclusion, and implementing a coping questionnaire to assess patent preferences for dealing with agitation helped to decrease the use of restraint and seclusion.

Definitions

1. Seclusion
   a. Open seclusion: The therapeutic isolation of a patient. Methods of open seclusion include quiet time alone in a patient's room, in an unlocked time-out room, or in a partitioned area. Open seclusion represents the least restrictive form of seclusion. Most regulations referring to seclusion relate specifically to locked seclusion only.
   b. Locked seclusion: The therapeutic isolation of a patient in a locked room designed specifically for the purpose of confining an agitated individual.

2. Physical Restraint: A confining apparatus commonly composed of leather or canvas. When properly applied, restraints maximally restrict physical movement without threatening the integrity of the limb or body part being restrained. Restraint configurations include the following:
   a. Bilateral wristlets and anklets; also known as four-point restraint.
   b. Camisole controlling the upper half of the body with or without bilateral anklets.
   c. Chest strap with either of the above.
   d. Whole body restraints, such as safety suits, which contain the patient's entire body with the exception of the head.
   e. Posey vests—used on medical floors, these vests are applied to the torso and tied to the bed, to prevent patients from climbing out of bed

Please note that each of these restraints may not be available at all hospitals; residents should become familiar with the restraints used at their particular facilities.

Indications and Contraindications

INDICATIONS

Prevention of imminent harm to the patient or to others when other means are ineffective
Prevention of substantial damage to the physical environment
Indications for seclusion without physical restraint:
- Decreasing stimulation for an agitated, potentially violent patient
- Fulfilling a patient's request in appropriate circumstances, such as self-awareness of poor impulse control or low frustration tolerance

CONTRAINDICATIONS

For the convenience or comfort of staff
To punish a patient
Absolute contraindications specific to seclusion:
   The acutely suicidal patient (without constant observation)
   The patient with unstable medical status
   The delirious or otherwise neurologically impaired patient whose clinical status may decline when stimulation is reduced
   The restrained patient who cannot be adequately monitored for aspiration or circulatory impairment
Relative contraindications specific to seclusion:
   The self-mutilating patient (without constant observation)

The patient with a seizure disorder
The hyperactive patient at risk for exhaustion
The developmentally disabled patient (discussed next)

Special Considerations

DEVELOPMENTAL DISABILITIES

Patients with documented developmental disabilities are at higher risk for injury during restraint and seclusion procedures and during the actual period of the restraint and/or seclusion. Such patients may have underlying physical anomalies, particularly craniofacial and cardiac, that can further endanger their safety during restraint and seclusion procedures. Developmentally disabled persons may not be able to understand why such interventions have been imposed and may not be able to communicate their discomfort while in restraints or while being secluded.

CHILDREN

Mechanical restraint and locked seclusion are not generally used for young or small children. A technique called therapeutic holding is often used to help control agitated and dangerous children. This typically entails hugging a child from behind, whereby his or her arms are held securely to each side. This technique requires training, and the physician on call should be familiar with the procedures used at his or her facility.

VICTIMS OF ABUSE

Patients with a personal history of abuse may experience restraints and locked seclusion as especially traumatic, particularly if some aspect of their initial traumatic event is re-created during the sequence of the locked seclusion or restraint procedure. Qualitative research shows that patients report retraumatization with use of restraints and may perceive the practice itself as unethical. Staff members should be sensitive to issues pertaining to patients who are victims of abuse.

DELIRIOUS PATIENTS

The use of restraints has been identified as a significant predictor of mortality in patients with delirium and may also exacerbate patients' disorientation. Restraints should be avoided when possible by using verbal redirection and one-to-one monitoring. A study of intubated patients in the intensive care unit (ICU) showed that those who received pharmacologic treatment of their delirium within 24 hours of onset spent a shorter median time in restraints, were extubated sooner, and had a shorter ICU/hospital length of stay.

ELDERLY PATIENTS

The use of physical restraints has been identified as a significant predictor of length of hospital stay for patients 60 years and older.

PATIENTS WITH SIGNIFICANT MEDICAL CONDITIONS

The risks and benefits of restraint use should be carefully considered in patients with significant medical conditions that may become aggravated with the use of restraints. For example, restraints that are fastened tightly may cause a patient on warfarin to bleed.

Physician Response

Seclusion and restraint are often initiated on an emergent basis by nurses or other trained staff on the psychiatric ward. In such cases, continuation of the seclusion or restraint will require a physician's face-to-face assessment, documentation, and written order. The physician should monitor the status of the patient with a face-to-face examination at least every 4 hours; a shorter time interval is preferred and can help to reduce the time spent in restraints. Again, it is important for physicians to be familiar with the guidelines of each facility where they will be on call regarding the time parameters for physician notification and response. Most organizations have a time limit beyond which delays must be explained in the documentation.

The treatment team may look to the physician to make a judgment regarding whether or not seclusion and restraint should be used and, if so, what type of seclusion or restraint should be used. The following questions should be considered to guide the decision-making process surrounding the implementation of seclusion and/or restraint and should be addressed in documentation of the event:

1. Is the seclusion or restraint proportional to and suitable for the patient's mental status and behavior?
2. Is the patient being treated with respect?
3. Has the patient's autonomy been respected?
4. Is the seclusion or restraint the least restrictive alternative to maintain safety and to achieve therapeutic goals?

Procedure for Locked Seclusion and Restraint

Locked seclusion and/or restraint procedures are undertaken when a patient remains agitated and potentially dangerous after less restrictive measures have failed. Subduing a dangerous individual should be a team effort involving a sufficient number of adequately trained professionals such as nurses, physicians, mental health technicians, and often security personnel. The physician on call must be notified immediately so that he or she may go to the area as quickly as possible.

TEAM

The team consists of trained staff members. The team leader instructs the others throughout the procedure while maintaining truthful and reassuring dialogue with the patient. The patient's experience of seclusion and restraint is related to caregivers' attitudes toward the patient, to the degree to which the patient has been educated on the use of seclusion and restraint, and to the level of confidence the patient has in treatment providers. A staff member with whom the patient is more familiar may be perceived by the patient as more comforting and therefore may be a good choice for the team leader.

Ideally, one team member may be assigned to each of the patient's limbs, and a fifth is assigned to protect and control the patient's head. One team member (a nurse) should be assigned to provide the necessary medications. The exact number of staff required for the procedure depends on individual factors such as patient size and level of agitation. All of the assignment decisions should be made before the procedure is implemented.

After a leader has been chosen, he or she should assign tasks among the remaining staff. An individual who is too agitated and volatile to comply with less restrictive alternatives will generally resist seclusion or restraints. The presence of a large team and backup such as hospital security or police is referred to as a "show of force." This is often helpful in encouraging compliance. Some facilities require the presence of hospital security or police before the initiation of seclusion and restraint procedures, although whether such persons may participate in the actual procedure varies among facilities. Sometimes the team decides on a prearranged signal to begin the procedure. If necessary, the leader may use this signal to indicate the initiation of physical force to achieve seclusion or restraint.

LOGISTICS

Before the patient is approached, the environment must be cleared of other patients and physical hazards. A team member should prepare a bed or stretcher suitable to accommodate mechanical restraints, with restraints on standby. Injectable medication should be drawn and made available as indicated. To maximize safety, all staff involved should remove any ties, scarves, dangling jewelry, and similar items and wear latex gloves. Face masks for the team members, particularly the one assigned to the patient's head, may be useful in the event the patient starts spitting.

APPROACH

When approaching the patient, the team members should gather around the leader and calmly present themselves in a confident yet caring, nonthreatening, nonprovocative manner. The leader should provide the patient with a simple explanation of why seclusion or restraint is required. The leader should explain the risks of using restraints, the alternatives to restraints, and explain the criteria necessary for the restraints to be removed. Only the leader should be speaking to the patient at this time. The patient should be given the option to voluntarily comply with the least restrictive measure clinically appropriate to the situation. The patient should be allowed a limited amount of time to follow directions. This conversation may not be possible due to the patient's level of agitation. The length of this discussion should be assessed by the leader on a case-by-case basis.

Negotiating with the patient at this point is ill advised. Doing so may lead to further escalation and violence.

IMPLEMENTATION

If the patient does not comply, the leader should give the prearranged signal, indicating that the team will proceed with the use of force to achieve seclusion or restraint. Ideally, four team members should then take hold of and control each limb as previously assigned. The patient should then be carefully brought to the ground, in a supine position, on a padded surface if available. The head should be controlled, using caution to avoid skull, neck, and facial injuries while attempting to protect staff from biting or spitting. Special attention to safety is imperative, particularly when dealing with physically challenged, elderly, pregnant, and developmentally disabled patients, who may be more vulnerable to injury in the process.

The patient should then be transferred to the seclusion room or the area where restraints are applied. Head, trunk, and extended legs are lifted simultaneously on the count of the team leader. Extended arms are held securely to the sides of the patient as he or she is moved and placed on a bed or stretcher.

Intramuscular medication should be injected at the point of maximal immobilization. This often occurs during the period after the takedown and the application of restraints.

If the patient has been brought to the seclusion room without the application of restraints, team members should release the limbs sequentially after the administration of intramuscular medication, as indicated. The staff members should be careful to assess the patient's status as each limb is released and should be careful to keep an eye on the patient as they leave the seclusion room.

Of note, most staff injuries related to patient care occur during the implementation of seclusion and restraint. The incidence of these injuries can be decreased with improved training programs for staff in the area of violence prediction, violence assessment, restraint and seclusion procedures, and self-defense.

DEBRIEFING

A debriefing session should follow as soon as possible after the procedure. This involves a gathering of all the staff involved in the seclusion and/or restraint procedure for the purpose of discussing the events. Debriefings serve to:

- Analyze and critique the intervention process
- Discuss feelings and concerns about the incident
- Solidify the cohesion of the team
- Prevent future misuse of imposed restrictions (this includes either implementing seclusion and restraint when not appropriate or avoiding these modalities when they are indicated)
- Allow for team assessment in the event of a staff injury

PATIENT

Although it is the safety of the patient, other patients, and the staff that is of utmost importance, the physician and the staff should proceed with as much care and compassion as possible. What is accurately perceived as necessary by the staff may be perceived as embarrassing, humiliating, and frightening for the patient, even when he or she believes the intervention to be necessary. Staff should help patients to discuss the experience. A dialogue with the patient should begin while he or she is still in restraints. It is also important to be prepared to discuss the intervention with other patients on the unit who will likely react differently according to their own personal histories with restraints and seclusion. Those patients who have never been restrained or secluded often feel safer seeing a potentially violent patient removed from the open space of the ward. Those who have been restrained or secluded in the past may feel angry when they see another patient undergoing a similar procedure.

Documentation

Seclusion and restraint procedures command the same intensity of charting as do other emergency patient care situations.

HOSPITAL FORMS

Hospitals will either use paper or electronic medical records (EMRs). If an EMR is used, electronic orders and templated notes may fulfill the institution's initial charting obligations. On-call physicians should verify which electronic order and documentation is required by their institution. The nursing staff is an excellent resource and may be able to help the physician become familiar with the process.

NOTE

An event note with the physician's observations is extremely important even if it is not required. The following information should be included in the documentation of a seclusion or restraint procedure, regardless of the charting format:

- The patient's last name and first name
- Chart or medical record number
- Date and time of incident
- The time of the physician's arrival on the scene
- Justification for a late arrival on the scene if it is longer than the required time after notification; the nursing staff is required to note the time of physician notification, and it is wise for the physician to do so as well
- The precipitating event, in a detailed fashion, specifying dangerous behavior
- Failure of the patient to respond to less restrictive measures such as verbal redirection and/or offers of oral medication
- The restrictive measures implemented (e.g., locked seclusion, four-point leather restraints)
- Clinical justification for these measures, which includes pertinent findings on mental status examination and specific behavior
- Length of time the restriction will be imposed; this must include the starting and ending times
- Behavioral goals to be met by the patient to have the restriction lifted, such as the ability to stay in an open room calmly for 20 minutes; this must also be verbalized to the patient. Plan for helping patient regain control to discontinue restraints

- Patient response to the procedure; again, an attempt should be made to continue a dialogue with the patient while in restraint or seclusion
- The name and (electronic) signature of the physician
- It is also useful to document that the patient and his or her environment have been checked and that potentially dangerous materials have been removed
- Documentation of family notification if prior consent given

ELECTRONIC OR WRITTEN ORDER

The order for seclusion or restraint must include the date and time the restriction was imposed and the time it will be lifted. Phrases such as "2 hours" are not considered sufficiently specific. Indicate exactly the type of restriction to be implemented and the justification for its use (e.g., for assaultive or self-injurious behavior). Some states require release criteria to be included in the written order. Seclusion and restraints may never be ordered on an as-needed basis.

Continuation and Discontinuation of Restrictions

The physician should be aware of the hospital's and jurisdiction's policies regarding requirements for one-to-one observation and for the frequency with which physicians must see or enter notes on a patient. These patients are usually placed on one-to-one observation given the need to monitor patient safety.

Periodic progress notes should include a mental status examination; references to the patient's physical stability, including vital signs and ability to tolerate restraints; and the patient's progress toward meeting the expectations that will facilitate the lifting of restrictions. Restrictions may be removed once a secluded or restrained patient has fulfilled preestablished criteria and appears clinically stable such that he or she no longer presents a threat to self, others, or the environment.

An individual in locked seclusion or restraints should gradually have restrictions lifted contingent on the ability to maintain calmness and safety. The suggested procedure for ending seclusion is to open the seclusion room door for 15 to 30 minutes while asking the patient to stay inside.

Safety Warnings

Leaving only one extremity in restraint can lead to avoidable patient injury and is not permissible in many jurisdictions. Restraints should be periodically checked by nursing staff.

Some situations involving mechanical restraints or seclusion affect the patient's temperature regulation. This can add to the effects of antipsychotic medications on temperature regulation, potentially leading to hyperthermia or neuroleptic malignant syndrome.

Suggested Readings

Bai X, Kwok TCY, Ip IN, Woo J, Chui MY, Ho FK. Physical restraint use and older patients' length of hospital stay. *Health Psychol Behav Med.* Jan 2014;2(1):160–170.

D'Orio BM, Purselle D, Stevens D, Garlow SJ. Reduction of episodes of seclusion and restraint in a psychiatric emergency service. *Psychiatric Serv.* 2004;55:581–583.

Fisher WA. Seclusion and restraint: a review of the literature. *Am J Psychiatry.* 1994;151:1584–1591.

Flammer E, Steinert T, Eisele F, Bergk J, Uhlmann C. Who is subjected to coercive measures as a psychiatric inpatient? A multi-level analysis. *Clin Pract Epidemiol Ment Health.* Jul 2013;9:110–119.

Grover S, Ghormode D, Ghosh A, et al. Risk factors for delirium and inpatient mortality with delirium. *J Postgrad Med.* Oct–Dec 2013;59(4): 263–270.

Hellerstein DJ, Staub AB, Lequense E. Decreasing the use of restraint and seclusion among psychiatric inpatients. *J Psychiatr Pract.* Sep 2007; 13(5):308–317.

Jonikas JA, Cook JA, Rosen C, Laris A, Kim JB. A program to reduce use of physical restraint in psychiatric inpatient facilities. *Psychiatr Serv.* 2004;55:818–820.

Michaud CJ, Thomas WL, McAllen KJ. Early pharmacological treatment of delirium may reduce physical restraint use: a retrospective study. *Ann Pharmacother.* Mar 2014;48(3):328–334.

Scanlan JN. Interventions to reduce the use of seclusion and restraint in inpatient psychiatric settings: what we know so far a review of the literature. *Int J Soc Psychiatry.* Jul 2010;56(4):412–423.

Strout TD. Perspectives on the experience of being physically restrained: an integrative review of the qualitative literature. *Int J Ment Health Nurs.* Dec 2010;19(6):416–427.

Assessment of Capacity and Other Legal Issues

This chapter discusses issues of capacity, competency, informed consent, and confidentiality, as well as types of psychiatric admissions, involuntary treatment, and discharge. State laws vary, so the physician should be familiar with the statutes and institutional policies that govern the legal aspects of psychiatry in their jurisdiction of practice. The hospital administrator or legal representative will often be able to provide information about state requirements.

Capacity and Competency

The terms "capacity" and "competency" are often used equivalently in the hospital setting; confusingly, even the seminal article that guides psychiatrists' assessment of capacity (by Appelbaum and Grisso, written in 1988) uses the two terms interchangeably, but they actually represent different concepts. Capacity describes a person's ability to make informed decisions about treatment. It is task-specific and can change over the course of illness. Innumerable factors, such as a person's response to stress, the medications that he or she is receiving, or an underlying and potentially treatable mental or medical illness can impair someone's capacity. The assessment of decisional capacity can be a time-consuming task and often requires the analysis and integration of ethical, legal, and clinical issues.

Competency is a legal term that is considered the legal correlate to capacity. It refers to the minimum cognitive ability required to carry out a legally recognized act, medical or nonmedical—for example, managing property, entering a contract, or giving informed consent. The law presumes that all patients except minors are competent unless there is convincing evidence otherwise. Although the consulting psychiatrist will be asked to perform a "competency evaluation," only a judge can determine competency; instead, the consultant may provide an estimate of what a judge might decide by assessing decisional capacity.

CAPACITY CRITERIA

To have capacity, a patient must be able to demonstrate the following four skills:

1. Communicate a choice: The patient must be able to convey a preference with respect to his or her care. This concept requires that the patient is able to maintain choices long enough for them to be implemented; a patient who frequently reverses his or her decision may lack this skill. Memory impairments, thought disorders, and extreme ambivalence may underlie a patient's inability to communicate a stable choice.

2. Understand relevant information: The patient must be able to receive and retain the information that is provided. He or she should be able to describe the details of the treatment, its risks and benefits, possible alternatives, and why it is necessary or recommended. The patient should also understand that he or she is the one responsible for making the decision. Commonly, a consultant may find that the patient does not understand the proposed intervention because he or she has not been adequately educated by the primary team on the choice at hand. However, if the team has indeed informed the patient of risks and benefits, cognitive impairments, such as in memory, attention, or intelligence, may prevent a patient from demonstrating this ability.

3. Appreciate the situation and its consequences: Appreciation of the situation implies that the patient can assess, according to his or her own values, the impact of his or her current condition. It differs from the previous skill in that the patient should understand how the current situation will influence not only acute outcomes, but also his or her future quality of life, with or without treatment. Collateral information, when available, should be used to assess whether the patient's current decision is consistent with his or her previous cultural, social, and/or religious beliefs. Distortions in thinking that can be found in illnesses, such as depression or psychotic disorders, for example, may impair a patient's appreciation of a given situation and its consequences.

4. Manipulate information rationally: The patient must be able to use logical thought processes to compare the risks and benefits of various treatment options and reach a decision. After assessing this skill, the clinician should be able to understand why the patient chose one option over another. Underlying psychiatric illnesses, such as psychosis or depression, and transient states, such as panic or anger, may limit a patient's ability to think through a situation logically.

The strictness with which the criteria for decisional capacity are interpreted often depends on the risk that the patient assumes with his or her decision; the higher the risk, the more stringently the criteria are applied. This is also known as the sliding scale approach. For example, the risks of refusing vital signs are generally lower than the risks of refusing amputation of a gangrenous limb, so the capacity standard will be lower in the former case.

It is important to remember that a competent patient has the right to self-determination and to make a decision with which his or her physicians or family members disagree. In 1914, in *Schloendorff v. New York Hospital,* Justice Cardozo wrote, "every human being of adult years and sound mind has a right to determine what shall be done with his or her body."

INFORMED CONSENT

A concept related to decisional capacity is informed consent. Derived from the ethical principle of autonomy, it is the process by which a patient agrees to or refuses a medical intervention. To give informed consent, a patient must first have capacity to make the decision. The patient must also consent to the procedure knowingly and voluntarily. To agree to treatment knowingly, a patient must be provided with all of the relevant information regarding his or her condition, including the diagnosis, risks, and benefits of the recommended treatment options, alternative treatment options (or no treatment), and the prognosis. To agree voluntarily to treatment, a patient must not be coerced into treatment. Coercion can be subtle, for example, by neglecting to disclose or realistically state the risks and benefits of various treatment options.

There are four exceptions to the requirement of informed consent in a treatment setting:

1. Incapacity (alternate decision maker required): As discussed, if a patient lacks capacity, he or she cannot consent to an intervention; surrogate decision makers are discussed later in this chapter.
2. Medical emergency (no consent required): However, even in this context, if the treatment team has prior information that the patient would refuse a life-saving intervention, the treatment team may not act against the patient's previously voiced wishes (e.g., in the care of a Jehovah's Witness who previously expressed that he or she would refuse a blood transfusion).
3. Patient waiver (patient waives right to informed consent): In this case, the patient must have previously made his or her desire to avoid hearing about risks and benefits of treatment

interventions known. Decisions are deferred to the judgment of the physician or another party.

4. Therapeutic privilege (when revealing information to the patient would clearly harm that patient): Under this exception, a physician would have to determine that the process of informed consent would be preventatively deleterious to the patient. Laws regarding this exception vary between jurisdictions.

CAPACITY CONSULTS: TREATMENT REFUSAL AND ACCEPTANCE

Treatment refusal is a common reason for a team to request a capacity consult, but it is NOT the job of the physician on call to obtain consent from the patient or to convince the patient to consent to treatment. Rather, the consultant must assess whether the patient has the capacity to make a decision and thus to provide informed consent or refusal.

Rarely, the situation may arise in which treatment acceptance results in a capacity consult. In this case, the treating physician has concerns that the patient has consented to a treatment but may not have the capacity to do so. For example, a team may request a consult to evaluate a patient for somatization disorder prior to an exploratory surgery meant to investigate symptoms that remain unexplained. The same criteria for assessing capacity apply. In the situation of questionable capacity to consent, the patient may be overestimating the benefit-to-risk ratio of the intervention, whereas a patient refusing treatment may be underestimating the benefit-to-risk ratio of the recommended intervention.

QUESTIONS FOR THE TEAM

The following are questions to consider asking the treating physician when he or she initiates a request for a psychiatric consultation regarding decisional capacity:

- What is the specific decision in question?
- If it involves a procedure or treatment, what are the details, risks and benefits, and likely outcomes of that procedure or treatment, and what are the alternatives?
- What is the urgency of the procedure?
- Is the patient suffering from a medical condition that may be impairing his or her cognition?
- Has the physician, family, or any staff member noted abnormalities in the mental status of the patient?
- What is the physician's and other health professionals' sense of the patient's decisional capacity?

- Which medications are the patient taking?
- Has the physician attempted to obtain informed consent?
- What exactly was the patient told about the procedure?
- Does the patient have a legal guardian?
- Who is the next of kin?
- Does the patient have a living will or advance directives? Is there a health care proxy?

When a decisional capacity assessment is requested, the evaluating physician should ensure that the request refers to a specific patient decision, such as refusing a medical procedure or signing out against medical advice. Different decisions require different levels of capacity, so a patient may demonstrate capacity for one task while lacking it for another.

Similarly, because of the narrow definition of decisional capacity and its potentially fluctuating nature, the treating physician and other health professionals must be informed that the psychiatric assessment will be valid only for the decision for which it was requested and for the time period during which the evaluation was performed. Therefore, if the treating physician does not feel that the recommended treatment is sufficiently urgent to pursue an alternate decision maker, a consult may be more appropriate when the clinician feels the clinical situation dictates that he or she do so.

The referring physician should also delineate the plan of action in the event that the patient is found either to have capacity or not. This discussion will clarify the urgency of providing the recommended treatment and will help to prioritize on-call tasks. In turn, considering both scenarios will help to determine the standard of capacity. For example, if the patient is found not to have capacity, is the referring physician willing to locate an alternate decision maker to proceed with the treatment urgently, or is he or she willing to forego treatment until the patient's capacity is restored? These situations of intermediate urgency are the ones most often encountered by the on-call psychiatrist because physicians usually do not consult for a determination of capacity if emergent intervention is indicated, and they often do not ask for a consult if they feel the recommended treatment is trivial.

EVALUATING THE PATIENT

The assessment of the patient should begin with a thorough history including a review of the patient's chart, laboratory test results, and medications. A detailed mental status exam is also warranted. When treatable illnesses such as depression, delirium, psychosis, and pseudodementia are present, lack of decisional capacity may be temporary. If possible, it is best to attempt to treat the underlying condition, restore capacity, and then allow the patient to make decisions about health care. However, in some cases the urgency of the treatment and the risk of delay may not allow time to fully treat the underlying illness.

The assessment should be focused on the decision in question and the patient's ability to become engaged in the decision-making process. When possible, it is often helpful to conduct a capacity evaluation with the primary team present, as the treating physician can give the most accurate information about why an intervention is being offered, its risks, benefits, and alternatives. The following is a list of questions that can help in assessing the patient's understanding and preferences.

- What is the patient's understanding of the medical problem?
- What is the patient's understanding of the physician's recommendations?
- What is the patient's understanding of the physician's rationale?
- What is the patient's choice?
- What is the patient's rationale for the choice?
- What does the patient anticipate as the consequences of exercising his or her choice?
- What is the patient's understanding of the risks and benefits of the recommended treatment? Of alternative treatments? Of no treatment?

COMMUNICATING THE ASSESSMENT

When the assessment has been made, findings should be discussed with the primary team and clearly documented in the patient's chart. If the patient has decisional capacity but refuses treatment or disagrees with the treatment team's recommendations, it may be helpful to explain the concept of self-determination and the rights of the patient to the treatment team in a nonconfrontational and clear manner. After a patient is found to lack decisional capacity, it is the duty of the treatment team to find out whether the patient has a health care proxy or any advance directives that might help to dictate how to proceed. Advance directives are legal documents created when the patient was competent; examples include forms such as a living will, health care proxy, and durable power of attorney over health care.

A living will is the most familiar of the advance directive documents. These documents are very specific and refer to situations such as administering cardiopulmonary resuscitation, giving medications, and providing or withdrawing life-supporting measures (a Do Not Resuscitate order is a form of an advance directive). Unfortunately, advance directives are often vague and may be easily contested if there is concern that the directives may not be in the best interest of the patient. In the United States, only approximately 20% of patients have any form of advance directives or health care proxies.

A health care proxy form or a durable power of attorney for health care are advance directives that empower another person to make decisions for the patient. In the absence of both of these documents, the primary team should investigate if the patient has a legal guardian already appointed. In most cases, the surrogate decision maker is tasked with choosing a course of action that, to the person's best knowledge, is what the patient would have chosen for himself or herself if he or she had the capacity. This concept is known as the substituted judgment standard. In some exceptional cases, such as when a court-appointed legal guardian has no knowledge of what the patient would have wanted, or in the treatment of minors, the surrogate decision maker makes the decision in the patient's best interest. This guideline is known as the best interest standard.

In many cases, there are no advance directives and no appointed legal guardian. Most states have statutory surrogate laws that allow a family member to make decisions for an incapacitated patient, often in a hierarchical order of which family member should be consulted first (e.g., a spouse, then an adult child, then a parent). In some cases, when surrogate decision makers disagree, or if treatment interventions are complex and unclear, a formal guardian may be appointed by a court.

The primary team must rely on the laws of the state and the policies and procedures of the facility in which the patient is being treated in determining a surrogate decision maker and deciphering how to proceed. In the case of an emergency (generally described as threatening life or limb), there is no requirement to find a surrogate decision maker until the emergency has passed. If the team has any uncertainty about identifying a surrogate decision maker, they should contact the hospital administrator or legal representative. If administrative consent is required, it is helpful to also discuss the case with the hospital's risk management department.

Psychiatric Admission, Treatment, and Discharge

ADMISSION

There are four basic types of admissions to a civil psychiatric facility, whether an inpatient psychiatric ward or a psychiatric state hospital. Each state may have different laws governing the mechanisms of admission; different hospitals across the state use one or more of these mechanisms. The on-call consultant should be aware of the local laws and facility policies governing the admission of psychiatric patients.

1. Informal (pure) admission: Informal admission is the same as a general hospital admission and constitutes the patient's verbal agreement to be admitted. The patient is free to enter and leave at will, which includes being discharged immediately on request. Most psychiatric hospitals do not use this mechanism of admission.

2. Voluntary (conditional) admission: A competent person seeking psychiatric care may apply in writing for admission to most psychiatric facilities. The patient requires examination by a physician or mental health professional to be admitted. Once admitted to the facility, there is a period of time (dictated by state statute, usually three to five days) during which the patient may be detained against his or her will to assess for safety in the event he or she requests discharge. If discharge is considered unsafe by the treatment team, the team may take the patient to court for an involuntary civil commitment hearing. This procedure is explained to the patient through a formal notice of status and rights when he or she signs in to the hospital.

3. Emergency admission: In the case of the emergency admission, the patient is in need of immediate hospitalization (usually because the patient is deemed a danger to himself, herself, or others outside of the hospital) but is unable or unwilling to make the decision to enter the hospital voluntarily. This type of admission is time-limited and is usually of shorter duration than an involuntary admission.

4. Involuntary admission: A patient must have a mental illness to be considered appropriate for involuntary psychiatric admission; beyond this, criteria vary from state to state, but common criteria include dangerousness to self or others or inability to meet one's basic needs. In addition, in many states the patient must be unwilling to sign in voluntarily or lack the appropriate capacity to do so.

In the case of involuntary admission a physician, friend, relative, or, in some jurisdictions, a community agency director may submit an application for admission to the courts. When a patient is involuntarily admitted, the physician is not "committing" him or her; rather, the doctor is initiating a hospitalization that will eventually bring the patient before the court to determine further retention or release. During this time, the patient must have access to legal counsel and be provided with a formal notice of legal status and rights. A judge can release the patient at any time if it is determined that the commitment criteria are not met. This type of admission is also time-limited and varies by state.

Occasionally, a patient will present to an emergency room requesting psychiatric admission, but the consulting psychiatrist will not feel that an admission would be necessary or even helpful for that patient. There is no requirement to admit a patient merely because he or she requests admission. In such situations, it is important to document the reasons why hospitalization is being refused (see "Discharge"). Alternatively, if a patient refuses voluntary admission and the psychiatrist feels that an admission would be helpful, the psychiatrist should not threaten the patient with an involuntary admission unless the psychiatrist feels confident that that patient actually meets the criteria for that status.

INVOLUNTARY TREATMENT

Psychiatric patients have a right to refuse treatment even if they have been hospitalized against their will. This right may be overridden only under special circumstances. In most jurisdictions, nonemergent forced treatment requires an administrative or judicial hearing. Nearly all states allow for exceptions when emergency circumstances arise. An emergency is said to exist when a patient suffering from a mental illness poses an imminent risk of bodily harm to self or to others in the treatment setting. Forced treatment to prevent such harm is permitted when it represents the least restrictive method of intervention in an emergency. A physician who orders a treatment to be administered against the wishes of a patient should carefully document his or her findings of a direct examination of the patient, the basis for the decision, and how the treatment is the least restrictive alternative to maintain safety.

DISCHARGE

The on-call physician will be asked to evaluate patients requesting discharge from medical or psychiatric settings against medical advice. In these cases, the consultant will need to evaluate the patient's decisional capacity to leave the hospital using the guidelines outlined earlier in this chapter. If the patient is not dangerous, is competent, and is admitted voluntarily to a medical floor, it is often appropriate to allow the discharge. A patient admitted to a psychiatric floor and admitted on a conditional voluntary status may be held against his or her will for as much time as is allowed by law to determine whether the discharge is safe. Making these decisions involves knowing the laws specific to the jurisdiction of the treatment facility.

Alternatively, the physician on call may be asked to discharge a patient against his or her wishes. These circumstances include administrative discharges, such as when a patient knowingly violates a rule like smuggling illicit drugs into the hospital or has been restored to health but refuses to leave. Documentation of the situation should be thorough, and it should include the opinions of consultants and other professionals whenever possible. The patient should be provided with other options for care such as a referral to a more appropriate treatment facility. The patient should be told that he or she may return to the emergency room for reevaluation because emergency care cannot be denied.

It is important to remember that the legal criteria regarding determination of capacity and involuntary commitment and treatment are open to some degree of interpretation. The ambiguity of these concepts permits the necessary flexibility to adapt one's professional judgment to a variety of clinical situations but may simultaneously lead a clinician to doubt whether he or she is using them properly. When in doubt regarding a decision, the consultant should discuss the case with a more experienced clinician or an institutional administrator for guidance, and always clearly document the rationale for the decision.

Confidentiality

Confidentiality is the obligation of the physician not to share information obtained from the patient in the course of evaluation and/or treatment unless the patient gives permission to do so. Exceptions to the duty of confidentiality include the following:
- Emergency situations for urgent interventions
- Mandated reporting of child abuse or suspected child abuse
- Competency proceedings
- Communication with other treatment providers
- Duties to inform third parties about dangerousness to self or others

The Health Insurance Portability and Accountability Act (HIPAA) was signed into law by Congress in 1996. The purpose of this law is to clarify when patient information can be shared without the patient's consent. Given that HIPAA allows for the consultant to speak with family members in the case of an emergency as well as with other providers, most on-call tasks that require breaking patient confidentiality are permissible; however, the consultant should become acquainted with these regulations. Most institutions provide HIPAA compliance training. The federal government also maintains a comprehensive website that may serve as a reference.

The American Psychiatric Association guidelines suggest that confidentiality may be broken when a patient is likely to commit suicide or murder and can be stopped only by notification of police. Confidentiality may also be broken when an impaired person may endanger the lives of others, as in the case of a pilot or a bus driver. In many jurisdictions, *Tarasoff* and related "duty to warn" court cases have established that a physician has the duty to warn or to protect potential victims from harm. The psychiatrist may be required to notify the police and/or the potential victim of danger threatened by a patient who is being released from or has left a facility without permission.

Suggested Readings

Appelbaum PS, Grisso T. Assessing patients' capacities to consent to treatment. *N Engl J Med.* 1998;319(5):1635–1638. https://doi.org/10.1056/NEJM198812223192504.

Brendel RW, Schouten R, Levenson JL. Legal issues. In: Levenson JL, ed. *The American Psychiatric Publishing Textbook of Psychosomatic Medicine: Psychiatric Care of the Medically Ill.* 2nd ed. Washington, DC: American Psychiatric Publishing, Inc; 2011:19–32.

Default Surrogate Consent Statuses. American Bar Association website. http://www.americanbar.org/content/dam/aba/administrative/law_aging/2014_default_surrogate_consent_statutes.authcheckdam.pdf. Published June 2014. Accessed 27.11.16.

Goldstein M. Assessment of competency and other legal issues. In: Bernstein CA, Ishak WW, Weiner ED, Ladds BJ, eds. *On Call Psychiatry.* 2nd ed. New York, NY: WB Saunders; 2001:27–34.

HIPAA Privacy in Emergency Situations. U.S. Department of Health and Human Services website. http://www.hhs.gov/sites/default/files/emergencysituations.pdf. Published November 2014. Accessed 27.11.16.

Kaplan H, Price M. The clinician's role in competency evaluations. *Gen Hosp Psychiatry.* 1989;11:397–403.

Leo RJ. Competency and the capacity to make treatment decisions: a primer for primary care physicians. *Primary Care Companion J Clin Psychiatry.* 1999;1(5):131–141.

Schwartz HI, Mack DM. Informed consent and competency. In: Rosner R, ed. *Principles and Practice of Forensic Psychiatry.* London, England: Arnold; 2003:97–106.

Schwartz HI, Mack DM, Zeman PM. Hospitalization. Voluntary and involuntary. In: Rosner R, ed. *Principles and Practice of Forensic Psychiatry.* London, England: Arnold; 2003:107–115.

Simon RI. Legal and ethical issues. In: Wise MG, Rundell JR, eds. *Textbook of Consult-Liaison Psychiatry in the Medically Ill.* 2nd ed. Washington, DC: American Psychiatric Publishing; 2002:167–186.

Sprehe DJ. Geriatric psychiatry and the law. In: Rosner R, ed. *Principles and Practice of Forensic Psychiatry.* London, England: Arnold; 2003:651–660.

State-Specific Data. Treatment Advocacy Center website. http://www.treatmentadvocacycenter.org/browse-by-state. Published September 8, 2015. Accessed 30.11.16.

Tarasoff v. Regents of the University of California, 551 P.2d 334 (1976) 872–873.

The Difficult Patient

Introduction

Few calls inspire more dread in the on-call psychiatrist than those regarding a "difficult patient." It can be tempting to quickly determine via phone that a clash between a patient and treatment team is not driven by mania, delirium, or psychosis and then try to "cancel" the consult. However, it is with these patients, perhaps more than any other, that we have the opportunity to repair a broken patient-team relationship to allow optimal medical care to proceed. Sometimes the patient-team relationship has fractured to such a degree that we are consulted to determine the capacity of a patient who is demanding to leave against medical advice. Those on the other end of the phone may be angry, frustrated, demoralized, exhausted, or afraid. As the psychiatrist consultant, our first priority in these consults is to support the team and ensure the patient's and staff's immediate safety. Our second aim is to identify sources of conflict between the patient and the team and to formulate a plan of action with treatment recommendations for acute stabilization. During this step, we supportively diffuse tensions and validate each side by playing to their strengths (see examples later). Our third goal is to educate and align the patient and team, providing a framework for future interactions. Depending on the acuity of the consult, not all of these steps may be completed overnight, but your goal should be to set the groundwork for ongoing effective communication between the two parties.

The Consult

By the time a consult for a difficult patient is placed, the staff and patient have likely hit an impasse in communication and expectations. Those calling may have difficulty expressing the reasons for the consult, but you can begin to collect clinical data during this initial conversation. If the patient is aggressive or suicidal, for example, you may hear a frightened call for help. If the request sounds exhausted or depleted, the patient may be emotionally demanding, clingy, or dependent. If the request sounds angry and frustrated, it may mean the patient has become hostile and team members are feeling manipulated. Requests may be vague or confusing if the patient's perception of reality is altered (e.g., due to denial, psychosis, or cognitive limitations). It may be apparent to you that staff is split in disagreement or are having difficulty coping with their own reactions to the patient (e.g., anger towards the patient without recognizing why, seeing the patient as wholly bad or wholly good, distorting or denying the current situation, becoming passive aggressive, projecting emotions onto the patient). These observations will all help to shape your initial approach and interaction.

Make sure to talk with the team directly regarding their concerns. Listen for the way they characterize the problem. Then, assess acuity as quickly as possible by asking questions such as:

- What is the patient's behavior at this very moment and when did it start?
- Is this an abrupt behavioral change?
- Is he/she alert and oriented? Assaulting staff? Screaming and threatening? Pulling out intravenous (IV) lines? Or is he/she lying in bed asleep?
- Are staff feeling scared?
- If the patient is agitated, has anyone attempted verbal redirection? Is it working?
- Has the patient been offered stat doses of as needed medications? Which ones?
- If the patient is not responding to redirection and sounds acutely dangerous, have hospital police been called?
- Is one-to-one arm's length observation necessary?

After asking these questions, you should be able to determine whether the patient's presentation is acute or nonacute. If you are unclear about this, make your way to the patient and staff to further assess.

If the presentation sounds acute, make sure hospital police have been called and additional support is available before ending the call and going to see the patient. If your hospital has a behavioral emergency system in place (e.g., a behavioral code), tell staff to activate it while you make your way there. If you foresee intramuscular (IM) medications or behavioral restraints becoming necessary due to acute dangerousness, inform staff to draw up requested medications and obtain restraints. Ask about the patient's most recent vital signs, orientation, medical problems, substance use history, and current medical stability. Confirm any medication allergies and review current medications.

If the patient's presentation sounds subacute, assess if the team is worried that things will soon escalate. Often, staff has a sense for this. If immediate escalation is of less concern, attempt to ascertain a concrete consult question—does the team want a recommendation for as needed medications? Are they concerned about the patient's capacity regarding specific decision-making? Would they like assistance creating a behavioral plan for a patient with poor boundaries? With a little help, the reason for consultation should become clearer. However, at times, things may not be obvious until you see the staff and patient in person.

En route to meet with the team, consider possible factors at play. You may already have recognized certain behavioral patterns through the consult request. Often, "difficult" patients have personality traits that make it harder for them to tolerate the acute stress of being ill in the hospital. However, not all difficult patients have personality disorders and not all patients with personality disorders are difficult patients! "Difficult" patients may simply find it exceedingly challenging to tolerate the loss of control that comes with being hospitalized. When the stress of their poor coping is placed on an already overworked and depleted medical staff, often the patient becomes increasingly agitated and the staff becomes increasingly alienated. Think about what assistance you can offer both sides:

- If the patient's problem behavior involves aggression or self-destructive threats or acts:
  1. evaluate for potential violence and the source of the patient's anger/fear and
  2. recommend social, chemical, and/or physical restraints for safety.
- If the patient's problem behavior involves denial of his or her illness, demanding requests related to his or her care, or other difficulties in understanding his or her medical problems in a way consistent with the team, focus on:
  1. performing reality testing to understand the patient's perspective and decide what it stems from (psychotic process? other cognitive disorder? personality disorder?)
  2. explain the patient's reality to staff and offer suggestions for effective communication.
- If the patient is manipulative, dependent or rejecting:
  1. clarify expectations and set clear limits while validating his or her perceived experience (e.g., "It can be so hard to be in the hospital" or "I can see why you are frustrated," linked with "We want to make sure you are safe and receiving the best possible care, so that is why I am recommending x and y")
  2. validate the team's frustration, allowing them to offset their guilt by realistically assessing the patient's behavior and

giving the patient permission to set limits (e.g., "You've done a great job handling a very difficult patient situation. I think we can make things easier for you by x and y")

3. work with the team to think of ways to help the patient feel more empowered in the hospital.

BEDSIDE

Before meeting with the patient at the bedside, check in with nursing or medical staff nearby to get an updated account of the patient's behavior and verify what has already been done. Ask them what their goals are and clarify what they want to achieve short and long term with the patient. Let them know you will check back in after assessing the patient.

When approaching the patient, the first and primary goal is safety of the patient, the team, and the milieu. Sometimes we are called to help contain the "unruly" patient who is disrupting a busy emergency department, only to find on assessment that he or she is delirious due to medical illness or substance withdrawal. As with any consult, you should immediately rule out life-threatening conditions such as delirium, alcohol withdrawal, other substance intoxication or withdrawal, physical pain, and medication side effects.

By the time you arrive on the scene, things may have already escalated to a degree where medication or even physical restraints may be immediately necessary. On the other hand, some patients will still be in the early process of escalating, and you will have more of a chance to establish an alliance through a calm, nonjudgmental approach. Here your relationship with the patient often benefits simply because you are a new face in the room. Acknowledge the stresses he or she is facing and validate his or her emotions. You may identify splitting ("all good" or "all bad"), projective identification (e.g., patient's bad feelings about staff have become reality as the patient treats staff poorly), or denial and idealization (e.g., fear about a medical condition causes a patient to leave against medical advice, or patient becomes overattached, thinking you will "save" him/her from the current predicament). Your job as an on-call psychiatrist is not to confront these defenses no matter how tempting, as that is the purview of long-term outpatient psychiatric treatment and would most likely worsen the difficult patient's behavior in this setting. However, by taking note of them, you can formulate a dynamic assessment of the patient-team relationship, which will guide your treatment recommendations.

Avoiding confrontation of defenses does not mean that we should enable the patient in their maladaptive patterns. Instead, it allows for alliance building to precede the discussion of how the patient and his or her team can move forward. After establishing rapport and exploring the patient's concerns, set ground rules for moving ahead. Be firm but nonpunitive and explain that these plans will help the patient to receive the best possible care, which is what they deserve. If entitlement and narcissism are problems, appeal to them! If possible, find a compromise that will enhance communication between both parties and allow the next steps to proceed.

After meeting with the patient at the bedside, approach the primary team and offer your assessment, recommendations, and support. All providers have emotional reactions to their patients, but physicians in other specialties may not have as much experience processing these feelings or using them as diagnostic tools. Often doctors may be embarrassed, ashamed, or scared by negative feelings they are experiencing towards a patient, and it can be helpful to normalize these emotions. Identify and praise the helpful things the team has done or attempted to do and validate expressed frustrations.

MANAGEMENT

The focus of management in on-call situations with a difficult patient is to stabilize the acute situation and open lines of communication between the patient and the team.

- Assess the degree of acuity of the patient's presentation, as described previously. If the patient is beyond verbal redirection, call for hospital police assistance and/or a behavioral code and consider the following:

  Haloperidol 1 to 5 mg by mouth or IM every 4 hours as needed for acute agitation

  Olanzapine 2.5 to 5 mg by mouth or IM every 4 hours as needed for acute agitation (may be available in dissolvable formulation which eases administration; when using IM, DO NOT administer IM benzodiazepine within 1 hour before or after, due to risk of dangerous hypotension)

  Lorazepam 0.5 to 2 mg by mouth or IM every 4 hours as needed for acute agitation (may give with antipsychotic to minimize the latter's side effects and provide additional sedation; avoid if benzodiazepine use disorder; may wish to avoid if actively intoxicated due to risk of respiratory depression, unless patient is closely monitored)

  Behavioral restraints and/or Posey vest (medical restraint)

  One-to-one monitoring

- If patient has not escalated beyond engaging in discussion and can respond to verbal redirection, approach him/her calmly, leaving plenty of space, and make empathic, validating statements expressing interest in what is wrong. Sometimes verbal redirection is enough on its own; other times, the patient's behavior has been disruptive and dangerous enough to warrant offering of medication.

If the patient is able to respond to verbal redirection, build rapport and then offer options for the next steps (e.g., "I think it would help to take some medicine to relax. Would you prefer to have it by mouth or in a shot?" or "I'm sorry to wake you in the middle of the night, but we need to place this IV line so we can give the best medical care possible. Would you prefer to have the IV in the right or left arm?")

Set limits with the patient after tensions are diffused, clearly stating that dangerous behavior cannot be allowed as it is the top priority to keep the patient, other patients, and staff safe.

After implementing immediate management, discuss your recommendations with staff (both nursing and medical) and validate their frustrations and efforts thus far. Review the way in which specific patient care recommendations are intended to target specific behaviors and be sure to ask if the staff has additional questions at this point.

Concluding Thoughts

Calls for the difficult patient put the spotlight on the psychiatric consultant, and in this role we may be able to help repair a patient-team relationship. Assess the acuity, provide support to the primary team, and assess the context as quickly as possible. Patterns will emerge to clarify the conditions leading to the problem. By approaching both the patient and the team without judgment and with empathy, rapport can be established and a plan can be built. Identify but do not challenge the patient's behavioral style (primary defense mechanisms utilized), and seek out the healthier aspects of the patient and the team. After this validation has occurred, firm, nonjudgmental limit setting is often successful. When the situation is stabilized, acknowledge the importance of continued communication and reassessment, work on signing out to the day team a concise but cohesive case assessment so that appropriate follow-up steps can be taken.

Suggested Readings

Geringer E, Stern T. Coping with medical illness: the impact of personality types. *Psychosomatics*. 1986;27:251–261.

Perry S, Gilmore M. The disruptive patient or visitor. *JAMA*. 1981;245:755–757.

Zerbo E, Cohen S, Bielska W, Caligor E. Transference-focused psychotherapy in the general psychiatry residency: a useful and applicable model for residents in acute care clinical settings. *Psychodyn Psychiatry*. 2013;41(1):163–181.

Zimmerman D, Groves J. Difficult patients. In: Stern T, ed. *Massachussetts General Hospital: Handbook of General Hospital Psychiatry*. St Louis, MO: WB Saunders; 2010:511–526.

Emergency Evaluation of Children and Adolescents

The evaluation of children and adolescents differs from that of adults in several ways. Consult questions may include evaluation of a newly emergent psychiatric condition, assessment of psychological response to a serious medical condition, management of agitation, assessment of suicidality, or assistance in managing difficult family dynamics (Box 8.1). Importantly, an understanding of the overall functioning of the child or adolescent requires a comprehensive assessment of the family, school, and social relationships. For this reason, other sources of information, such as parents or legal guardians, social workers, teachers, and other professionals or organizations involved in the care of the patient play an essential role of the work-up of children and adolescents. Depending on state laws and the age of the child in question, approval of the patient's parent or guardian may be required for decisions regarding disposition or medication interventions.

BOX 8.1	Reasons for Consultation

Suicidal ideation, suicide attempt, or self-harm behaviors
Agitation, aggressive behavior, or violent ideation
Evaluation of new-onset depressive, manic, or anxious symptoms
Evaluation of new-onset psychotic symptoms
Evaluation of adjustment reaction in setting of medical illness
Pharmacologic management of previously diagnosed psychiatric conditions
Evaluation of acute mental status change
Evaluation of neurodevelopmental disorder
Evaluation of substance use
Concern for abuse or neglect
Management of difficult family dynamics

PHONE CALL

The on-call psychiatrist may be consulted to evaluate a child or adolescent in the emergency room, on a medical floor, or on an inpatient unit. The call may be as ambiguous as "We have a child for you to evaluate." As with other calls for a consultation, it is important to clarify the reason for the consultation.

Questions

1. Where is the patient?
2. What is the age of the patient?
3. Who brought the patient to the hospital, and why? Will they be available to speak in person at the time of evaluation? If not, can their contact information be recorded and provided to the on-call psychiatrist?
4. Has the patient had a physical examination and/or laboratory tests done? If so, what specific tests were performed, and are there any abnormalities?
5. Does the patient take medications? If so, which ones and at what dosages?
6. Has the patient abused drugs or alcohol? Was a toxicology screening done?
7. Does the patient require one-to-one observation, seclusion, or restraint?

Requests for Staff Before Consultant Arrives

1. Have the patient placed in a room in which he or she will be safe. One-to-one observation may be required if the patient is assaultive, aggressive, suicidal, or an elopement risk. Consider the layout of the area in which the patient will be waiting for evaluation to ensure that it is adequate for the safety of the patient and appropriate for the patient's age.
2. Request that the patient be searched for weapons and other instruments that may cause injury. However, it is important to ensure that the search be done with sensitivity to the age of the patient.

ELEVATOR THOUGHTS

Whom will you interview first?

In general, parents or guardians are interviewed first when the patient is a child, whereas the adolescent patient is interviewed before his or her parents or guardians.

Which conditions and behaviors are emergencies that require hospitalization?

Children and adolescents who are at imminent risk of harm to themselves or others should be hospitalized. Examples include patients with recent serious suicidal or self-injurious behavior, those who endorse significant suicidal ideation with plan or intent, and those who engage in violent or aggressive behavior. Children and adolescents who are impulsive, psychotic, or live in an abusive environment are also at elevated risk for engaging in harmful behaviors and may also require hospitalization.

Is the adult accompanying the patient the legal guardian? If not, who is?

It is important to attempt to establish contact with the patient's legal guardian. The guardian must be informed about the results of the psychiatric evaluation and should be involved in treatment decisions. This individual's consent may be helpful in facilitating inpatient hospitalization and may be essential in approving medication regimen changes.

MAJOR THREAT TO LIFE

Safety

To complete a comprehensive evaluation, both the evaluating physician and the patient must be in an environment that is free of distractions and dangerous furnishings or medical equipment. A safe setting is necessary to protect the physician, the patient, anyone accompanying the patient, and others in the area. Restraint is sometimes necessary to prevent aggression or elopement. Chemical and physical restraint should only be used if less restrictive means, including verbal deescalation, have failed. Although several first- and second-generation antipsychotics have been approved for children with autistic, mood, psychotic, and tic disorders, none have been approved for the use of chemical restraint in children. Because physical restraint has the potential to be traumatic to a child or adolescent, its use must be considered carefully. Finally, the evaluating physician must assess immediately for primary medical emergencies including medical illness, medication side effect, head trauma, overdose, and alcohol or drug intoxication or withdrawal.

Suicidality

Suicide is the second leading cause of death in American youth aged 10 to 19 (Box 8.2). A psychiatric evaluation of a child or adolescent is incomplete without an assessment of suicide risk, even if suicidality is not the chief complaint. Some examples of pediatric screening tools that have been used in emergency psychiatric settings include the Reynolds Suicide Ideation Questionnaire, the Columbia Suicide Severity Rating Scale, and the Ask Suicide-Screening Questions.

BOX 8.2	Common Psychiatric Emergencies Seen in Children and Adolescents

Violence toward others or weapon possession
Suicidal ideation, suicide attempt or gesture
Physical abuse or neglect
Sexual abuse or rape
Psychosis
Anxiety
Conversion disorder
Eating disorders
Substance abuse
Behavioral disorders
Fire-setting
Running away
School refusal
Acute mental status change

In determining a young patient's risk of suicide, the evaluating psychiatrist should consider both chronic and acute risk factors, as well as collateral information. An individual's chronic risk of suicide is elevated by a family history of suicide, personal history of physical or sexual abuse, and prior suicide attempts. Acute risk factors include substance abuse or intoxication, mania, depression, psychosis, impulsivity, and severe psychosocial stressors. In the case of recent suicide attempts or current suicidal ideation, lethality of the method and intent to die should be considered. Access to firearms and other weapons should always be investigated. However, attention-seeking or manipulative self-harming behavior should not be discounted because individuals without true suicidal ideation may inadvertently endanger their lives in an effort to have their distress taken seriously.

Homicidality and Aggression

The psychiatrist who is called to evaluate aggression or violence in a young person should consider biologic, psychological, and social contributions to the patient's presentation, as well as collateral information. These risks are elevated in young patients with a history of aggressive behavior toward people or animals, fire-setting, truancy or serious rule violation, running away from home, and use and access to firearms and other weapons. Children and adolescents with poor frustration tolerance, behavioral dysregulation, and impulsivity are at increased risk for violence and aggression. Acute elevations in risk can also be caused by undiagnosed medical conditions, such as altered mental status due to a neurologic condition or toxic metabolic state, intoxication or withdrawal, or acute psychiatric states of mania and psychosis. The evaluating physician should attempt to identify stressors or triggers for violence or increased aggression. Finally, collateral information from parents or legal guardians, school officials, or residential facility staff is essential to fully assess the risk of violence.

ASSESSMENT

Always remember to introduce yourself to the patient and adults at the bedside before you start asking questions. When interviewing a child, beginning with noninvasive questions (i.e., name, age, school, hobby, sport, or favorite television show) often helps to foster an alliance. It is important to ask about psychotic symptoms with vocabulary that children can understand (ask them if their ears or eyes ever play tricks on them). If they endorse auditory hallucinations, ask children if they ever feel like they have to obey the voices that nobody else hears. Psychotic symptoms often present differently in children than in adults and may manifest, for example, only as unpredictable or unusual behavior. An adolescent patient may be more comfortable speaking candidly if they are interviewed privately and reassured of confidentiality regarding nonlife-threatening issues. If there is any suspicion of abuse or neglect or if the parent appears to be attempting to influence the child's response, arranging for the child to speak to the clinician privately—once a rapport has been established—is essential. Refer to Table 8.1, which provides an expanded outline for the initial evaluation.

TABLE 8.1	Emergency History for Child and Adolescent Psychiatry
Demographics	Age, guardian, living arrangements, social agencies
History of present illness	Mood and psychotic symptoms, substance use, behavioral dyscontrol, physical/sexual abuse, environmental factors
Psychiatric history	First psychiatric presentation, previous diagnoses and symptoms, previous hospitalizations, outpatient treatment, medication trials, substance use history
Suicide attempts/ self-harm	Character of attempt (e.g., firearms, overdose, hanging), impulsive or planned, reaction to discovery, remorse, child's concept of death
Violence/legal history	Aggression, conduct disorder, truancy, legal involvement
Medical history	Diagnoses, medications, allergies, head trauma, seizure history
Family history	Psychiatric diagnoses, suicides, substance abuse
Personal history	Developmental milestones, mental retardation, school performance, social relations

On mental status exam, special attention should be paid to level of consciousness, evidence of psychosis, mood lability, suicidality, aggression, and impulsivity. The physical examination must include vital signs, careful investigation of head trauma, signs of physical or sexual abuse, signs of an eating disorder, toxic metabolic states, and intoxication/substance abuse. Laboratory tests should include a complete blood count, electrolytes including calcium, renal function tests, liver function tests, urine and blood toxicology, and blood alcohol level. In the case of first-episode psychosis, erythrocyte sedimentation rate, antinuclear antibody, thyroid stimulating hormone, human immunodeficiency virus screening, ceruloplasmin, vitamin B12, treponemal antibody test, and neuroimaging are also recommended. In young women of childbearing age, a pregnancy test is warranted.

The evaluating psychiatrist should review prior psychiatric assessments, as well as documentation from the current hospital presentation (Emergency Department notes, notes from the primary treatment team, social work notes, nursing notes), medication lists, laboratory studies, and imaging. The psychiatric evaluation of a young person will include information from collateral sources, such as a parent or legal guardian, school authorities, residential treatment facility, and other medical or mental health care providers.

MANAGEMENT

The basic tenet guiding management decisions is the safety of the patient. The disposition decisions in pediatric patients are often more conservative than for adults. In general, patients evaluated by a resident physician should be discussed with a supervisor, attending physician, or a child and adolescent psychiatric fellow. Disposition may also include reporting to child protection/welfare agencies. Reporting the suspicion of child abuse or neglect to the appropriate agency should be reviewed in advance with a supervisor and social worker, who can also help with the management of difficult family reactions.

Admission or Discharge

If the decision is made to admit the patient, a detailed discussion with the parent or legal guardian about the reasons for admission can facilitate voluntary admission. State laws vary as to how children can be admitted to a psychiatric unit; in general, the parent or guardian can sign the patient in "voluntarily" even if the child is objecting. Taking time to educate and have this discussion with the family can also assist in forming an alliance with the patient. If the patient has the potential to become assaultive or attempt elopement, informing the patient of the decision to admit may be deferred until after the full evaluation, family discussion, and paperwork have all been completed. In these situations, alerting hospital security or initiating one-to-one observation may be warranted before informing the patient of the need for admission. If any medical issues require further monitoring, the patient should be admitted to a pediatric unit. A low threshold should be maintained for one-to-one observation, especially if the patient is to be admitted to a nonpsychiatric floor. Clear recommendations should be given for as-needed medications.

If the decision is made to discharge the patient, a follow-up appointment with an outpatient mental health worker or crisis clinic is necessary. If the patient had been evaluated for suicidal intent or attempt, injury prevention education is essential prior to discharge. The discharge plan should include ensuring adequate supervision and support for the patient, as well as instructing caretakers to remove or disarm all firearms and remove all substances of abuse. If the patient has been evaluated for aggression and violence, the safety of potential targets of violence must be addressed prior to discharge. If the patient was evaluated for potential abuse, the multidisciplinary team including a social worker, pediatrician, and child protective services should be in agreement with the discharge plan.

Laws regarding admission of minors to psychiatric facilities vary by state; however, in general, the guardian of a minor can voluntarily admit the child to a psychiatric unit, even if the child disagrees. If the parent/guardian disagrees with a decision to admit the patient, state laws vary as to the requirements for involuntary admission, but a parent refusing to admit a child who is acutely dangerous to himself or herself or others may constitute medical neglect and referral to protective services may be indicated. In many cases involving child protective services or children in residential treatment settings, it can be very difficult to determine who actually has the legal right to make medical decisions for the patient. Consent for admission is separate from consent for medication, and, in most states, parent/guardian consent is required for medication administration except in cases of emergency, when parent/guardian notification is still required. These are difficult questions that will require supervision from attendings and possibly hospital administration and risk management.

Treatment of Acute Agitation

The management of agitation in children and adolescents should be guided by the likely or presumed cause of agitation. Common causes of agitation in this population appear in Table 8.2.

TABLE 8.2	Common Causes of Agitation in Children and Adolescents

Neurologic/Structural: hemorrhage/hematoma, contusion, tumor, seizure/
  postictal state, stroke
Infection: meningitis, encephalitis, brain abscess, sepsis
Metabolic derangements: hyper/hypoglycemia, hyponatremia, hypercalcemia,
  changes in oxygen levels, encephalopathy, thyrotoxicosis/hypothyroidism
Primary psychiatric: depression, psychosis, bipolar disorder, anxiety,
  externalizing behavioral disorders, intellectual disability
Toxic: intoxication/withdrawal, poisoning, medication side effect

Nonpharmacologic Management of Agitation

Management of acute agitation should be as conservative as possible while maintaining the safety of the patient and others. Verbal deescalation should be the first strategy to defuse agitation. Identifying the source of stress will often help to guide the intervention (e.g., separating an agitating parent or providing a quiet place for psychotic overstimulation or intoxicating substance metabolism). If the patient remains dangerously agitated, medications or seclusion and restraints may be required. Seclusion and restraint policies vary by institution and should be reviewed with hospital staff. Most states require parent/guardian notification regarding involuntary medication, seclusion, or restraint.

Pharmacologic Management of Agitation

If medications are required, a conservative approach is recommended. Young children rarely require medications because temper tantrums are usually short lived and because children generally respond to verbal reassurance and removal of the agitating stimulus. Prior to initiating any medication, the physician must review allergies, medical conditions, prior adverse reactions to medications, and other medications serving as contraindications for use. The following medications are commonly used for agitation in children and adolescents.

ANTIHISTAMINES

Diphenhydramine (Benadryl). Administer 25 to 50 mg by mouth (PO) every 2 to 4 hours until therapeutic effect is observed. This agent may be used in infants greater than 20 lb. Children may respond to 25 mg, but adolescents may require the 50-mg dosage. For severe agitation, intramuscular (IM) formulation may be used in similar dosages. Diphenhydramine has a generally favorable side-effect profile and is therefore first line for treatment of agitation in children. However, rarely, children may have a paradoxical reaction leading to hyperactivity, increased agitation, or even hallucinations.

BENZODIAZEPINES

Lorazepam (Ativan). Administer 0.05 to 0.1 mg/kg (usually 1 to 2 mg) by mouth (PO) every 4 to 8 hours until therapeutic effect is observed. Onset of action is 20 to 30 minutes in PO formulation and 5 to 10 minutes in IM or intravenous (IV) formulation. This medication may be used in children older than 12 years for agitation not responding to diphenhydramine. For severe agitation, IM formulation may be used in similar dosages. For patients younger than 12 years or with pervasive developmental disorders or traumatic brain injury, benzodiazepines may cause disinhibition and may compound agitation, so they should be avoided. Other adverse effects include respiratory depression and sedation.

FIRST-GENERATION ANTIPSYCHOTICS

Haloperidol (Haldol). Administer 0.05 to 0.15 mg/kg (usually 2 to 5 mg) PO every hour as needed until therapeutic effect (or adverse side effects) is observed. Onset of action is 45 to 60 minutes in PO formulation and 20 to 30 minutes in IM formulation. This agent is approved to be used in children 3 years and older for severe behavioral problems and hyperactive behavior, schizophrenia, and psychosis. For acutely dangerous agitation, IM formulation may be used in half-strength of the PO dosage. Adverse effects include extrapyramidal symptoms, neuroleptic malignant syndrome, hypotension, and QTc prolongation.

Chlorpromazine (Thorazine). For children and adolescents weighing less than 100 pounds, administer 0.55 mg/kg PO every 4 to 6 hours until therapeutic effect (or adverse side effects) is observed. For adolescents weighing more than 100 pounds, administer 30 to 800 mg/day PO in two to four divided doses, starting at lower doses and titrating as needed (usual dose is 200 mg/day). Onset of action is 30 to 60 minutes in PO formulation. This medication is approved to be used in children aged 1 to 12 years for schizophrenia, bipolar disorder, severe behavioral problems, and hyperactive behaviors with conduct disorders. Adverse effects include orthostatic hypotension and anticholinergic symptoms.

SECOND-GENERATION ANTIPSYCHOTICS

Risperidone (Risperdal). Administer 0.25 to 2 mg PO every 4 to 6 hours until therapeutic effect (or adverse side effects) is observed. Risperidone comes in tablet, orally disintegrating tablet, and liquid formulations. Dosages between formulations are equivalent. This medication is approved to be used in children aged 5 to 16 for autism-irritability, in children older than 10 years for bipolar disorder, and in children older than 13 years for schizophrenia. Adverse effects include extrapyramidal symptoms, neuroleptic malignant syndrome, and QTc prolongation.

Olanzapine (Zyprexa). Administer 2.5 to 5 mg every 4 to 6 hours until therapeutic effect (or adverse side effects) is observed. Olanzapine comes in tablet, orally disintegrating tablet formulation, and IM formulations. Onset of action is 15 to 45 minutes in IM formulation. This medication is approved for use in children 13 years or older for bipolar I disorder and schizophrenia. IM formulation has not been studied in patients younger than 18 years. Adverse effects include QTc prolongation, extrapyramidal symptoms, neuroleptic malignant syndrome, bradycardia, hypotension, and anticholinergic symptoms. It is not recommended to combine this medication with benzodiazepines.

Suggested Readings

Allen NG, Khan JS, Alzahri MS, Stolar AG. Ethical issues in emergency psychiatry. *Emerg Med Clin North Am.* 2015;33(4):863–874. https://doi.org/10.1016/j.emc.2015.07.012.

Carubia B, Becker A, Levine BH. Child psychiatric emergencies: updates on trends, clinical care, and practice challenges. *Curr Psychiatry Rep.* 2016;18(4):41. https://doi.org/10.1007/s11920-016-0670-9.

Chun TH, Katz ER, Duffy SJ, Gerson RS. Challenges of managing pediatric mental health crises in the emergency department. *Child Adolesc Psychiatry Clin N Am.* 2015;24(1):21–40. https://doi.org/10.1016/j.chc.2014.09.003.

Freudenreich O, Schulz SC, Goff DC. Initial medical work-up of first-episode psychosis: a conceptual review. *Early Interv Psychiatry.* 2009;3(1):10–18. https://doi.org/10.1111/j.1751-7893.2008.00105.x.

Marzullo LR. Pharmacologic management of the agitated child. *Pediatr Emerg Care.* 2014;30(4):269–275. https://doi.org/10.1097/PEC.0000000000000112. quiz 276–8.

Masters KJ, Bellonci C, Bernet W, et al. Practice parameter for the prevention and management of aggressive behavior in child and adolescent psychiatric institutions, with special reference to seclusion and restraint. *J Am Acad Child Adolesc Psychiatry.* 2002;41(suppl 2):4S–25S.

The Agitated Patient

"Agitation" is a word commonly used in the colloquial setting; however, people often use it to mean different things. Per Cummings et al., "There is no consensus definition of agitation and no widespread agreement on what elements should be included in the syndrome." Therefore it is important to ask the person(s) reporting that a patient is agitated to clarify exactly what he or she means by "agitation." Clinically, psychiatrists often refer to agitation as a state of heightened affect, characterized by excessive motor and/or verbal activity. Motor activity may include grabbing, throwing, and pacing. Excessive verbal activity may refer to cursing, screaming, etc. A patient's agitation can stir up anxiety in staff and in other patients. Often, a call for agitation represents a call to help manage the agitated patient, as well as a call to help the staff deal with anxiety from interacting with the patient. Staff may be uncomfortable dealing with agitated patients and may look to you for reassurance and guidance. Agitation has numerous etiologies, ranging from complicated medical problems such as organic brain syndromes, to primary psychotic disorders, to substance abuse/withdrawal, to personality disorders such as antisocial personality disorder and borderline personality disorder. Your primary goal on arriving is to assess for potential dangerous behavior and to create a safe environment for everyone. Secondarily, your goal is to evaluate the patient to diagnose and treat the underlying cause of the agitation.

PHONE CALL

Questions

1. What is the nature and duration of the agitation? That is, what happened and what is the patient doing now?
   - Is the patient currently a threat to self, staff, or other patients? If yes, order stat oral (PO)/intramuscular (IM) medications, and request additional help, including hospital security.

- If administering stat medication, attempt to ascertain allergies, current medications, and known medical issues.
- Is the patient jeopardizing his or her medical care and/or attempting to leave the hospital against medical advice? If yes, alert hospital security to prevent elopement prior to your evaluation.
- Has the patient displayed similar behavior in the recent past? If so, try to get details about how it was managed and think about speaking with staff familiar with the patient.

2. What is the patient's age, reason for hospitalization, and medical history?
   - What are the vital signs?
   - What are the allergies?
   - What is the QTc from a recent electrocardiogram (EKG)?
   - Does the patient have medical problems, specifically cardiac problems?
   - Has there been a change in the level of consciousness?
   - What medications is the patient on? Was any new medication recently started?
3. What is the patient's psychiatric history?
4. Does the patient have a history of substance abuse?

Orders

1. If there is an acute danger to the patient or staff members, you will need to notify the staff over the phone that you may need to order medication and/or physical or chemical restraints as soon as you have seen the patient and that a psychiatric code should be called to alert additional staff that help is needed.
2. Order appropriate observation and measurement of vital signs and level of alertness.
3. For an alert, cooperative patient, consider ordering oral medication as needed (PRN) to help with symptomatic relief until you can evaluate the patient, but do evaluate the patient as soon as possible. Order low doses so that the patient will be alert for an evaluation when you arrive at the site.

Inform RN

"Will arrive in…minutes."

In addition, ask the registered nurse (RN) to page or call the patient's primary medical doctor or team, if at all possible, to inform you of the patient's medical conditions and baseline behavior.

ELEVATOR THOUGHTS

What causes agitation?

The timing of the onset of the agitation provides important information regarding the underlying etiology. A more acute onset may suggest a medical problem or an acute intoxicated or withdrawal state (this is possible even if a patient has been in the hospital for days). Manic symptoms usually escalate over time, and a schizophrenic decompensation usually follows a prodromal period; however, exceptions do occur. Substance withdrawal syndromes usually occur 1 to 7 days after admission and are generally accompanied by changes in vital signs.

In addition, a patient may become agitated in cases in which communication between the treating team and the patient is jeopardized. Occasionally, patients who want or expect to be discharged from the hospital may become agitated when told by their primary team that they should remain in the hospital longer for more treatment, or when they have returned from court and commitment over objection has been upheld.

An assessment of the level of consciousness may also help to elucidate the underlying cause of an agitated state. Patients who are agitated because of a primary psychiatric illness should not have fluctuations in the level of consciousness and should be fully alert. Patients who are agitated because of a primary medical illness often will have fluctuations in their level of consciousness and may not be alert.

A good history and physical examination (including a full neurologic exam) will help to elucidate the underlying cause of an agitated state. Someone with multiple medical problems or taking multiple medications is more likely to have a general medical condition causing the agitation. Likewise, someone who appears to be in physical distress usually has a medical condition causing the agitation. Be sure to assess fall risk and rule out recent head injury as a cause of symptoms. If there is any doubt that the patient has had a recent head injury or that the patient has an acute neurological problem or dementia contributing to the agitation, order a noncontrast head computed tomography (CT) scan.

Psychiatric Causes of Agitation

- Psychotic disorders
- Mood disorders
- Anxiety disorders
- Personality disorders
- Major neurocognitive disorder

Substance Use Disorders (See Later)

Medical Causes of Agitation

1. Systemic
   a. Delirium
   b. Metabolic
      i. Electrolyte imbalances
      ii. Diabetes (particularly a hypoglycemic episode)
      iii. Hypoxia
      iv. Acute intermittent porphyria (rare!)
   c. Endocrine
      i. Thyroid and adrenal conditions
      ii. Carcinoid syndrome
   d. Organ failure
      i. Hepatic encephalopathy
      ii. Uremic encephalopathy
      iii. Respiratory failure
      iv. Cardiovascular conditions
         1. Congestive heart failure
         2. Coronary artery disease
         3. Paroxysmal supraventricular tachycardia and other arrhythmias
2. Drugs
   a. Drugs of abuse
      i. Alcohol intoxication, delirium, and withdrawal (one of the most common causes of postoperative agitation is alcohol withdrawal)
      ii. Stimulant intoxication and withdrawal, including cocaine and amphetamines
      iii. Sedative, hypnotic, and anxiolytic withdrawal and delirium
   b. Idiosyncratic or toxic effects of medications
      i. Corticosteroids
      ii. Anticholinergic medications
      iii. Anticonvulsants
      iv. Antihistamines
      v. Antimalarials
      vi. Antibiotics
      vii. Others: lidocaine, meperidine, metoclopramide, podophyllin, procaine penicillin, propoxyphene withdrawal, pyridostigmine, and sulfonamides
   c. Idiosyncratic or side effects of psychotropics
      i. Benzodiazepine withdrawal or disinhibition (especially in patients with organic disease)
      ii. L-dopa
      iii. Antidepressants: tricyclic, selective, and nonselective serotonin reuptake inhibitors and monoamine oxidase inhibitors

       iv. Antipsychotics: agitation versus extrapyramidal adverse effects and akathisia

       v. Psychostimulants

  d. Poisonings

       i. Carbon monoxide

       ii. Insecticides

3. Central nervous system

  a. Trauma

       i. Subdural and epidural hematoma

       ii. Hemorrhage

       iii. Traumatic brain injury sequelae

  b. Vascular conditions

       i. Transient ischemic attack

       ii. Stroke

       iii. Vasculitis: systemic lupus erythematosus and polyarteritis nodosa

  c. Infections

       i. Meningitis

       ii. Encephalitis

       iii. Human immunodeficiency virus (HIV)- and acquired immunodeficiency syndrome (AIDS)-related conditions

       iv. Lyme disease

  d. Epilepsy

       i. Complex partial seizure disorder

       ii. Postictal states

  e. Dementia: age and diagnosis are important ("sundowning" is a common cause of agitation in older patients but is a diagnosis of exclusion)

       i. Alzheimer disease

       ii. Multiinfarct dementia: hypertension, stepwise progression, and focal neurologic signs

       iii. Normal-pressure hydrocephalus: dementia, gait apraxia, and incontinence

       iv. Parkinson disease

       v. Other: vitamin B12 deficiency, Wernicke-Korsakoff syndrome, Huntington disease, Pick disease, and multiple sclerosis

       vi. Neoplasms

       vii. Hypertensive encephalopathy

MAJOR THREAT TO LIFE

The most common immediate risk with an agitated patient is the potential for aggression from lack of behavioral control. Agitated patients can have tremendous strength and can hit or throw things, making it dangerous to be in their presence.

Agitation may be the first sign of a potentially life-threatening medical condition (e.g., intracranial bleeding or tumor, pulmonary embolism, myocardial infarct, hypoglycemia, neuroleptic malignant syndrome).

Agitation can also be physically uncomfortable for the patient. For example, akathisia can even increase the risk of suicide.

Untreated agitation can lead to serious medical complications, including exhaustion, dehydration, rhabdomyolysis, renal failure, and even death.

BEDSIDE

Depending on the degree and nature of the agitation, there may or may not be time to go through the medical chart. The patient should be evaluated first to assess whether there is time to review the patient's medical records. Have a member of the team review the records and report findings if you need to attend to the patient immediately.

Quick-Look Test

The patient should be initially viewed from a distance. If at all possible, it is helpful to meet the patient early. If the patient appears to be in control and able to cooperate, you can approach cautiously to perform an evaluation or tell the patient that he or she may need to wait a few minutes (while you observe). If the patient appears to be in distress or has a significant amount of psychomotor activity, you should assume that the situation is dangerous and prepare for it before approaching the patient.

Some guidelines include the following:

1. Make sure there are a sufficient number of trained staff members available to help physically control the patient. A show of force may help to prevent aggressive behaviors.
2. Do not wear loose hair, hanging clothing (ties), or exposed jewelry that a patient can grab.
3. Assess the environment for dangerous objects and remove them.
4. Do not place yourself in a situation or room in which the patient can trap or assault you. Stand closer to the door than the patient stands or evaluate the patient in an open space.
5. Separate the agitated patient from an overstimulating situation. This includes roommates, family members, or staff with whom the patient does not feel comfortable.
6. Avoid getting too close to the patient.
7. Use clear, calm, and direct language to avoid ambiguity. Identify yourself; if the patient appears disoriented, state the place where you are and that you are here to help the patient. Be empathic: try to help the patient feel that he or she is being heard and understood.

8. Maintain a dialogue with staff. They may be feeling anxious about the situation too and are looking to you to familiarize them with how to manage the situation. Talk to the staff about what you believe is going on with the patient and what you suggest is the best way to handle the situation. This reduces anxiety, fosters alliances, keeps everyone on the same page, and avoids any confusion later on.

MANAGEMENT

Medical Interventions

If the patient is experiencing obvious physical symptoms (e.g., cyanosis, shortness of breath, pain, sweating, tremulousness), diagnosis and articulating the problem and immediate intervention will reduce the patient's level of agitation. Obtaining vital signs is absolutely necessary with the physically compromised patient. A hypoxic patient should respond to oxygen, and a hypoglycemic patient should respond to glucose, while you call for medical backup or consultation.

Verbal Deescalation and Reorientation

If the patient is able to cooperate with an interview, he or she can be evaluated in a quiet, open area that is easily accessible to nursing staff. Sometimes an agitated patient can get relief by explaining what he or she is experiencing or from a calming, supportive interaction. In the case of delirium, reorient the patient to the date and place.

Environmental Modifications

If agitation has occurred on a psychiatric unit, time in a quiet room can be considered. In any circumstance, it is prudent to remove dangerous objects from the room. Some patients may also benefit from a one-to-one staff member, sitter, or another patient care tech nearby to monitor behavior and safety. In some cases a patient may benefit from a room closer to the nursing station or further from the exit.

Oral Medications

Often PO medication PRN can be helpful in relieving agitation in a nonacute situation. Refer to medication guide later.

If the patient resists your efforts and continues to be agitated, consider seclusion, restraint, and/or need for IM medications. Patients have a right to hear the risks, benefits, and alternatives of your treatment; however, sometimes, the patient is too agitated to participate in this conversation. Always document the circumstances of the situation, and state that either the risks/benefits/

alternatives to the chosen treatment were explained to the patient, or state that an attempt was made to explain these to the patient, but the patient was too agitated to participate in a discussion at that time.

Intramuscular Medications (i.e., Chemical Restraint)

If the patient is out of control or unable to respond to the previously mentioned measures, the situation can quickly become dangerous, and physical or chemical restraint may be necessary to keep the patient and the environment safe. This is common with acutely manic or psychotic patients. Refer to medication guide later.

Physical Restraints

For agitation that poses imminent risk of danger that is not responsive to verbal deescalation and medications, physical restraint may be indicated. Patients on medical and surgical units sometimes exhibit agitated behavior that compromises their medical care. Once this is evident, restraint is indicated. Hesitation may jeopardize the patient's safety and care. See the Seclusion and Restraints chapter for information and guidelines.

Continued Management

Communicate with the treating staff. Hold a debriefing to state what worked well, and what could be improved, in managing the situation. Also be sure to ask about and address staff members' concerns and anxiety, because the staff may have felt threatened from the patient, and will have to interact with the patient in the future.

After emergency measures are carried out, carefully read the chart and follow up with the staff and the patient to determine further treatment. This should include gathering a complete psychiatric and medical history. Any interventions should reinforce the existing treatment plan.

A physical examination should be performed, with attention to neurologic assessment.

Laboratory tests should be ordered and followed up to facilitate treatment of underlying medical conditions. Consider obtaining the following:

- Complete blood count with differential
- Electrolytes
- Liver function tests
- Thyroid function tests
- Serum alcohol and urine toxicologies
- Arterial blood gas
- Medication levels (if suspect, hold medication until further notice)

- Electrocardiogram (ECG)
- Electroencephalogram (EEG)
- Skull or head imaging

Do not hesitate to call other consultants if you suspect medical conditions.

If the agitation is thought to be due to medication toxicity, consider discontinuing, tapering, or changing medications. Stopping or decreasing doses of medications may not immediately relieve the agitation, and therefore psychotropic medications may initially be required to control the agitation. In some cases, more aggressive interventions may be indicated (e.g., toxic lithium levels may require intravenous fluids or even renal dialysis). Sudden discontinuation of certain medications may have deleterious effects. To ensure good follow-up, document your consultation and the rationale for your decisions and speak with the primary team directly to let them know your suggestions.

In cases of suspected overdose, follow protocols for the specific substance.

MEDICATING THE PATIENT

As described previously, prior to medicating the patient, attempts should be made to verbally deescalate the patient, both by yourself and by staff members who may have/be able to form a connection with the patient. However, if the patient is acutely dangerous, it is important to ensure the safety of all of the patients and the staff by medicating the patient, as necessary.

Common PRN medications for managing agitation include haloperidol 5 mg and lorazepam 2 mg PO q6h PRN agitation. However, if needed, haloperidol 5 mg PO can be given as often as 15 minutes, with a maximum daily dose of 20 mg, and lorazepam 2 mg PO can be given as often as every 2 hours, with a maximum daily dose of 12 mg. This should both calm and sedate the patient within approximately 30 minutes (haloperidol can take 30 to 60 minutes and lorazepam can take 20 to 30 minutes to have therapeutic effect). Instead of haloperidol, olanzapine 5 to 10 mg PO or risperidone 1 to 2 mg PO q6h PRN can be used, along with a short-acting benzodiazepine. Although, if needed, olanzapine 5 to 10 mg PO can be given every 2 hours, with a maximum daily dose of 20 mg, and risperidone 2 mg PO can be given every 2 hours, with a maximum daily dose of 6 mg. However, the patient's medical conditions must be considered. If the patient has multiple medical comorbidities, especially cardiac in nature, or is elderly, reduced dosing should be considered, such as haloperidol 2.5 mg PO or risperidone 1 mg PO or olanzapine 2.5 mg PO or quetiapine 25 mg PO q6h PRN, along with lorazepam 1 mg PO q6h PRN. Many antipsychotics, such as haloperidol, should be avoided if the QTc is greater than 480, especially if it is 500 or more; safer choices for a prolonged QTc include olanzapine and quetiapine. To ensure that the patient is not "cheeking" medication, consider giving the liquid formulation (such as the liquid formulation of risperidone) or the orally disintegrating form (such as Zydis instead of olanzapine, and risperidone M-tabs) of the medication. If the patient's level of agitation is severe, consider giving IM medications for agitation, usually of the same doses that are listed previously for the oral doses. However, higher doses of antipsychotics, in both PO and IM form, may be used if needed. Haloperidol IM can be given as frequently as 5 mg q1h for agitation; olanzapine can be started at 10 mg IM and the second injection of 5 to 10 mg IM may be given 2 hours after the first injection, with a maximum daily recommended dose of 20 mg unless patient is extremely agitated in which case it is permissible to administer greater than 20 mg in 1 day. HOWEVER, do not give olanzapine IM concurrently with IM benzodiazepine, because doing so could cause cardiorespiratory depression and excessive sedation, and fatalities have occurred when olanzapine and benzodiazepines have been administered concurrently. Do not give IM olanzapine within 1 hour preadministration or postadministration of a benzodiazepine.

IM medications generally work at least as quickly, if not faster, than PO medications; however, each patient is different, and the time to onset can vary.

The following are alternative or backup medications:

- Chlorpromazine 25 to 50 mg IM can be administered. Extreme caution should be used with IM chlorpromazine because of the potential for orthostatic hypotension; therefore monitor vital signs. Do not give IM injections more than 50 mg.
- Diphenhydramine 50 mg PO or IM can be given to patients sensitive to antipsychotics or benzodiazepines. It can also be used to control agitation in children.

As described previously, if these measures are not effective, consider medical etiologies and also that the patient may need seclusion and possibly restraints.

It is best to stay on the unit until the agitation has been resolved to observe the mental status of the patient and to support the staff and to lead a debriefing session.

Suggested Readings

Cummings J, et al. Agitation in cognitive disorders: International psychogeriatric association provisional consensus clinical and research definition. *Int Psychogeriatr.* 2015;27(1):7–17.

Eli Lily and Company. Zyprexa: Highlights of prescribing information. 23 Jan 2017. Retrieved from < http://pi.lilly.com/us/zyprexa-pi.pdf >.

Marder SR, et al. Case reports of postmarketing adverse event experiences with olanzapine intramuscular treatment in patients with agitation. *The Journal of Clinical Psychiatry*. 2010;71(4):433–441.

Sanofi-aventis New Zealand limited. Largactil data sheet. 5 Aug 2016. Retrieved from < http://www.medsafe.govt.nz/profs/Datasheet/l/largactiltabinjsusp.pdf > .

Stahl SM. *Essential Psychopharmacology Online.* Retrieved from http://stahlonline.cambridge.org.ezproxy.med.nyu.edu/prescribers_guide.jsf.

Wilson MP, et al. Western Journal of Emergency Medicine. 2012. The psychopharmacology of agitation: consensus statement of the American association for emergency psychiatry project BETA psychopharmacology workgroup. *Western Journal of Emergency*. 2012;13(1):26–34.

The Anxious Patient

When receiving a call for anxiety, it is useful to distinguish between fear, anxiety, and panic. These are all states characterized by a feeling of apprehension and are often accompanied by physiologic signs of autonomic arousal. Fear is a normal response to a realistic and a clearly identified source of danger. It is adaptive in that it activates the body's autonomic system in preparation for a "flight-or-fight" response in case of dangerous or life-threatening situations. Anxiety refers to a more sustained, generalized apprehension without any identifiable stimulus. Anxiety is pathologic in nature when characterized by uncertainty and excessive worries with many physical symptoms of arousal. When anxiety is intense and rapid in onset, it can take the form of a panic attack, which is experienced as a state of sudden terror and feelings of imminent death or losing control, along with a number of physical symptoms.

In the evaluation of the anxious patient, one should attempt to understand the patient's anxiety symptoms and search for any potential source of the anxiety. Rule out any underlying medical or drug-related etiology before attributing anxiety to a known psychiatric disorder. Anxiety of sufficient intensity that necessitates an emergency room visit or a call from staff nurses requires careful assessment and treatment.

PHONE CALL

Questions

1. What are the patient's presenting symptoms and the duration of anxiety?
2. What is the patient's age and reason for hospitalization?
3. What are the vital signs?
4. What medications is the patient taking?
5. Is the patient taking any alternative medicine therapies or nutritional supplements?

6. Does the patient have a history of a psychiatric disorder?
7. Does the patient have a history of drug or alcohol abuse?

Orders

1. The most important aspect of assessment over the telephone is to determine if the patient is in a life-threatening situation. Order the vital signs if they were not already taken.
2. Order other tests based on the patient's additional symptoms. For example, if the patient also complains of shortness of breath, order a pulse oximeter, or, if the patient has accompanying chest pain, order an electrocardiogram (ECG).
3. Although it is not usual practice to order medications over the telephone, this may be indicated in certain situations. For example, a wheezing patient with a known history of asthma may benefit from as-needed (PRN) medications for asthma before the arrival of the psychiatrist.
4. Place the patient in a safe and quiet environment, and make sure the patient is being closely monitored.

Inform RN

"Will arrive in…minutes."

After the telephone call, prioritize the timing of arrival depending on the severity of the patient's symptoms. If the cardiovascular or respiratory system is the suspected etiology, see the patient immediately. If the patient's vital signs are stable, there are no acutely concerning physical symptoms, and the situation is not life threatening, arrival is less urgent.

ELEVATOR THOUGHTS

What causes anxiety?
- Medical and drug-related causes (Tables 10.1 and 10.2)
- Primary psychiatric disorders
    Generalized anxiety disorder (GAD)
    Obsessive-compulsive disorder (OCD)
    Panic disorder and agoraphobia
    Social phobia
    Specific phobia
    Posttraumatic stress disorder (PTSD) and acute stress disorder
    Adjustment disorder with anxious mood
    Anxiety secondary to psychotic symptoms
    Anxiety in the context of depressive disorders
    Personality disorders

TABLE 10.1	Physical Causes of Anxiety-Like Symptoms

Type of Cause	Specific Cause
Cardiovascular	Angina pectoris, arrhythmias, congestive heart failure, hypertension, hypovolemia, myocardial infarction, syncope (multiple causes), valvular disease, vascular collapse (shock)
Dietary	Caffeine, monosodium glutamate (Chinese restaurant syndrome), vitamin-deficiency diseases
Drug related	Akathisia (secondary to antipsychotic drugs), anticholinergic toxicity, digitalis toxicity, hallucinogens, stimulants (amphetamines, cocaine, related drugs), withdrawal syndromes (alcohol, sedative-hypnotics), bronchodilators (theophylline)
Endocrine	Adrenal gland dysfunction, menopause and ovarian dysfunction, parathyroid disease, pheochromocytoma, premenstrual syndrome, hyperthyroidism, hypothyroidism, carcinoid, insulinoma
Hematologic	Anemias
Immunologic	Anaphylaxis, systemic lupus erythematosus
Metabolic	Hyperkalemia, hyperthermia, hypocalcemia, hypoglycemia, hyponatremia, acute intermittent porphyria
Neurologic	Encephalopathies (infectious, metabolic, toxic), essential tremor, intracranial mass lesions, cerebral anoxia, postconcussive syndrome, seizure disorders (especially of the temporal lobe), vertigo, myasthenia gravis, pain
Respiratory	Asthma, chronic obstructive pulmonary disease, pneumonia, pneumothorax, pulmonary edema, pulmonary embolism, hyperventilation, hypoxia

Modified from Rosenbaum JF. The drug treatment of anxiety. *N Engl J Med*. 1982;306:401. Copyright 1982 Massachusetts Medical Society. With permission.

TABLE 10.2	Drugs That May Cause Anxiety

Stimulants
Amphetamine
Aminophylline
Caffeine
Cocaine
Methylphenidate
Theophylline

Sympathomimetics
Ephedrine
Epinephrine

Phenylpropanolamine
Pseudoephedrine

Drug Withdrawal
Barbiturates
Benzodiazepines
Narcotics
Alcohol
Hypnotic sedatives
Clonidine

Anticholinergics
Benztropine mesylate (Cogentin)
Diphenhydramine (Benadryl)
Meperidine (Demerol)
Oxybutynin (Ditropan)
Propantheline (Probanthine)
Tricyclic antidepressants
Trihexyphenidyl (Artane)

Dopaminergics
Amantadine
Antipsychotics
Bromocriptine
Levodopa (L-dopa)
Levodopa-carbidopa (Sinemet)
Metoclopramide

Miscellaneous
Baclofen
Cycloserine
Hallucinogens
Indomethacin

From Goldberg RJ. *Practical Guide to the Care of the Psychiatric Patient.* St. Louis: Mosby–Year Book; 1995.

MAJOR THREAT TO LIFE

Anxiety is a symptom in certain life-threatening medical conditions, such as pulmonary embolism or myocardial infarction. Therefore it is imperative to rule out any medical causes of anxiety because they may result in significant morbidity or mortality if left untreated. In addition, anxiety is a physiologic symptom of alcohol or benzodiazepine withdrawal, which can result in death if not recognized and treated. Untreated anxiety of psychiatric etiology can be disabling and can lead to impaired judgment. When anxiety becomes intolerable, as can happen in panic disorder and akathisia, it has been associated with suicidal behavior.

Quick Look Test

Does the patient appear to be in acute medical distress?

- If so, collect a set of vitals, fingerstick, and consider pulmonary, cardiologic, or neurologic etiologies.

What are the patient's facial expression, posture, and mannerisms?

- These may give indications of the patient's level of anxiety.

Is the patient breathing in a fast and shallow manner, clutching his or her throat? Is the patient holding his or her chest or abdomen, sweating, or holding on to an object, fearing that he or she might collapse? Is the patient describing dizziness, faintness, fear of going crazy, or even fear of dying?

- These patients are generally receptive to any support that can be offered, and even in the midst of a panic attack, they will be able to verbalize their symptoms. Still, be sure to carefully examine the patient because these symptoms can mimic medical problems. If panic seems likely, the patient may be able to engage in deep breathing exercises.

Is the patient pacing? Is the patient fidgety and unable to sit or stand still?

- These signs indicate that a patient may be experiencing akathisia.

Is the patient tearful, intense, or labile, but not acutely distressed?

- This may indicate generalized anxiety, fear, or worry; in this case the patient will likely be receptive to an interview.

On occasion, the patient may appear to be calm, relaxed, and able to describe symptoms in a coherent manner because some acute anxiety attacks are self-limited. For example, this presentation may be a defining feature of a panic attack. Do not be misled by rapid relief from symptoms and withhold treatment or a careful examination.

Airway and Vital Signs

Although the nurse should have already taken vital signs, it is advisable to order vital signs to be taken frequently. This may calm the patient as well. Repeat vital signs may point to an association with a specific medical condition (e.g., pheochromocytoma).

Selective History and Chart Review

New and acute-onset of anxiety merits a full psychiatric and medical evaluation.

Obtain a full history of the present illness:

- Does the patient report excessive worries, ruminating thoughts, intrusive or obsessive thoughts, compulsions, or specific fears?

- Does the patient experience panic? If so, obtain information about symptoms, duration, and frequency.
- Has there been recent trauma or the onset of new life stressors?
- Does the patient demonstrate evidence of a mood disorder or a psychotic illness?
- Has the patient experienced recent insomnia or agitation?

Obtain a pertinent past psychiatric history:

- Does the patient have a history of primary anxiety disorders, including GAD, OCD, PTSD, social phobia, and panic disorder?
- Does the patient have a history of a mood disorder or a psychotic illness?
- Is there a family history of anxiety?

Obtain information about psychiatric medications, keeping the following in mind:

- Has the patient recently been started on or had a change of a serotonin reuptake inhibitor (SSRI) preparation? Initiation of SSRIs, intended to treat depression or anxiety, may cause severe intolerable anxiety in the beginning phase of treatment, particularly if too high a dose is given.
- Is this a discontinuation syndrome? Medically or surgically hospitalized patients may have had medications discontinued prior to hospitalization or may forget to fully report medications to their primary team. Abrupt discontinuation of sedatives like benzodiazepines can provoke withdrawal symptoms that can cause anxiety. The shorter the half-life of the benzodiazepine and the longer the patient has been on the medication, the more severe the withdrawal symptoms after discontinuation. Discontinuation of antidepressants (particularly venlafaxine and paroxetine) can also precipitate a discontinuation syndrome, which includes symptoms of dizziness, lethargy, headache, irritability, paresthesias, and anxiety.
- Is the patient exhibiting akathisia caused by a new medication or by a change in the dosage of an existing medication? Akathisia is characterized by a subjective feeling of physical restlessness, especially in the lower extremities, and an inability to sit or stand still, and can be distinguished from anxiety based on history, patient characterization, and observation. Both antipsychotics (aripiprazole in particular) and to a lesser extent selective SSRIs are known to potentially cause akathisia.
- If available, consult a registry of controlled substance prescriptions, which may guide both diagnosis and management.

Carefully screen for substance use:

- Does the patient smoke, and is adequate nicotine replacement being given in the hospital?
- What is the pattern of alcohol use and benzodiazepine treatment, and is the patient at risk for withdrawal?

- Does the patient use illicit drugs?
- Some patients who abuse substances may be reluctant to disclose their history. It is helpful to inform these patients of the need to know of any recent use or cessation of use (especially of alcohol) to prevent any serious and potentially life-threatening withdrawal effects.
- Inquire about the use of over-the-counter products (e.g., cold remedies), dietary supplements for weight loss or weight gain, herbal medications, and other alternative or "natural" products that often contain stimulants and sympathomimetics, such as ephedrine (look for ingredients called ephedra or ma-huang).
- Keep in mind that substance use disorders are also highly comorbid with anxiety disorders, so it is also important to search for anxiety symptoms that predated any substance use.
- Order a urine toxicology test if not yet performed.
  Perform a brief test of orientation.

In the medical evaluation, carefully rule out any suspected medical etiology. Perform any relevant physical examination or laboratory tests as indicated. Review the medical history, medications, and recent laboratory results. The following questions may be helpful:

- Does the patient present with any symptoms or history suggestive of a medical cause of anxiety, as listed in Table 10.1?
- Does the patient have a history or physical signs of substance abuse or withdrawal?
- Is the patient overusing medications that can produce anxiety, such as bronchodilators?
- Is the patient experiencing side effects secondary to drug interactions? For example, potent inhibitors of the cytochrome P-450 system (e.g., cimetidine or fluoxetine) may increase the plasma levels of other drugs such as digoxin.
- Have there been recent changes in medications or dosage adjustments that might be responsible for the onset of anxiety?
  Order laboratory tests and other exams as indicated, which may include:
- Orthostatic vital signs
- Complete blood count (CBC)
- Basic metabolic panel (BMP)
- Urine toxicology
- Thyroid stimulating hormone
- ECG

Mental Status Examination

The full mental status examination is important, but some features are more relevant for the diagnosis of anxiety. An anxious patient's appearance, posture, gestures, and facial expressions are revealing.

Motor behavior may reveal agitation and restlessness. Also note any sweating or tremulousness (speech may be stammering or stuttering). Mood and affect usually reflect anxiety. Thought processes usually remain logical. Any perceptual disturbances suggest the use of substances or the possibility of a psychotic process. Psychotic symptoms may also induce anxiety. Patients experiencing panic attack or symptoms of PTSD may report depersonalization and derealization. Always screen for the presence of any suicidal ideation or plan because suicide is not uncommon in patients with severe anxiety. Sensoria are generally clear unless the patient has anxiety associated with delirium. Severe anxiety can impair concentration, which will affect other parts of the cognitive examination. The patient's insight and judgment may also appear impaired secondary to the level of distress.

Selective Physical Examination

The physical examination can be helpful in identifying a potential medical etiology for anxiety symptoms. The physical examination should focus on the patient's somatic complaints and evidence of any preexisting medical condition that may cause anxiety. A neurologic examination, including examination of the pupils, deep tendon reflexes, and tremors (and tongue fasciculations), can elicit signs of substance abuse or withdrawal. Patients with akathisia have characteristic signs, such as swinging of one leg while sitting, rocking from foot to foot, or "walking on the spot" while standing.

MANAGEMENT

Nearly all patients with anxiety will benefit from a calm and supportive bedside presence and from a soothing and nonstimulating environment, if this can be arranged in the often chaotic hospital setting. Sometimes the simple act of sitting down at a patient's bedside, turning off the television, and directing full attention towards the patient for several minutes can help reduce acute distress. Many patients will also respond to therapeutic interventions such as cognitive reframing, progressive muscle relaxation, paced breathing, and general reassurance and validation. It is also important to bear in mind that consultations may be requested to help manage strong affect from both the patient and the primary treatment team. It is not uncommon for anxious patients to elicit intense reactions (e.g., annoyance, frustration, helplessness) from those directly responsible for his or her care. In these situations, it can be helpful to remain calm and measured and to encourage clear communication between the team and the patient.

Optimal management of anxiety in the hospital setting depends in large part upon identification of the underlying etiology. If a primary medical cause is suspected, this should be addressed quickly and as clinically indicated. For medication-induced anxiety, the dose of the offending agent can be lowered or stopped entirely after discussion with the primary team to ensure that the risks and benefits of changing or discontinuing the medication are thoroughly considered. If anxiety is thought to be secondary to substance intoxication or withdrawal, addressing those conditions is what is clinically indicated (e.g., treating alcohol withdrawal with benzodiazepines, allowing for metabolism of cocaine). For anxious patients with a primary psychiatric disorder, ensuring optimal treatment of the psychiatric condition is central.

For many patients, medication will be necessary (in addition to other interventions) to obtain adequate control of acute or severe anxiety. Before starting or recommending any medication, one should always be aware of potential drug-drug interactions, adverse effects, and contraindications.

- **Benzodiazepines** are extremely effective anxiolytics, although they are not without risks (behavioral disinhibition particularly in the elderly or medically ill, oversedation, respiratory depression, increased potential for falls, development of tolerance) and should typically be avoided in patients with delirium or with active substance abuse issues. See Table 10.3 for information about specific properties and comparative doses of commonly used benzodiazepines. Typical choices for acute anxiety include lorazepam (0.5 to 2 mg PO/IM/IV), clonazepam (0.25 to 1 mg PO), or alprazolam (0.25 to 1 mg PO). Clonazepam and alprazolam are also available in rapidly disintegrating tablets for faster onset of action. Lorazepam (along with oxazepam and temazepam, although these are not widely used in the acute setting) is preferred in patients with hepatic dysfunction because it does not undergo oxidation and does not have active metabolites, so its half-life is not affected by liver disease. Consider benzodiazepine use particularly in anxiety secondary to initiation of SSRI treatment or in akathisia in patients who do not respond well to other treatments.
- Other medications to consider for acute use include **antihistamines** (e.g., diphenhydrame 25 to 50 mg PO or IM PRN, hydroxyzine 25 to 100 mg PO or IM PRN), particularly in patients with respiratory issues, given minimal risk of respiratory depression and in patients with substance abuse issues. Keep in mind that these medications also increase anticholinergic burden and may lower the seizure threshold. **Gabapentin** (typically 100 to 300 mg PO PRN or three times daily [TID] standing) can be helpful particularly in patients with substance use disorders (of note, there are data to suggest that it may help treat alcohol dependence) or in patients with hepatic

TABLE 10.3 Pharmacology of Benzodiazepines

Pharmacology of Benzodiazepines

Drug	Adult Oral Total Daily Dose (mg)[a]	Comparative Potency (mg)[b]	Onset After Oral Dose (Hours)	Metabolism	Elimination Half-Life (Hours)[c]
Used Primarily to Treat Anxiety Symptoms/Anxiety Disorders					
Alprazolam	0.5–6	0.5	1	CYP3A4 to minimally active metabolites.	11–15
Alprazolam extended release	0.5–6 once daily	0.5	1		16 (older adults) 20 (hepatic impairment)
Bromazepam[d]	6–30	7.5	1	CYP1A2. No active metabolite.	22 (obesity) 8–20
Chlordiazepoxide	5–100	10	1	CYP3A4 to active metabolites.	30–100
Clonazepam	0.5–4	0.25–0.5	0.5–1	CYP3A4. No active metabolite.	18–50
Clorazepate	15–60	7.5	0.5–1	CYP3A4 to active metabolite.	36–200
Diazepam	4–40	5	0.25–0.5	CYP2C19 and 3A4 to active metabolites.	50–100
					Prolonged in older adults and renal or hepatic impairment
Lorazepam	0.5–6 0.5–4 (hypnotic)	1	0.5–1	Non-CYP glucuronidation in liver. No active metabolite.	10–14

Oxazepam	30–120	15–30	1–2	Non-CYP glucuronidation in liver. No active metabolite.	5–15
Prazepam[d]	15–30 (hypnotic) 15–60	15	2–3	CYP3A4 to active metabolites.	30–200 Prolonged in older adults
Used Primarily to Treat Insomnia[e]					
Estazolam	1–2	0.3	0.5–1	CYP3A4 to minimally active metabolite.	10–24
Flurazepam	15–30	5	0.5–1	CYP3A4 to active metabolites.	40–114 120–160 (older adults)
Nitrazepam[d]	5–10	5	0.5–1	Non-CYP acetylation in liver. No active metabolites.	24–30
Temazepam	7.5–30	5	0.5–1	Primarily non-CYP glucuronidation in liver to minimally active metabolite.	40 (older adults) 8–15
Triazolam	0.125–0.25	0.1	0.25–0.5	CYP3A4. No active metabolite.	2–5
Quazepam	7.5–15	5	1	CYP3A4 and non-CYP metabolism in liver to active metabolites.	28–84 190 (older adults)

[a]Range of usual total dose for treatment of adults with anxiety or panic disorder typically given in divided doses two to four times daily.

[b]Important: Data shown are approximate equal potencies relative to lorazepam 1 mg orally and are NOT recommendations for initiation of therapy or for conversion between agents.

[c]Half-life of parent drug and pharmacologically active metabolite, if any.

[d]Not available in United States.

[e]Range of usual hypnotic dose for adults, given at bedtime.

Data on drug metabolism and activity of metabolite(s) are for assessment of potential for CYP drug interactions and risk of accumulation. Risk of accumulation is greater, and dose reduction is necessary for older or debilitated adults and for patients with renal or hepatic insufficiency.

dysfunction because it is excreted unchanged by the kidneys. The dose of gabapentin must be adjusted according to creatinine clearance. **Beta-blockers** are useful in treating anxiety secondary to hyperadrenergic states (e.g., hyperthyroidism) and for treating medication-related akathisia (in addition to stopping or changing the offending agent), although it is important to consider any medical contraindications to use such as bradycardia or asthma. **Clonidine** can also be used in the treatment of akathisia, although it is important to be aware of potential cardiovascular side effects.

- **Antipsychotics** are clearly indicated when the anxiety is related to psychosis (e.g., paranoia, distress from hallucinations) or in delirious patients who are anxious and distressed. These medications can also be helpful in patients whose anxiety takes on a quasipsychotic appearance, such as patients with extreme perseveration or severe affective dysregulation, even in the absence of an underlying primary psychotic disorder; in these cases in particular, one should carefully consider the risks and benefits of using the medication and use low doses of the antipsychotic to start.

- **SSRIs** or **serotonin and norepinephrine reuptake inhibitors (SNRIs)** are safe and effective first-line treatments for most primary anxiety disorders and for anxiety related to depressive disorders, although these medications will usually not be immediately effective and can cause acute worsening of anxiety in the initial phases of treatment. It is acceptable to start the patient on one of these medications as long as it is possible to observe for an initial response and side effects for at least a few days and if there is appropriate posthospitalization follow-up. Remember, it is important to "start low and go slow" when using the medication to treat anxiety (e.g., consider using sertraline 25 mg versus 50 mg, escitalopram 5 mg versus 10 mg).

- **Buspirone** can be an effective agent for GAD and is well tolerated in the elderly and medically ill. However, as with SSRIs, it is generally not useful in acute settings because of its lag time of 3 to 4 weeks for a full therapeutic effect.

The Violent Patient

Being called to manage a violent patient can be one of the most anxiety-provoking and difficult tasks asked of a psychiatrist. Often, the phone call is from a nurse or another physician who is frightened of a patient and in a situation that is out of their control. The call may be from the emergency room of a hospital or from an inpatient psychiatric or medical unit. As a psychiatrist on call, you are expected to be the team leader in a multidisciplinary approach to help maintain the safety of the patient and those in the immediate vicinity. You may feel that you are expected to single-handedly make the patient nonviolent and make the staff and other patients feel safe and comfortable again. Because violent behavior or threat of violent behavior is often already in progress at the time you receive the call, you are asked to arrive right away and have immediate solutions. Behavioral emergencies are complex and difficult, as they require ongoing evaluation and changes in management strategy as new information becomes available. There is a sense of urgency; however, we often do not know a diagnosis, and there is limited time for decision making.

To be effective at helping to restore a safe environment, it is essential that you take a moment to collect your thoughts and prepare yourself to interact as calmly, clearly, and directly as possible with people who are upset and dangerous. Remember that you are being called on to do your best to prevent any harm to yourself and others, and you will need the support of other staff members. This chapter helps you to approach and manage the violent patient in a stepwise fashion beginning with the initial phone call through the bedside evaluation and management.

PHONE CALL

Questions

These questions are in the order that you might ask them when called to deal with a violent patient. Depending on the acuity of the situation, you may have to ask some of these questions on the scene. The answers will determine how you will manage the situation, as seen later in the "Bedside" and "Management" sections.

1. Where is the patient located? (emergency room, inpatient psychiatric unit, inpatient medical unit)
2. What is the patient doing right now?
3. Does the patient appear threatening, or has he or she verbally threatened violence or already behaved in a violent manner?
4. Has anyone been injured, and, if so, how badly?
5. Have security personnel been called, and are they at the scene?
6. Does the patient have access to weapons of violence, including hospital furniture and medical equipment?
7. Is the patient psychotic or delirious? What is/are the patient's psychiatric diagnosis/diagnoses, including substance abuse?
8. Does the patient have any medical illnesses?
9. Are medications and restraints ready for immediate use?

Orders

1. Call hospital police to the area if this has not been done already.
2. Have as-needed (PRN) medication, both orally (PO) and intramuscularly (IM), available to be administered, even if the patient has already received PRN medication (the patient may need more than the first PRN dose). If there is no standing order for PRN medication, haloperidol (Haldol) and lorazepam (Ativan) should be ready for use on arrival.
3. Remove any potentially dangerous materials and attempt to keep other patients away from the vicinity of the patient.
4. Have restraints and the seclusion room ready for use if necessary.

Inform RN

"Will arrive in … minutes."

This situation should become your top priority, and you should make every attempt to make it to the scene as quickly as possible.

ELEVATOR THOUGHTS

What issue(s) might be at the root of a patient's violent or potentially violent behavior?

- First attempt to rule out medical illnesses leading to agitation including delirium (from multiple medical etiologies including infection, electrolyte abnormalities, myocardial infarction), agitation associated with dementia, and cognitive deficits including developmental disabilities
- Next consider agitation and violence stemming from substance intoxication (cocaine, amphetamines, and phencyclidine [PCP]) or withdrawal (alcohol, opiates, and benzodiazepines)

- Then consider different psychiatric etiologies including:
  - Psychosis (paranoia, command or noncommand hallucinations)
  - Manic symptoms (grandiosity, psychomotor agitation, irritability, psychosis)
  - Akathisia (feeling of inner restlessness and a need to be in constant motion) from antipsychotic medication
  - Impulsivity/explosiveness
  - Dissociative state
  - Poor frustration tolerance/needs not being met or perceived as not being met
  - Avoidance of an undesirable situation (e.g., incarceration, transfer)

Again, take the time on the way to the scene to assess your own demeanor, take a deep breath, and remember that you will be most helpful and a more effective team leader if you are a calming, rational presence.

BEDSIDE

Chart Review

If on arrival to the scene you have a moment to review the patient's chart to get a sense of the patient's history or hospital course, take this opportunity to look for the following information:

- Vital signs
- Current medications
- The patient's age
- Circumstances of presentation to the hospital
- Medical and psychiatric diagnoses
- History of violence

If you are unable to view the chart before seeing the patient, ask these questions of the staff on your way to seeing the patient.

Quick Look Test

Are there enough staff members/security personnel to make you feel reasonably safe approaching the patient?

Are there enough staff, equipment, and medications to safely restrain the patient if necessary?

Has the area been cleared of other patients and any furniture or other objects that could be used as weapons? Is the patient in possession of any potential weapons?

Is the patient visibly agitated?

How is the patient responding to your arrival? Is he or she verbal? Assuming an aggressive physical or verbal stance? Speaking or behaving in a disorganized manner?

Does the patient appear physically ill?

Vital Signs

Although you should not attempt to approach the patient to take vital signs until you are certain that you or anyone else can do so safely, note possible indications of abnormal vital signs, including diaphoresis, pallor, unsteady gait, or dyspnea. As soon as possible, take vital signs to help determine if the etiology of the violent behavior could be from medical problems or alcohol or drug withdrawal.

Approaching the Patient

Make sure that you are not carrying any objects that could be used by the patient as a weapon. Remove all dangling jewelry and identification badges, pens, sharp objects, stethoscopes, and neckties. Make sure your hands are free. Stand as far from the patient as necessary for you to feel safe, at least a body's length from a patient. It is recommended that you stand to the side as opposed to facing in a full-frontal position. This lessens the surface area for an attack on your person. Never turn your back on the patient.

Make sure that the patient is not holding any weapons and has been searched for weapons. If either of these is not the case, making sure the patient has no weapons is the first order of business. This is especially important in the emergency room, where searching a patient, especially an agitated and uncooperative patient, may not have been done adequately. Security officers should be responsible for making sure the patient is not carrying weapons. In the interim, ask the patient to keep his or her hands free and in sight.

Approach the patient only when you feel comfortable that you have enough staff present to protect your safety and that you have done the previous "quick look" tests. You must feel safe, because the violent patient will likely sense your fear and level of confidence. Often, the violent patient is out of control and your feeling safe and in control may allow the patient to feel safer and more in control. Try to see the patient in as open and secure an area as possible. You and the staff should be standing together and closer to any exit than the patient. Although an open area is preferable to allow the patient to feel less trapped, security is paramount, so you and the staff must be able to exit a dangerous room if absolutely necessary and the violent patient must be prevented from leaving the secured area.

Approach the patient from the front or side, not the back. Maintain adequate distance as violent patients may need more room than others to feel comfortable. Mirror body language to demonstrate empathy (sit if patient is sitting, walk alongside if patient is pacing). Avoid confrontational stances (such as sustained eye contact, crossed arms, hands behind back or in pockets) and hold a neutral tone and relaxed body posture. Identify yourself and your objectives in simple terms. You may need to repeat yourself several times, as patients in an emotionally aroused state will have diffi-culty retaining information.

Selective History and Mental Status

You are now ready to attempt to obtain a history from the patient. This history must be concise and direct, but your level of firmness with the patient will depend on the acuity of the situation. If you have not introduced yourself to the patient before, introduce your-self and let the patient know that you and the staff are there to see if you can help him or her in any way. Ask the patient if there are any problems that need to be addressed. Say why you have been called and reiterate that you have come to address the patient's concerns, that you would like to fix any problems if you can, and that your most important role is to make sure that the patient and others remain safe. Listen to the patient's concerns. If there is anything that you do not understand, ask for clarification.

You will need to perform a focused mental status examination after you have approached the patient. Assess the patient's level of psychomotor agitation, volume and rate of speech, and degree of irritability. If the patient's thought process is disorganized or the patient is otherwise grossly psychotic, you will need to minimize the history you take from the patient and move toward managing the behavioral disturbance. If the patient is not psychotic or delir-ious, violent threats or behavior is more likely to be the result of feeling that his or her needs are not being met. Engaging the patient to obtain more history may be helpful in calming the patient and letting the patient know that someone is listening to what he or she has to say. Make note of any specific verbal threats or gestures the patient makes. You will later need to document exactly what the patient has said or done that is dangerous and has required the appropriate interventions to maintain safety. Find out why the patient is in the hospital or emergency room and what are the patient's most serious immediate problems. Ask who is available to help the patient and what the immediate and more chronic precipitants are for the present violent or threatening behavior. Remember that getting this history requires that you and the staff are safe. These important elements of the history may need to be garnered after the acute situation is managed.

INITIAL MANAGEMENT

Your management of the situation will depend on the answers to the previously mentioned questions that you have been asking yourself, the staff, and the patient. You must decide how much the patient's medical illness, current mental status, and other such factors are contributing to the situation.

If the patient is behaving violently, is agitated, or has just behaved violently, you must first assess if the patient is responding to verbal redirection. Ask the patient to stop what he or she is doing and stand or sit so that you can speak to him or her. If the patient will not respond to verbal redirection, and you cannot obtain more history to further pinpoint the etiology of the violence, medication should be offered first in oral form and then in intramuscular form.

If the patient can speak, you should first attempt verbal redirection and de-escalating techniques. The verbal approach includes introducing yourself and explaining what you are going to do using short and clear sentences, reorienting the patient, setting limits of what is acceptable and nonacceptable behavior, and allowing the patient to express feelings and concerns (including anger). Offering food, water, or assistance may be helpful. Always look for signs that may signal the patient is becoming more agitated. Preliminary signs include change in speech (speed, tone, volume, content), posturing and tension (clenched fists or jaw), and increased physical movement/restlessness, irritability, or hostility when answering questions.

If the patient does not respond to verbal redirection, then medication should be offered. Oral medications should be offered, but you should use your judgment as to whether that is the safest course of action. Oral medication may not have a rapid enough onset for most acutely violent situations and should be used only if you assess that the patient will remain behaviorally in control until the medication is absorbed and takes effect. The patient must be monitored and held if necessary while medication is being administered to ensure that the proper dose is given and to prevent anyone from getting stuck by a needle or by a patient trying to hit the person administering the medication. Deciding to give medication by injection may be a difficult decision to make, but remember that you are taking this action to maintain the safety of the patient and everyone around the patient.

When choosing a medication for behavioral emergencies, the most important factors to consider include whether there is availability of an IM formulation, the onset of speech, history of medical response, effectiveness at producing useful sedation, likelihood to produce intolerable or dangerous side effects, and patient preference.

Haloperidol and lorazepam used in combination (usually haloperidol 5 mg and lorazepam 2 mg) is often the first-line medication for agitation and violence related to psychosis, mood symptoms, or alcohol/substance intoxication/withdrawal, but various factors need to be taken into consideration. If there is evidence that the patient is medically ill or is elderly, the doses of these medications should be adjusted downward and vital signs should be monitored frequently if not continuously (e.g., haloperidol 2.5 mg and loraze-pam 1 mg). Care must be taken using benzodiazepines in patients with organic brain syndromes, mental retardation, dementia, or delirium, because the patient may become disinhibited and confused paradoxically. If the patient is behaving violently because of an alcohol or drug withdrawal syndrome as evidenced by his or her history, autonomic instability, or other signs of withdrawal, the appropriate withdrawal protocol should be implemented immediately (e.g., symptom-triggered therapy with benzodiazepines).

While mood stabilizers are not used as first-line treatment in emergency situations, valproic acid to manage further episodes of agitation/violence due to mania may be considered. In these cases, treatment begins with 20 mg/kg while checking blood levels after 5 days. For more rapid action, can use a loading dose of 20 to 30 mg/kg.

Common formulations of antipsychotics are detailed as follows.

In liquid or rapidly disintegrating form:

Risperidone 1 mg/mL solution

Olanzapine 5 mg disintegrating tablet

Aripiprazole 1 mg/mL solution (5 to 10 mg is generally effective)

Aripiprazole 10 mg disintegrating tablet

Haloperidol 2 mg/mL solution

In IM form (dosing recommendations in parenthesis):

Haloperidol IM (2.5 to 5 mg)

Olanzapine IM (5 to 10 mg), use with caution in medically ill patients; do not administer IM olanzapine within 1 hour of benzodiazepines given the risk for cardiovascular/cardiopulmonary collapse

Ziprasidone (10 mg IM q 2 hours not to exceed 40 mg/day), use with caution in medically ill patients, since use is contraindicated in patients with recent myocardial infarction or in heart failure

In IV form:

Haloperidol IV (2 to 5 mg), note that IV haloperidol carries the highest risk for QTc prolongation and precipitation of torsade de pointes

Chlorpromazine IV (12.5 to 50 mg)

If there is an inadequate response with a single agent after 45 to 60 minutes, proceeding to the combination of a benzodiazepine and an antipsychotic or giving another dose of the initial agent alone are both reasonable options. If the patient was initially treated with a combination, then an additional dose of the combination is reasonable.

Safety and Tolerability Issues

In pregnancy, an expert panel preferred use of high-potency first-generation antipsychotics such as haloperidol due to larger studies conducted with this class and lack of teratogenicity.

In children, there was no first-line consensus for medication management of a violent child. Second-line options included an antihistamine or low-dose benzodiazepine.

Other factors to consider include whether the patient has a history of extrapyramidal side effects (EPS) (avoid high-potency antipsychotics such as haloperidol and fluphenazine), a history of substance dependence/drug-seeking behavior (avoid benzodiazepines if possible), a history of seizures (recommend benzodiazepines), or a history of cardiac arrhythmias or conduction defects (avoid antipsychotics).

Physical Restraints

Expert consensus is that restraints should be used as a last resort when all less restrictive measures have failed. Restraints are usually appropriate if there is acute danger to other patients, staff, or self. They are sometimes appropriate to prevent an involuntary patient from leaving prior to assessment or transfer to a locked facility. Restraints are not appropriate in certain situations, such as a lack of resources to adequately supervise restrained patient, to maintain an orderly environment, to prevent a voluntary patient from leaving, and if there is a history of self-injury with restraints. If it is necessary to physically restrain the patient or place the patient in seclusion, then this decision should be communicated to the family of the patient. The patient should be informed of what will happen ("we are going to hold you, we are going to put you on the bed and place restraints on each limb"). He or she should also understand the reasons for these steps ("in order to keep you and other patients/staff safe") as well as the expected duration of restraints/seclusion and requirements for discontinuing the intervention ("when you are more calm and not acting in a violent manner"). Every effort should be made to respect the patient's right's and privacy during this process. For further information, see the chapter on Seclusion and Restraint.

NEXT STEPS IN MANAGEMENT

The next step is to address any injuries sustained by the violent patient, other patients, or staff. Appropriate medical consults should be called and radiologic tests performed. Whether or not injuries have occurred, other patients and staff may need to have your attention and reassurance that the environment will remain safe. Placing the patient on one-to-one observation for assault precaution should be seriously considered, at least for a short period of time. The patient may benefit from having one-to-one observation if he or she is verbally redirectable or can use the one-to-one staff as someone to whom he or she can verbalize concerns.

Once the patient is calm, because he or she has been medicated or restrained or is not acutely violent, and is verbally redirectable, you can proceed to further investigation of the causes and precipitants of the violence. If the patient is medically ill, the patient's underlying problem may be causing the violent behavior. Delirious patients can be violent, and they may require short-term standing antipsychotic medication if the violent behavior cannot be controlled using PRN medication alone. Again, any alcohol or drug withdrawal syndromes should be aggressively treated.

If the patient can communicate coherently, he or she should be asked to try to describe the precipitants for the problematic behavior. Every effort should be made to accommodate reasonable requests or lessen stressors. The rules of the unit and the consequences of violent behavior, including the possibility of criminal charges, should be clearly stated. Wherever the patient is located, recommendations should be made if the patient again becomes agitated and threatening. The staff should be instructed specifically to monitor the patient closely for renewed expressions of anger and agitation. In the event of future threats of violence, the patient should be offered medication and the patient's needs should be addressed promptly and directly.

Make sure to check with staff to see that they feel comfortable with the resolution of the current situation. Ask them for their assessment, tell them what you believe are the precipitants and etiology for the patient's behavior, and make clear recommendations for future treatment.

You must document any violent activity or threats in the patient's chart and in any incident reports for the hospital. You should write clearly why you were called to see the patient; the specifics of violent acts or threats; how you dealt with that behavior, including assessment and treatment of any injuries; the risks of future violence; and your recommendations for further assessment and treatment. If you are serving as the psychiatric consultant, make sure you verbally communicate any urgent recommendations to the primary treatment team. Be specific about what laboratory tests (e.g., electrolytes, thyroid function tests) and other tests (e.g., electroencephalogram) should be ordered, how PRN medications should be used, and how any withdrawal symptoms should be treated. Any uncertainty about the patient's psychiatric diagnosis and current treatment (e.g., evidence that the patient has a bipolar disorder rather than schizophrenia and may benefit from valproic acid) should be included.

If the patient has made specific violent threats to someone who is not aware of those threats, you may be required by your state's law to report that dangerousness before the threatening patient is able to leave your institution. If at all possible, you should make the call to that person and explain the situation. If you cannot contact that person, you must make sure that you have documented your attempt. If you believe a patient is acutely dangerous, that patient should not leave the hospital. The patient's primary team should be made aware of the threat so that any appropriate warnings can be made.

Before leaving the vicinity, you may want to check on the patient one more time. Just making sure the patient has responded to your interventions can make the rest of your on-call experience safer for all.

REMEMBER

By definition, the violent patient can be a serious threat to his or her life as well as to staff and visitors. Violence in the hospital can cause serious and permanent injury to patients and staff. It is your responsibility to help the patient restore his or her composure in the least restrictive, yet safest, manner possible. Because it is impossible to assess impulsivity and dangerousness with certainty, take whatever measures are necessary to ensure patient and staff safety.

It is normal to struggle with managing violent patients, especially when first starting out. It is also normal to experience negative feelings towards the situation and even the patient. Try to be aware of your own responses and never feel embarrassed to ask for help and supervision to debrief.

Suggested Readings

Allen MH, Currier GW, Hughes DH, Docherty JP, Carpenter D, Ross R. Treatment of behavioral emergencies: a summary of the expert consensus guidelines. *J Psychiatr Pract.* 2003;9:16–38. Available from: http://www.ncbi.nlm.nih.gov/pubmed/15985913.

The Suicidal Patient

Helping a team manage suicidal patients is one of the most important tasks of the psychiatrist. It is also one of the most anxiety-provoking situations we face. Expect powerful emotional responses from the patient's family, hospital staff, and yourself. When on call in the hospital, you may be asked to assess suicidal patients in various settings including the emergency room, inpatient psychiatric unit, and inpatient medical or surgical services. Each situation comes with unique considerations and challenges.

The Consult

When the phone rings and the person on the other line tells you, "Our patient is reporting suicidality," many feelings may arise, including anxiety, fear, frustration, and annoyance. On one hand, suicide is a "true" psychiatric emergency, and completed suicide can be difficult to predict and prevent (making care of the suicidal patient an art as much as a science). At the same time, it is not uncommon for patients to report suicidality when the primary motivation is secondary gain. This phone call can help you begin to formulate the patient's complaints and can guide emergent management.

PHONE CALL

Questions

1. Has a suicide attempt been made, and if so, is the patient medically stable?

    If you are being called by staff from an inpatient psychiatry unit, you are probably the first physician who is being notified about the case. Determine if there is active bleeding, if there has been a toxic ingestion, if there are vital sign abnormalities or changes in mental status, or if there is any other cause for immediate medical attention. If so, you will want to contact the medical or surgical consult teams as quickly as possible.

2. What brought the patient to the hospital?

   Once you have established medical stability, you will want to obtain more detailed information about the case on the phone. For patients in a medical unit or in the emergency department, acute medical issues have probably been addressed, and you may be told "patient has been cleared for admission (or transfer) to psychiatry" before the consult has even begun. It is crucial to be vigilant of medical issues that may not have been considered by the medical teams, to rule out the possibility of an illicit ingestion, and to confirm that there have been no recent mental status changes. Remember that suicidality in the context of new onset confusion in a medically hospitalized patient is delirium until proven otherwise.

3. What does the patient look like right now?

   Always make sure to begin assessing the physical safety of the patient during this phone call. A disorganized, psychotic patient reporting suicidality in the context of psychosis, or an agitated, impulsive, intoxicated patient, may warrant social or chemical restraints urgently. It may be prudent to ask that the patient be placed on one-to-one observation immediately (see "Orders"), and you can ask that the primary team institute this monitoring even before you reach the patient to begin your clinical assessment.

Orders

With a suicidal patient, your first decision is determining whether or not the patient needs a higher level of observation than is standard. Though you are the psychiatrist, you will likely be working in tandem with other physicians and hospital staff who may be able to give you important input. Discuss with the nurse or primary physician whether the patient has a specific plan for suicide and active intent or has expressed passive suicidal ideation. If the former is true, consider starting one-to-one observation prior to your assessment and asking the nurse to remove any potentially dangerous objects from the patient's room. If the latter is true, you can probably defer the decision about one-to-one observation until you meet the patient. If unsure, err on the side of caution and recommend a one-to-one. Though close monitoring is a limited hospital resource, it is certainly better to be cautious and recommend a high level of observation, particularly as this can be easily discontinued after your assessment. Regardless of your decision, make sure to communicate the rationale for your recommendation to the nurse or primary physician, particularly your assessment of the safety risk.

While you are on the phone getting the initial consult, consider if the immediate administration of as-needed (or PRN) medications might be necessary. If the patient appears acutely psychotic—particularly if he or she is reporting command auditory hallucinations or exhibiting other gross impairments in reality testing—the patient may benefit from an immediate dose of antipsychotic medication. Antipsychotics should be offered in oral form; however, they can be given via intramuscular injection or intravenous push if oral is refused and there is an acute risk of danger towards the patient or staff. If the patient is complaining of intolerable anxiety (e.g., a patient who informs a nurse that he or she is having a panic attack and sees suicide as the only way out), a benzodiazepine such as low-dose lorazepam (orally or intramuscular/intravascular if needed) may be highly effective. The expeditious and judicious use of medication can sometimes relieve a patient's suffering so a more effective interview can be performed. If the patient becomes too sedated to be interviewed, it will be necessary to frequently reassess the patient until an interview can be performed.

Inform RN

"Will arrive in … minutes."

As suicidality constitutes a potentially life-threatening emergency, this patient should probably be triaged to the top of your list.

ELEVATOR THOUGHTS

What is underlying this patient's complaint of suicidality?

Suicidality can present as a symptom of many psychiatric and nonpsychiatric disorders. Even before you reach the patient, begin to think about how you will assess for different categories of illness.

1. In assessing for **affective disorders,** you will want to ask about current and past manic and depressive symptoms, remembering that the treatment of unipolar and bipolar depression will be different.
2. **Substance use disorders** can increase suicidality and are a major risk factor for completed suicides.
3. Patients with **psychotic spectrum disorders,** including schizophrenia and schizoaffective disorder, may present with suicidality, and patients with recently diagnosed psychotic disorders may be at particularly high risk.
4. Also assess for **cognitive disorders** including major and minor neurocognitive disorder, delirium, and intellectual disability, as well as **anxiety.**
5. Patients with **personality disorders** frequently present with suicidal ideation. Patients with narcissistic traits may make serious attempts when faced with losses or injuries to their self-esteem, while patients with borderline personality disorder may present after a suicide attempt or suicidal gesture with

nonsuicidal self-injurious behavior (e.g., cutting, nonmedically significant overdose), especially in the context of loss or absence of a love object. While patients with personality disorders often induce strong negative countertransference feelings in the psychiatrist as well as other hospital staff, it is important to be aware of these feelings and avoid acting on them, as this population is vulnerable to completed suicide. Thorough risk assessment is always warranted, even if the patient may not benefit from a long-term inpatient hospitalization.

A report of suicidal ideation may also represent an individual's attempt to manage a psychosocial stressor, such as homelessness or relationship conflict. It is important to consider if secondary gain is present, and if so, to discuss viable alternatives to inpatient psychiatric hospitalization. Remember, malingering is a diagnosis of exclusion, and a report of suicidality can be a mark of underlying psychiatric illness, even if a patient is not actively suicidal.

Remember that a patient who is threatening suicide and has a plan is a patient in crisis requiring your immediate attention. Factors that increase a patient's risk for a suicide attempt include previous suicide attempt, which is the most powerful predictor, as well as a history of self-injurious behavior, age above 45 years, male sex, substance abuse, history of violent behavior, past psychiatric hospitalizations, and family history of suicide. Other factors that increase a patient's risk for a suicide attempt include insomnia, panic attacks, medical illness, particularly a newly diagnosed severe medical illness, intoxication, and uncontrolled pain. Evaluating for the presence of these risk factors is integral to the development of a thorough risk assessment and guides further management.

BEDSIDE

Remember, you begin your assessment of the patient from first glance at the bedside, and a lot of important information may be available even before words are exchanged.

1. Always make sure that you conduct your interview in an **environment** where both you and the patient feel safe. Particularly when you are concerned about the possibility of an overdose or other suicide attempt, immediately rule out medical emergencies when you arrive at the bedside.
2. Review **vital signs,** assess for altered mental status, and examine for physical injuries.
3. Consider the patient's **affect and appearance.** Does the patient appear distressed, anxious, internally preoccupied, confused, or medically ill? What is the patient wearing, and what is his or her level of grooming? If you are concerned about his or her safety and worried about elopement, you might want to make sure the

patient changes out of his or her street clothes and into hospital garments.

4. Pay attention to his or her **behavior:** Is the patient sitting calmly or yelling and pacing? Is the patient engaged in a gregarious conversation, only to immediately begin sobbing when you enter the room? Do you receive a report from the team that the patient has recently been angry, demanding, or described as "manipulative" by the staff? Also, take immediate note of the environment at the bedside. Are there objects nearby that could be used for self-harm or violence?

INTERVIEW

Technique

When interviewing a suicidal patient, keep in mind that it is essential to establish a good therapeutic alliance with the patient. Even in the acute setting, an empathic and straightforward approach can go a long way in encouraging the patient to communicate openly and specifically about his or her suicidal ideas or plan.

Initially, introduce yourself and explain why you have been called. Ask basic questions about the patient's age and reason for presentation or hospitalization. One successful approach is to ask a general question about what the patient has been doing or feeling recently, and follow the patient's lead. Should you find the patient reluctant to talk, try to gain some rapport through an exploration of his or her life and medical history. If you quickly assess the patient to be floridly thought-disordered or psychotic, a highly structured interview may help you get the information you most need. If the patient is generally organized, you may get more information by taking a conversational approach.

Selective History

Recent history: What has been happening? Have there been any recent stressors, including medical illnesses or untreated pain? Any recent panic attacks? Does this time period correlate with an important anniversary or painful event? Is there a sense of hopelessness, guilt, or demoralization? Has the patient been feeling sad, blue, or "down in the dumps"? Have there been changes in sleep or appetite?

Suicidal ideation: Ask the patient about his or her exact thoughts about suicide. How long has the patient been having suicidal thoughts? When did they start? Is there more of a wish to be dead than an active plan? If there is a plan, get the details. Does the patient have the means to carry out the plan? (Are there firearms in the home? Are there syringes, catheters, or other hospital supplies at the bedside that might be used in an attempt?) If the patient did not follow through with the plan, why not? Explore the patient's ideas about what would happen after his or her death. Does he or she have fantasies of reuniting with a loved one? Have there been any "final acts" such as giving away possessions or saying goodbyes?

If there has already been an attempt, probe for details surrounding the event. Was the act impulsive or planned? Was there a note left? Did the patient try to prevent others from finding him (i.e., turned off phones, locked doors)? What did the patient imagine would happen after the act?

Finally, remember to assess for protective factors—what reasons does the patient have for living? For example, religiosity, stable employment, children at home and pregnancy, strong family support, and a history of stable relationships all diminish the likelihood of attempting or completing suicide. Other strengths include a good therapeutic relationship with a current provider and evidence of treatment compliance. However, even with mitigating factors, there is no guarantee that the patient will not attempt to harm himself or herself.

Substance abuse: Is the patient abusing alcohol, cocaine, opiates, benzodiazepines, or other drugs? If so, how much is consumed daily? When did the abuse begin, and when was the last use? You may elicit more information with a question such as "How much do you drink a day?" rather than "Do you drink alcohol?" If the patient actively abuses drugs or alcohol, suicidal ideation may manifest itself as a form of substance-induced mood or withdrawal-induced dysphoria (the latter is particularly relevant in crack cocaine withdrawal).

History of suicide attempts or gestures: As with any history, find out as many details as possible. Did the patient think the attempt would be successful? What treatment was necessary afterward (intubation, dialysis, charcoal/lavage, surgery)? Did the patient contact someone in the process (make a phone call after swallowing pills, write a suicide note), or was he or she found by accident? Does the patient regret not having succeeded? Try to determine the nature of the attempt—premeditated versus impulsive versus manipulative.

History of self-injurious behavior: Some patients resort to impulsive self-injurious behaviors such as self-mutilation, burning, or taking minor overdoses as a way of regulating their internal states. Although usually not lethal, it is the psychiatrist's job to treat these as psychiatric emergencies, because such acts can unintentionally cause serious injury or death.

Past psychiatric history: Obtain information about previous hospitalizations and treatments. Is there a history of depression, or of a manic episode, especially one with irritable or mixed features leading to risky behaviors? Is there any history of psychosis? In addition to lending data for diagnosis, such information may offer insight into the reasons for suicidality, for example, experiencing command auditory hallucinations to hurt oneself.

Medical history: Obtain a thorough medical history, including current health and medications taken. Many patients with untreated postsurgical or other pain may feel suicidal and articulate these thoughts only when expressing relief at being alive once their analgesia has reached an adequate and comfortable level. Are you concerned that the patient may be delirious or is exhibiting altered mental status? Review laboratory studies that have been completed and consider additional tests that would be helpful. Is the patient recently postpartum? This places them at higher risk for suicide. And lastly, have there been any recent medication changes that may be contributing to the presentation (i.e., interferon can cause severe depression; steroids can mimic almost any psychiatric disorder; antipsychotic medications can cause akathisia, which is a risk factor for suicide; there is some evidence in children and adolescents that initial titrations of selective serotonin reuptake inhibitors [SSRIs] can cause an increase in suicidal thoughts)?

Family and social history: Is there a family history of psychiatric illness or of suicide? What is the quality of the patient's interpersonal relationships and his or her social safety net? What is the work history, and has there been a recent decline in work habits? Difficulties in these arenas may help clarify the seriousness of the attempt.

Mental Status Examination

A full, current mental status examination is always a vital part of the assessment. Areas of focus include appearance, behavior, lability of mood, and level of psychomotor activity. Is the patient withdrawn, unkempt, or profoundly motorically retarded? Is the speech slowed or pressured? Is the patient sad, anxious, or constricted? Does the patient suffer from a thought disorder or from perceptual abnormalities? Are there any auditory hallucinations, particularly command auditory hallucinations? Is the patient's reported mood congruent with the observed affect? Ask specifically about the content of the voices and if the patient can resist them. Assess suicidal ideation in depth, as discussed earlier. Evaluate the patient's insight and judgment, with particular attention to his or her level of impulsivity.

MANAGEMENT

Regardless of the underlying diagnosis, the safety of the patient is paramount. If the evaluation takes place in the emergency room, you must decide whether to admit the patient based on your assessment of the current level of risk. If you feel the patient poses an acute danger to himself or herself, you can admit the patient on a voluntary or involuntary basis. Should you feel that admission is not indicated, confirm or arrange for prompt outpatient follow-up. Prior to allowing a potentially suicidal patient to leave the emergency room, it is prudent to corroborate the history and follow-up plan with a collateral source such as a family member or outside therapist. It is important to document that you have discussed the case with your supervisor and that a risk assessment has been performed (including some consideration of the previously mentioned risk factors) and clearly state why you feel the patient does not present an acute risk of self-harm.

If the patient is already admitted to a medical or surgical service, you must decide whether the patient should be placed on one-to-one observation. Should the patient be an active risk, initiate one-to-one observation or consider transferring the patient to a psychiatric floor. Always make sure the patient's current environment is safe (e.g., remove objects that can be used as weapons from the room and remove clothing and property to prevent elopement).

Treatment starts during the interview. A supportive style, with emphasis on encouraging the patient to share concerns, often proves therapeutic. The patient may benefit from a variety of PRN medications, including those for insomnia, anxiety, or agitation.

In general, starting an antidepressant medication can be deferred until either diagnostic or treatment arrangements have been clarified. Recommend a psychiatric medical work-up to expedite the initiation of pharmacotherapy. Routine tests include complete blood count with differential, electrolytes, liver function tests, thyroid function, rapid plasma regain for syphilis, vitamin B12, folate, electrocardiogram, urine bHCG (if the patient is female), and urine toxicology.

If you believe that the depression at hand stems from a medical illness, discuss this with the treating or consulting internist for follow-up. Should you find psychotic symptoms on examination, prescribing an antipsychotic (and discussing with the patient the risks and benefits of antipsychotic medications to the extent possible) may facilitate a more rapid recovery.

Should the suicidal ideation stem from a substance use disorder, or acute intoxication or withdrawal, emergent monitoring and management of withdrawal is critical. As always, prescribe psychotropic agents with addictive potential carefully to this patient population.

It is crucial for the on-call doctor to remember that suicide, despite our best efforts, cannot always be prevented or predicted, and even the most competent doctor may be unable to accurately assess suicide risk. Still, also remember that if there is doubt about the patient's safety, err on the side of caution. A one-to-one can easily be discontinued, and a patient admitted to a psychiatric unit can be discharged if suicidality resolves.

Suggested Readings

American Foundation for Suicide Prevention. Available at http://www.afsp.org.

APA Practice Guidelines: Practice Guidelines for the Psychiatric Evaluation of Adults, 3rd ed. July 2015. Available at http://psychiatryonline.org/action/showCitFormats?doi=10.1176%2Fappi.books.9780890426760.pe02.

Grant CL, Lusk JL. A multidisciplinary approach to therapeutic risk management of the suicidal patient. *J Multidiscip Healthc.* 2015;8:291–298.

Hom MA, Stanley IH, Podlogar MC, Joiner TE. Are you having thoughts of suicide? Examining experiences with disclosing and denying suicidal ideation. *J Clin Psychol.* 2017;73:1382–1392.

Tanguturi Y, Bodic M, Taub A, et al. Suicide risk assessment by residents: deficiencies of documentation. *Acad Psychiatry.* 2017;41:513–519.

Waern M, Kaiser N, Renberg ES. Psychiatrists experiences of suicide assessment. *BMC Psychiatry.* 2016;16:440.

The Psychotic Patient

When considering the psychotic patient in the hospitalized setting, it is helpful to recall that while psychosis is a characteristic of some psychiatric disorders (e.g., schizophrenia, schizoaffective disorder, mood disorders with psychotic features), not every patient with psychosis has a primary psychiatric condition: indeed, psychosis is a general descriptive term for a phenomenon that may be present in multiple medical and substance-related conditions, many of them life-threatening, in addition to psychiatric disorders. Patients with psychosis can present with a broad range of signs and symptoms that may include hallucinations or other misperceptions, delusions, disorganized or illogical speech and thinking, blunted or inappropriate emotional expression, difficulties with self-care, behavioral disturbances, and sometimes agitation or aggression. Because there are many etiologies for psychosis, your role is to help determine the cause of the psychosis (medical illness, substance- or drug-related, or psychiatric) and to provide a management strategy to the referring physician.

PHONE CALL

Questions

1. What specific behavior is the patient exhibiting at this time?
2. Is the patient physically agitated, behaving aggressively, or making threats to harm himself or herself or to others?
3. When did the symptoms begin?
4. What are the reasons for hospitalization?
5. What are the patient's medical illnesses?
6. What medications is the patient taking, and have there been any recent changes?
7. Have there been any recent changes in the level of arousal or any episodes of confusion or disorientation?
8. Does the patient have a history of psychotic episodes or any known psychiatric history?
9. Does the patient have a history of substance use?
10. What are the patient's vital signs?

Orders

1. Order the appropriate level of monitoring for the situation. Remember that behavior associated with psychosis is very unpredictable. One-to-one observation may be necessary until you can assess the situation personally.
2. If the patient is reported to be extremely agitated or behaving dangerously, you should consider ordering an as-needed medication such as an antipsychotic or a benzodiazepine to optimize the safety of the patient and those caring for him or her and to be able to safely perform an assessment.
3. In the case of behavior acutely dangerous to either the patient or others, you need to personally evaluate the situation before verbally ordering the nurse to implement physical restraints or seclusion. (Most institutions have their own protocols for restraint and seclusion and for the assistance of hospital security. You should be familiar with these procedures and consider their implementation.) This makes seeing the patient a priority and something to be done immediately.

Inform RN

"Will arrive in … minutes."

ELEVATOR THOUGHTS

What causes psychosis?
   See Tables 13.1, 13.2, and 13.3.

MAJOR THREAT TO LIFE

Psychosis may be associated with multiple severe and potentially life-threatening medical conditions, such as alcohol or benzodiazepine withdrawal, delirium, hepatic encephalopathy, thyrotoxicosis, and many others, all of which need to be urgently diagnosed and appropriately addressed. Psychosis can also be exacerbated by toxic levels of various medications such as antiarrhythmics, anticonvulsants, or anesthetic agents. Regardless of etiology, psychosis can cause disinhibition, impaired reality testing, paranoia, and disorganized thinking and behavior, all of which can result in agitation, physical aggression, or self-injurious or suicidal behavior, particularly in an unfamiliar or frightening hospital setting.

BEDSIDE

Quick Look Test

Does the patient look calm, distressed, or agitated?

TABLE 13.1	Psychiatric Disorders

Psychiatric Disorders	Associated Findings
Schizophrenia	>6-month disturbance characterized by delusions, hallucinations, disorganized speech/behavior, negative symptoms
Schizophreniform disorder	Symptoms of schizophrenia persisting longer than 1 month but less than 6 months
Brief psychotic disorder	Time limited (1 day to 1 month) psychotic symptoms
Schizoaffective disorder	Episodes of both mood and psychotic symptoms together in addition to at least 2 weeks of psychotic symptoms in absence of mood symptoms
Delusional disorder	Nonbizarre delusions without presence of hallucinations, disorganization, or negative symptoms
Shared psychotic disorder	Delusions develop in individuals influenced by someone else with a similar delusion
Mood disorder	Psychotic symptoms occur only during a depressive or manic episode; often psychotic symptoms have mood congruent delusions and hallucinations
Borderline personality disorder	Transient stress-related paranoid ideation or severe dissociative symptoms
Schizoid personality disorder	Social isolation, no positive symptoms
Schizotypal personality disorder	Ideas of reference, magical thinking, unusual perceptual experiences
Paranoid personality disorder	Paranoid ideation without delusions
Psychosis not otherwise specified	Psychotic symptoms that do not meet criteria for specific psychotic disorder
Postpartum psychosis	Onset of episode within 4 weeks postpartum
Autoscopic phenomena	Hallucinations of one's physical self, such as near-death perceptual experiences
Cotard's syndrome	Delusions of nihilism
Capgras syndrome	Delusions of imposture
Obsessive-compulsive disorder	Repetitive, intrusive, and unwanted thoughts or rituals
Autism spectrum disorder	Onset during infancy/early childhood, absence of prominent positive symptoms, may have speech/behavioral abnormalities
Factitious disorder	Intentional symptom production for internal incentive
Malingering	Intentional symptom production for external incentive

TABLE 13.2	Drug-Induced Psychosis

Drug-Induced Psychosis	Associated Findings
Amantadine	Hallucinations
Anticholinergic drugs	Somnolence, tachycardia, flushed/fever, dry mouth, dilated pupils/blurred vision, nausea/vomiting, urinary retention/overflow incontinence
Anticonvulsant drugs	Nystagmus, drowsiness, tremor, ataxia
Antimalarial drugs	GI symptoms, impaired hearing, seizure, rash, blood dyscrasias
Bromides	Low or negative anion gap (Br recognized as Cl)
Belladonna alkaloids	Delirium with hallucinations and anticholinergic symptoms
Carbon monoxide	Confusion, agitation can persist if there was chronic exposure
Digitalis	ECG disturbances, visual disturbances
H_2 blockers	Hallucinations, bizarre behavior
Interferon	Psychotic depression
Isoniazid	Mood lability leading to agitation, delusions, hallucinations, with lactic acidosis
L-dopa	Hallucinations, delusions
Lidocaine	Paranoid delusions
MAOIs	Tyramine-induced ataxia, hypertension, tachycardia, hyperthermia, seizure
Methylphenidate	Agitation, paranoia, tactile hallucinations
Nitrous oxide	Metabolic acidosis, cyanotic appearance, dizziness, nausea, headache, dyspnea, seizure, coma
Phenylpropanolamine	Paranoia
Penicillin	Fear, auditory/visual/tactile hallucinations, paranoia/religious delusions
Podophyllin	Keratolytic agent that poisons mitotic spindle and causes intense vasospasm
Steroids	Hallucinations, delusions, mood symptoms
Sulfonamides	Associated with confusion, hallucinations, depression
Alcohol withdrawal	Delirium tremens-confusion, visual and/or tactile hallucinations, unstable vital signs occurring 3–5 days following reduction of alcohol consumption
Amphetamines	Paranoid ideation, agitation, psychotic sequelae can have long-term course
Cannabis	Perceptual distortions, paranoid ideation common, conjunctival injection
Cocaine	Paranoid ideation, visual and tactile hallucinations, formication
Ethyl alcohol	Hallucinations and delusions occurring in context of ongoing heavy drinking
Hallucinogens	Perceptual distortions
Phencyclidine	Severe agitation, nystagmus, tachycardia, diaphoresis
Ketamine	Dissociation, hallucinations, hypersalivation
Synthetic cannabinoids	Agitation, hallucinations, hypertension, tachycardia

ECG, Electrocardiogram; *GI*, gastrointestinal; *MAOIs*, monoamine oxidase inhibitors.

| TABLE 13.3 | Medical Conditions |

Medical Conditions (Selected List)	Associated Findings
Acquired immunodeficiency	Constitutional symptoms, syndrome (AIDS) opportunistic infections, dementia
Acute intermittent	Intermittent abdominal pain, porphyria autonomic and peripheral neuropathy, seizure, basal ganglia abnormalities, hyponatremia
B_{12} deficiency	Megaloblastic anemia, neurologic deficits, glossitis, GI disturbances
Creutzfeldt-Jakob disease	Cerebellar ataxia, tremors, dysarthria, emotional lability
Dementias (cortical and hallucinations when moderate to subcortical)	Severe dementia
Epilepsy	Episodic, EEG abnormalities
Herpes encephalitis	Flulike prodrome, headache, fever, seizures, temporal lobe abnormalities on EEG or imaging
Homocystinuria	Autosomal recessive, mental retardation, thromboses, ectopia lentis, abnormal body habitus
Huntington's disease	Choreiform movements, dementia, paranoid ideation, trinucleotide repeats on IT-15 gene
Hypothyroidism/myxedema	Auditory hallucinations, paranoid ideation, cold intolerance, weight gain, dry brittle hair, elevated TSH
CNS neoplasms	Neurologic findings, headache, psychotic symptoms based on site of lesion, positive CT findings
Neurosyphilis	Hyperactive reflexes, Argyll-Robertson pupil, dementia, positive RPR and VDRL
Normal pressure	Gait instability, dementia, bowel hydrocephalus incontinence
Pellagra	Niacin deficiency, peripheral neuropathy, memory impairment
Systemic lupus	Malar or discoid rash, photosensitivity, erythematosus (SLE) oral ulcers, arthritis, serositis, proteinuria, seizures, psychotic symptoms
Wernicke-Korsakoff	Persistent amnesia, persistent syndrome nystagmus, history of alcohol abuse

CNS, Central nervous system; *CT,* computed tomography; *EEG,* electroencephalogram; *GI,* gastrointestinal; *RPR,* rapid plasma reagin; *TSH,* thyroid-stimulating hormone; *VDRL,* Venereal Disease Research Laboratory.

Observe the patient's appearance and interaction with family members or caretakers present. Assess posture, grooming, personal hygiene, and clothing. Observe if there is fidgeting, pacing, hyperactivity, tardive dyskinesia, or catatonia. Loud speech, property damage, and combative behavior should also be noted. If the patient looks agitated, ask the nursing and medical staff to ensure a safe environment for the patient and others, calling for additional staff to use physical restraints if necessary.

Is the patient awake and alert or does he or she appear lethargic or obtunded?

Altered or fluctuating levels of arousal accompanied by disorientation or confusion may indicate delirium and should be urgently addressed.

AIRWAY AND VITAL SIGNS

What is the heart rate and blood pressure?

Tachycardia or hypertension may be indicative of withdrawal states or other medical illnesses.

What is the temperature?

Fever may be a sign of sepsis, infection, or neuroleptic malignant syndrome.

SELECTIVE HISTORY AND CHART REVIEW

Discuss with medical and nursing staff the time course of symptoms and the behavior of the patient as observed. Note the time of onset of any vegetative symptoms, concomitant medical illnesses, and medications taken, including over-the-counter drugs. Obtain a thorough medical history and note the procedures performed and medications administered. Review the electronic record or old charts for psychiatric history and psychiatric consultations during previous medical hospitalizations. Interview family members or friends accompanying the patient for events leading up to the time of presentation, family history of neurologic or psychiatric illness, and patient's past psychiatric history, including alcohol and drug use.

SELECTIVE PHYSICAL EXAMINATION

A thorough physical examination with special emphasis on the neurologic evaluation should be performed.

SELECTIVE MENTAL STATUS EXAMINATION

Appearance: poor personal hygiene, bizarre or inappropriate dress

Psychomotor activity: agitation, pacing, combativeness, posturing, stereotyped movements, psychomotor retardation, tremors, perioral movements, restlessness, dystonias, dyskinesias

Speech: impoverished, mute to mumbling, loud or shouting, pressured

Affect: inappropriate, labile to constricted, angry, irritable, anxious, depressed, or euphoric

Thought processes: goal directed, coherent or incoherent, looseness of associations, flight of ideas, internal preoccupation, talking to oneself, thought blocking, disorganization, tangentiality, circumstantiality, echolalia, word salad

Perceptions: hallucinations (visual, auditory, tactile, or olfactory)

Thought content: paranoia, ideas of reference, magical thinking, delusions of grandiosity or persecution, obsessions or preoccupations, suicidal or homicidal ideation with plan or intent

Cognitive examination: if level of consciousness, orientation, or memory is impaired, delirium should be suspected.

Insight and judgment: often impaired

LABORATORY EVALUATION

Review laboratory tests, including blood chemistries, liver function tests, complete blood count, testing for infectious disease including syphilis and human immunodeficiency virus (HIV), thyroid function tests, B_{12}, folate, urinalysis, and blood and urine cultures if infection is strongly suspected. Urine toxicology tests may also shed light on drug use and withdrawal states. It may be necessary to perform a computed tomographic scan of the head and a lumbar puncture to rule out infectious and neurologic etiologies for an acute onset of psychotic symptoms. Work-up for the first episode of psychotic symptoms should include computed tomographic scan and an electroencephalogram.

MANAGEMENT

The etiology of the patient's psychosis will determine management. Medical and neurologic disorders should be referred to the appropriate consulting team. Treatment of the underlying cause of the psychosis will eventually lead to clearance of the psychotic symptoms. For instance, psychosis secondary to a delirium from a urinary tract infection will improve with a course of appropriate antibiotics, while psychosis secondary to delirium tremens from alcohol withdrawal will improve with benzodiazepine treatment.

For chronic psychotic symptoms, either from a psychiatric disorder or other chronic medical condition, consider an atypical antipsychotic medication. Discuss with the patient past medication trials and, if possible, coordinate care with outpatient medical and psychiatric providers. Generally start with lower initial doses in patients who are naïve to antipsychotics and in elderly patients. If there is a history of medication nonadherence, consider starting an antipsychotic for which a long-acting depot formulation is available, with an eye towards switching to the depot formulation once the appropriate dose is determined. Aripiprazole, risperidone, paliperidone, haloperidol, and fluphenazine are currently available as long-acting injectables. A long-acting formulation of olanzapine is also available, although it is not widely used because of the risk of postinjection delirium/sedation and related restrictions on distribution and use.

Be sure to assess the patient for dangerousness to self or others and discuss any safety concerns with the team. In addition to pharmacologic recommendations, be sure to make recommendations for providing a safe and supportive environment, including appropriate monitoring in case of suicidality, concern for elopement, or severe disorganization. For cases of agitation, please refer to Chapter 9. For cases where there is a question of capacity, please refer to Chapter 6.

In some cases, you may need to facilitate a transfer to the inpatient psychiatric service once the medical or surgical service medically clears the patient. You may offer a voluntary admission if you assess that the patient has the capacity to sign into the hospital and that he or she would benefit from an inpatient level of care due to the level of decompensation and impairment. You may be responsible for involuntarily hospitalizing the patient if there is sufficient concern about the patient's safety due to mental illness and if he or she either lacks the capacity to sign in and/or is refusing psychiatric admission. Most often, the threshold for involuntary hospitalization is imminent danger of harm to self or others or inability to care for self. Legal criteria and procedures vary by state, region, and country, so be sure to be familiar with those that pertain to where you practice.

The Confused Patient: Delirium and Dementia

A patient's confusion in the general medical setting is most often a result of delirium or dementia. Delirium indicates the presence of an acute underlying medical problem (or combination of problems). Less commonly, confusion may be due to conditions such as pseudodementia and amnestic syndrome. It is important to distinguish between delirium and dementia to initiate appropriate medical treatment while trying to reduce the anxiety and agitation often associated with the confusion. Remember that delirium and dementia can appear in the same patient and that demented patients are especially susceptible to delirium. When in doubt, it is always prudent to begin a work-up for delirium, because delayed medical treatment may lead to increased morbidity or even mortality and longer hospital stays.

Definitions

DELIRIUM

Delirium is an acute process that reflects medical problems, particularly in elderly, brain-injured, or acutely ill patients and in children.

Signs and symptoms of delirium include the following:
Inattention
Disorientation to person, place, time, or situation
Fluctuations in consciousness
Mood or speech that is inappropriate to situation
Hallucinations or delusions
Alterations in the sleep-wake cycle
Fluctuation in symptoms
Psychomotor agitation or retardation

Delirium is characterized by rapid onset, although sometimes the patient will show prodromal behavioral disturbances up to several days before frank delirium sets in. These can include irritability, anxiety, sleep disturbances, and lethargy.

Delirium usually has a fluctuating course ("waxing and waning") ranging from clouding of consciousness to coma interrupted by lucid intervals. It can have a duration lasting from minutes to weeks. Typically, symptoms of delirium worsen at night ("sundowning"). "Sundowning" is typical in the elderly and is characterized by disorientation at night, falls, wandering, illusions, or hallucinations.

Disturbances of the sleep-wake cycle and an increased or decreased level of psychomotor activity are hallmarks of the delirium, but features vary widely, often making the diagnosis more difficult.

Global impairment of cognition occurs, causing disturbances in memory, perception, and thinking. Delirious patients often have a reduced ability to remain focused, leading to easy distractibility. They may demonstrate disorganized thinking, incoherent speech, and sensory misperceptions, especially visual hallucinations and illusions.

The delirious patient can be either agitated or apathetic, reflecting psychomotor agitation or retardation. Patients may be restless, pick at their bedclothes ("floccillation" or carphology), or try to get out of bed. The physician on call is much more likely to be called for a delirious patient who is combative and agitated, whereas the "quietly" delirious patient may be overlooked or regarded as depressed and withdrawn.

Emotional disturbances appear in the form of depressed mood, anxiety or fear, paranoia, irritability, euphoria, or apathy. Lability of affect is manifested by rapid shifts between crying, laughter, fear, and anger. Thus, if a patient is described as confused or disoriented, especially with concomitant flux in mood or behavior, delirium is a likely diagnosis.

Sympathetic hyperactivity may occur, including tachycardia, diaphoresis, flushed face, dilated pupils, and elevated blood pressure.

DEMENTIA

Dementia is the decline of higher cortical functions, especially memory, thinking, orientation, comprehension, calculation, learning capacity, language, and judgment. The dysfunction is sufficient to impair activities of daily living and social activities. Although it can occur at any age, dementia is most common in the elderly. Alzheimer's dementia, the most common form of dementia, affects as many as 5.2 million Americans, or roughly 11% of the US adult population age 65 and older. The incidence doubles with every

5-year interval beyond age 65. It is the sixth leading cause of death in the United States and the fifth leading cause of death in Americans age 65 and older.

Unlike in delirium, consciousness is typically clear in dementia (i.e., the patient is alert). Depending on the etiology, dementia may have a sudden or insidious onset, be progressive with a long duration, be static, or have a remitting course.

Primary symptoms of dementia include memory loss, particularly difficulty in learning new information (immediate memory), recalling recent events (recent memory), and remembering past personal information (remote memory). Impairment in abstract thinking, judgment, and impulse control; neglect of personal appearance and hygiene; personality changes, anxiety, or depression; paranoid ideation; and irritability are all associated with dementia.

PSEUDODEMENTIA

Pseudodementia is a severe type of major depression with symptoms similar to dementia, such as withdrawal, decline in concrete thinking, and loss of memory. History of a previous mood disorder, recent emotional distress, and loss of short-term and long-term memory may help distinguish pseudodementia from dementia.

AMNESTIC DISORDER

Amnestic disorder is characterized by memory impairment with no other cognitive deficits that affect occupational or social functioning. Because amnesia may have psychological or organic etiologies, it is important to take a careful history. Electroconvulsive therapy, psychological stress, or a recent traumatic event all may contribute to amnesia.

PHONE CALL

Questions

1. How old is the patient?
2. What is the medical history?
3. What is the patient's diagnosis or reason for admission?
4. What are the vital signs? Has a finger stick glucose been done?
5. Is the patient agitated? Is he or she a threat to himself or herself or to others?
6. Is this an acute mental status change?

7. What is the level of consciousness?
8. Are there any associated symptoms or signs (e.g., chest pain, hallucinations, jaundice, or tremors)?
9. Have there been previous episodes of confusion?
10. What medications is the patient taking? Have any new medications been added or discontinued? Has there been a change in dosage or scheduling?
11. Does the patient abuse alcohol or drugs? If so, when was the last known use?

Orders

1. Ask the staff to provide one-to-one (1:1) observation if the patient is dangerous to himself or herself or to others.
2. Restraints can be applied if absolutely necessary.
3. You should attempt to see the patient before giving medication, but if the patient is acutely agitated and dangerous, haloperidol can be administered.

Inform RN

"Will arrive in … minutes."

ELEVATOR THOUGHTS

What are the causes of confusion in the patient you are about to see?

Delirium

There are many causes of delirium. They can be roughly categorized as those resulting from chronic cerebral disease, such as dementia, systemic illness, recreational drug or medication toxicity, and those resulting from drug or medication withdrawal. Sometimes, the cause may be a combination of these disturbances.

Generally, the most common causes of delirium are:

Hypoglycemia or marked hyperglycemia
Fever
Alcohol withdrawal
Drug reaction or intoxication
Polypharmacy (and drug interactions), including use of over-the-counter medications
Head trauma
Recent surgery, especially involving general anesthesia

The most common causes based on hospital location:

Emergency room: head trauma, drug intoxication, cerebrovascular accidents
Medical, surgical, and intensive care units (ICUs): fever, electrolyte imbalance, sepsis, alcohol withdrawal, postoperative states,

hypoglycemia, medication, polypharmacy, urinary tract infections

Psychiatric units: medication, drug intoxication, alcohol withdrawal, depression, catatonia, fever

Dementia

Alzheimer's disease (AD) and multiinfarct dementia are the two most common causes of dementia; however, it is useful to categorize the causes of dementia by those that are reversible and those that are irreversible.

Potentially reversible causes include:

Central nervous system infections, including human immunodeficiency virus (HIV), neurosyphilis, and tubercular and fungal infections (meningitis, viral encephalitis)

Normal-pressure hydrocephalus

Subdural hematoma

Vasculitis

Pernicious anemia

Bromide intoxication

Nutritional deficiencies

Potentially irreversible causes of dementia include the following:

Alzheimer's disease: two-thirds of all cases of dementia. AD has an insidious onset with progressive decline in functioning.

Multiinfarct dementia: second leading cause of dementia, multiinfarct dementia presents more acutely with an incremental stepwise loss of function. The medical conditions leading to multiinfarct dementia, such as diabetes, hypertension, cardiac disease, and embolic disease from prosthetic valves, may be controlled to prevent further episodes of infarct that may lead to progression of the dementia.

Huntington's chorea

Multiple sclerosis

Pick's disease

Parkinson's disease

Creutzfeldt-Jakob disease

Cerebellar degeneration

Postanoxic or posthypoglycemic states

Lewy body dementia

DIFFERENTIAL DIAGNOSES

Pseudodementia

In the setting of major depression, a patient may also present as confused. This presentation is known as pseudodementia.

Amnestic Disorder

If the confusion appears due to an amnestic disorder, consider the following in the differential diagnosis:

Head trauma or neurologic signs may indicate a brain tumor, a cerebrovascular accident, or seizures.

Alcoholism is a common cause of blackouts, seizures, or vitamin deficiencies (Korsakoff's syndrome).

Wernicke's encephalopathy may be revealed by the triad of ophthalmoplegia, ataxia, and delirium.

Psychogenic amnesia may arise as a defense or for secondary gain. Immediate recall and anterograde memory usually are not affected.

Psychogenic fugue, associated with alcoholism, involves loss of personal identity and/or remote memory.

Life-Threatening Causes Leading to Delirium

Although delirium secondary to any cause is a medical emergency, some causes are potentially life threatening. They include the following:

Intracranial hemorrhage
Sepsis
Shock
Narcotic overdose
Intracranial neoplasm
Delirium tremens (alcohol withdrawal)
Arrhythmias

REMEMBER

Often, an extensive work-up for delirium will not yield a definitive medical cause. Nonetheless, delirium is a clinical diagnosis, indicating one or more causes leading to brain dysfunction; these causes need not be identified to make a diagnosis of delirium.

BEDSIDE

Quick Look Test

Does the patient look calm, distressed, or agitated?

Observe the patient's appearance and interaction with others. If the patient is agitated, ask the staff to ensure a safe environment, using restraints if necessary.

AIRWAY AND VITAL SIGNS

What is the patient's heart rate?

Tachycardia may be indicative of withdrawal states or other medical illnesses.

What is the patient's blood pressure?

Hypertensive encephalopathy and hypotension from blood loss may lead to mental status changes. Hypertension may also be indicative of alcohol withdrawal.

What is the patient's temperature?

Fever may be a sign of sepsis or infection.

What is the patient's respiratory rate?

A rapid respiratory rate may indicate hypoxia secondary to pulmonary embolus or compromised pulmonary function.

SELECTIVE HISTORY AND CHART REVIEW

What is the history of this episode of confusion?

Ask staff about the time course and whether it has been episodic or continuous.

What preceded the episode?

Obtain a thorough medical history and note procedures and medications before the onset of confusion. Review the medication record to rule out errors in transcription or administration of as-needed medication.

What do the nursing notes reveal?

Review the nursing notes for documentation of a change in the patient's mental status, "sundowning," or the fluctuating nature of agitation or confusion.

Were there earlier psychiatric consultations?

Review old charts from previous hospitalizations to assess the patient's behavior in similar settings and situations.

What do friends and family know?

Interview those available as to observed changes in the patient before hospitalization.

SELECTIVE PHYSICAL EXAMINATION

Perform a thorough physical examination, with special emphasis on the neurologic component, to rule out underlying medical illness.

Delirium

SELECTIVE MENTAL STATUS EXAMINATION

A fluctuating level of consciousness may be noted as confusion alternating with lucidity or agitation alternating with stupor.

Psychomotor activity may include combativeness, picking at sheets, or drifting to sleep during the interview.

Speech may be mumbling, normal, or shouting.

Thought processes may be incoherent, rambling, or disorganized.

Altered perceptual states may be present, including hallucinations (visual, auditory, tactile, olfactory), paranoia, and illusions or delusions regarding procedures or staff.

Anxiety, irritability, depression or euphoria, nightmares, and insomnia with disorientation may occur.

LABORATORY TESTS

An array of tests may be necessary to isolate the underlying cause or causes of the confusion. These should include:

Complete blood count with differential

Complete metabolic profile including glucose, electrolytes, calcium, and phosphorous

Liver function tests

Cyanocobalamin

Folic acid

Erythrocyte sedimentation rate (remember that elderly patients normally have higher levels)

RPR test for syphilis

Thyroid function tests (measure thyroid-stimulating hormone level first)

HIV test

Arterial blood gases

Urinalysis

If fever is present, urinalysis and urine and blood cultures may reveal the source of the infection causing the fever. A chest x-ray film may reveal pneumonia.

Urine and/or serum drug toxicology tests may reveal drug use or withdrawal. A head computed tomography scan and/or lumbar puncture may be needed to rule out infectious or neurologic causes for an acute change in mental status.

MANAGEMENT

Structured Environment

Delirium is potentially reversible with treatment of the underlying medical disorder. In the interim, provide a safe and structured environment to limit harm to the patient or to others. If possible, the patient should be moved to a room where he or she will not be isolated and can be easily monitored. Staff should provide repeated explanations of procedures and tests, as well as clocks and calendars, to keep the patient oriented. The presence of family members and familiar objects is also reassuring to the patient.

Treatment of the Underlying Medical Disorder
Medication-Related Delirium

Medications are implicated in up to 30% of cases of delirium. Although almost any drug can contribute to delirium in susceptible individuals, certain categories of medications often lead to acute and even chronic states of confusion.

Drugs with known anticholinergic properties include long-acting benzodiazepines, opioids, tricyclic antidepressants, and some of the older antihypertensive medications such as reserpine and clonidine. In addition, H_2 blockers, other cardiac medications such as digoxin, nonsteroidal antiinflammatory drugs, antibiotics, and corticosteroids have been determined to contribute to delirium in the susceptible individual.

Treatment of medication-related delirium involves discontinuing the responsible medication(s). To reduce the likelihood of an adverse reaction, heed the adage, "start low and go slow."

Other Underlying Problems

Hypoxia, metabolic disorders, and endocrine abnormalities: Treatment of hypoxia, metabolic disorders, and endocrine abnormalities can often quickly clear delirium.

Infections: Infection leading to delirium can be as simple as a urinary tract infection in an elderly patient.

Postoperative status: Whether resulting from general anesthesia or an underlying medical complication, delirium is often found in the postoperative patient.

Toxins: Toxicologic tests may shed light on drug use and withdrawal states.

"ICU delirium" is defined by agitation associated with an intensive care setting. Control of the agitation in a timely manner is a priority, as are attempts to understand what may be contributing to the patient's delirium.

Medications to Treat the Underlying Disorder

As stated earlier, the most important treatment for delirium is determining and trying to eliminate the medical problem or problems leading to the syndrome. Therefore, any necessary medication changes toward that end, such as beginning antibiotics, lowering dosages, or changing maintenance medications, must be initiated.

Calming the Delirious Patient

Management with medications should be reserved for patients whose symptoms of delirium threaten their own safety or the safety of others or interfere with life-saving therapy.

Haloperidol is the agent of choice for calming the agitated, paranoid, or belligerent patient. Haloperidol should be administered 0.5–1.0 mg by mouth twice daily, with additional doses every 4 hr as needed, or if more rapid onset is required, 0.5–1.0 mg intramuscularly with observation for 30–60 min with repeat dose if agitation persists (maximum dosage 20 mg with 24 hour period). Atypical antipsychotics (e.g., risperidone, olanzapine, quetiapine) can also be used. Risperidone doses start at 0.25 mg, quetiapine doses start at 12.5 mg, and olanzapine doses start at 2.5 mg. While there is an intramuscular form of olanzapine, it should not be given within 1 hour of intramuscular or intravenous benzodiazepines. There is less experience with using atypical antipsychotics in delirium; keep in mind that while, in general, they are better tolerated, they can be more sedating and anticholinergic than haloperidol, which can be problematic in the medically ill. Prior to using antipsychotics, it is important to first check the corrected QT interval on the patient's electrocardiogram. Antipsychotics can prolong the QT interval, and QTc intervals of greater than 500 ms are associated with arrhythmias such as torsades de pointes. Serum potassium and magnesium levels should also be checked, as low levels predispose to torsades de pointes. In particular, intravenous haloperidol has been associated with torsades de pointes; continuous electrocardiographic monitoring, correcting electrolyte abnormalities, and avoiding other QTc prolonging drugs are recommended.

Benzodiazepines, similar to lorazepam, are only indicated in patients undergoing sedative or alcohol withdrawal, Parkinson's disease, and neuroleptic malignant syndrome; otherwise, studies show that benzodiazepines may worsen delirium and are contraindicated.

Both elderly and brain-injured patients should be treated with lower amounts of the medications initially. The drugs may be titrated upward as warranted.

Physical restraints should be avoided unless there is a threat to the patient's safety, the safety of others, or the integrity of the intravenous lines, tubes, or other connections. If physical restraints are required in an acute situation, their continued need should be frequently reassessed and removal of restraints should occur as soon as safely possible. Additionally, reasoning behind the necessity of physical restraints should be properly documented.

Dementia

SELECTIVE MENTAL STATUS EXAMINATION

Cognitive changes are notable over time, with loss of date, time, and memory for recent events occurring first, followed by loss of place and then person.

Learning new tasks may become impossible, followed by the inability to perform activities of daily living.

Aphasia, agnosia, and apraxia may be evident.

Loss of abstract thinking and judgment may lead to poor impulse control, indiscretions, and violations of social norms.

Affect may be labile with changes in personality.

Denial, angry outbursts, or anxiety may be present.

The patient may exhibit depression or psychosis with paranoia or delusions.

Psychomotor activity may be characterized by agitation, assaultive behavior, withdrawal, or retardation.

Remember that the mini-mental status examination is not diagnostic, but it can be used over a period of time to follow progression of dysfunction.

LABORATORY TESTS

To help clarify the patient's diagnosis, additional tests for dementia may include:

Blood chemistries

Vitamin B_{12}

Folate

Heavy metals

Testing for nutritional deficiencies

MANAGEMENT

Dementia is a disorder of brain function and cognition. It is occasionally reversible. Even when its progression is inevitable, steps may be taken to manage certain signs and symptoms that are distressing to the patient, his or her family, and staff caring for the patient.

Behavioral therapy, reality orientation, and environmental manipulations are three often-used management techniques.

Depression in the context of dementia symptoms may be the result of pseudodementia or it may be a mood disorder superimposed on true dementia. Cognitive dysfunction with pseudodementia can be expected to resolve with successful treatment of the depression, while it will persist in the demented patient even when the depression is successfully treated.

Treatment of the Underlying Medical Disorder

In some forms of dementia, treating the underlying cause often reverses the disorder.

Some underlying causes include the following:

Some nutritional deficiencies may cause dementia; supplement by adding nutrients to the daily regimen.

A history of drug and alcohol abuse may reveal delirium tremens or sedative-hypnotic withdrawal.

Subdural hematoma may be associated with a history of trauma or frequent falls.

Normal-pressure hydrocephalus may be diagnosed with the triad of dementia, incontinence, and gait apraxia. Obtain a neurology consult if this disorder is suspected.

Intracranial masses and lesions may be seen on head computed tomography scan.

Encephalitis, tertiary syphilis, and fungal meningitis may be revealed by lumbar puncture.

Pseudodementia is associated with a normal electroencephalogram; true dementia is not.

Medications

Superimposed psychiatric symptoms in the elderly demented patient may be targeted with medications.

Anticholinergic agents and benzodiazepines should be avoided because of the risk of delirium in the elderly.

Any psychotropic medications used in the elderly and brain-impaired should be initiated at one-third to one-half of the usual adult dose. They can be slowly titrated upward as clinically warranted to minimize side effects. Haloperidol may also be used IM or PO at 0.25 to 1.0 mg at bedtime or twice daily.

While antipsychotics have been commonly used to treat psychotic symptoms and agitation in elderly patients with dementia, the US Food and Drug Administration (FDA) has issued a "Black Box Warning" noting that multiple studies have shown an increased risk of death in this population when treated with antipsychotics, and that antipsychotics are not approved for dementia-related psychosis. However, one must weigh the risks against the benefits, especially when the treatment of neuropsychiatric symptoms is essential to both patient and caregiver safety and well-being. Treatment should aim to be brief, and attempts at discontinuation should occur with regularity. While atypical antipsychotics have been used commonly in this population, studies to date have not revealed a clear benefit over the use of haloperidol. It has been assumed that treatment with atypical antipsychotics might offer a benefit in terms of lower likelihood of tardive dyskinesia and extrapyramidal side effects to which elderly patients are particularly susceptible, although they may potentially have a risk of causing metabolic disturbances in glucose and lipid levels. Notably, most of the clinical trials cited by the FDA in the "Black Box Warning" involved atypical antipsychotics, although other studies were cited that suggest typical antipsychotics shared the same increased risk of mortality.

Insomnia may be treated with trazodone 25 to 50 mg PO at bedtime. As with other medications with anticholinergic properties, diphenhydramine should be avoided.

Physical Restraints

As with the delirious patient, the use of physical restraints is not indicated in the management of patients with dementia unless the patient poses an imminent danger to himself or herself or others.

Amnesia

SELECTIVE MENTAL STATUS EXAMINATION

Common manifestations include the following:
Loss of memory
Retrograde, anterograde, circumscribed amnesia
Confabulation
Denial
Apathy

MANAGEMENT

1. Treatment of the underlying medical disorder should resolve the amnestic disorder.
2. Furthermore, if no obvious cause of amnesia is identified, an amobarbital sodium interview or hypnosis may be recommended to the day team and may help to elucidate the origin of the patient's amnesia.

Suggested Readings

Brummel NE, Vasilevskis EE, Han JH, Boehm L, Pun BT, Ely EW. Implementing delirium screening in the intensive care unit: secrets to success. *Crit Care Med.* 2013;41(9):2196–2208. https://doi.org/10.1097/CCM .0b013e31829a6f1e.

Hebert LE, Weuve J, Scherr PA, Evans DA. Alzheimer's disease in the United States (2010-2050) estimated using the 2010 census. *Neurol.* 2013;80:1778–1783.

Inouye SK. Delirium in older persons. *N Engl J Med.* 2006;354:1157–1165.

Kalish VB, Gillham JE, Unwin BK. Delirium in older persons: evaluation and management. *Am Fam Physician.* 2014;90:150–158.

Lee PE, Gill SS, Freedman M, et al. Atypical antipsychotic drugs in the treatment of behavioural and psychological symptoms of dementia: systematic review. *BMJ.* 2004;329:75. UI: 15194601.

Miller MO. Evaluation and management of delirium in hospitalized older patients. *Am Fam Physician.* 2008;78(11):1265–1270.

Steinberg M, Lyketsos CG. Atypical antipsychotic use in patients with dementia: managing safety concerns. *Am J Psychiatry*. 2012;169 (9):900–906. https://doi.org/10.1176/appi.ajp.2012.12030342.

US Department of Health and Human Services. *National Alzheimer's plan*. https://aspe.hhs.gov/report/national-plan-address-alzheimers-disease-2016-update. Accessed November 25, 2016.

Movement Disorders

Psychiatrists on call often evaluate patients' complaints of stiffness, tremor, rigidity, and other abnormal movements. The causes vary, and the clinician should be prepared to manage both commonly encountered and reversible problems such as acute dystonia and more lethal conditions such as neuroleptic malignant syndrome (NMS). Although the more common problems represent some of the most dramatic presentations in the field of psychiatry, they can often be treated rapidly, effectively, and easily. In contrast, more subtle presentations of NMS and acute laryngeal spasm represent life-threatening emergencies that require careful diagnosis and management to minimize relatively high mortality rates. Proper management of NMS and laryngeal spasm entails rapid recognition and work-up and often transfer of the patient to an intensive care unit.

PHONE CALL

Questions

1. Is the patient stable? Does the patient have difficulty breathing? Are there changes in mental status?
2. What are the most recent vital signs (including temperature)?
3. When did the movement disorder start? Was the onset sudden or gradual?
4. Describe the movement disorder. Is it hyperkinetic or hypokinetic? Is it generalized or is it only in certain body regions?
5. Has the patient been given any medications recently? In particular, is the patient taking an antipsychotic or has there been a recent addition of an antipsychotic to the medication regimen?
6. Are there any other associated signs or symptoms, such as focal weakness, muscle spasms, dysphagia, drooling, or tremor?
7. Does the patient have any acute or chronic medical problems?

Orders

Attempt when possible to examine the dystonic patient immediately. The patient should be evaluated before giving any medications; however, the physician may want to ask the nurse to do the following:

1. In the case of suspected acute dystonia, prepare benztropine 1 to 2 mg IM or Benadryl 25 to 50 mg IM (in milder cases use PO).
2. If NMS is suspected (rigidity, vital sign abnormalities, difficulties in respiration, changes in mental status), hold all medications.

Inform RN

"Will arrive in ... minutes."

ELEVATOR THOUGHTS

See Table 15.1.

MAJOR THREAT TO LIFE

NMS
Laryngeal dystonia
Acute stroke

Neuroleptic Malignant Syndrome

NMS is characterized by rigidity, hyperthermia, mental status changes, elevated creatine kinase (CK) level, and autonomic instability. NMS is rare but life threatening, with mortality rates of 20%. Some patients have a variant of NMS in which only two or three of these features are present. Symptoms of autonomic dysfunction range from rapid and irregular heart rates and hypertension to tachypnea, diaphoresis, and urinary incontinence. Also pay attention to dysphagia, dysarthria, sialorrhea, akinesia, bradykinesia, tremor, and fluctuating level of awareness. The patient initially may be quite alert but may later become agitated or obtunded. Other neurologic features such as seizures, ataxia, and nystagmus can eventually develop.

NMS must always be considered when patients complain of rigidity; however, it is also a diagnosis of exclusion. Other disorders must first be considered, especially in the context of abnormal laboratory values. In cases of mild to moderate temperature elevations with variable rigidity, be sure to consider the medication and substance abuse history and possible toxic syndromes (anticholinergic-related or monoamine oxidase inhibitor [MAOI]–related serotonin syndromes).

TABLE 15.1 | **Common Movement Disorders**

Movement Disorder	Type	Description	Types	Treatment	To Be Aware
Tremor	Hyperkinetic	Involuntary, rhythmic oscillating movement that may involve the head, hands, limbs, lips, jaw, and voice	• Physiologic (low amplitude, rarely disruptive to daily activities) • Essential (low to medium amplitude) • Cerebellar (tremor occurs with movement) • Resting (drug induced or Parkinson's) • Psychogenic (suppressible with distraction)	• Physiologic—manage underlying problem (mental state, metabolic, medications) • Essential—treatments of choice are propranolol and primidone • Cerebellar—if acute onset, cause is stroke until proven otherwise, manage accordingly	
Tics	Hyperkinetic	Intermittent, sudden, brief, stereotyped movements or sounds that may involve head, face, trunk, or extremities	May consist of motor movements or sounds; may be simple jerklike movements or meaningless sounds or complex, coordinated sequences of movements or vocalizations	Treatment not usually urgent; patients often started on clonidine Refractory patients often require neuroleptics	Neuroleptic-induced tardive syndromes may also present with tics

Dystonia	Hyperkinetic	Sustained, spasmodic contractions that result in abnormal posturing of any voluntary muscle	Shocklike (myoclonic) or slow (athetotic) movements. Can be categorized as primary (familial, almost always focal) or secondary (due to neurodegenerative diseases, inherited forms, structural neurologic lesion)	Anticholinergic or antihistaminergic medications	Seizures can present with dystonic posturing as can neuroleptic-induced tardive dystonias. Forms of dystonia include: • Protruding tongue, difficulty swallowing, facial grimaces • Torticollis (head twisted to one side) • Retrocollis (head forced backwards) • Oculogyric crisis (eyes rolled upwards, sometimes laterally) • Laryngopharyngeal spasm (can cause sudden death)
Chorea	Hyperkinetic	Involuntary, irregular, sometimes dancelike movements that are brief and nonrhythmic. Movements mostly involve distal extremities but may involve tongue, face, trunk, or head	Can have multiple etiologies (metabolic, toxic, vascular, infectious). Psychotropic medications can cause chorea as a tardive syndrome. Prototypical illness associated with chorea is Huntington's disease	There is no treatment for Huntington's disease motor abnormalities; however, symptomatic treatment of behavioral and psychiatric comorbidities is important	Athetosis is similar to chorea but slower and more writhing in nature

		Description	Causes	Treatment	Notes
Hemiballism	Hyperkinetic	Uncontrollable large amplitude flinging of one extremity	Most common cause is contralateral subthalamic nucleus infarct	Valproate has been shown to be helpful in some patients with disabling hemiballism	Often coexists with chorea
Myoclonus	Hyperkinetic	Sudden, involuntary contractions of individual or groups of muscles	• Physiologic (e.g., hiccups and hypnic jerks) • Epileptic (e.g., juvenile myoclonic epilepsy) • Essential (no epileptic activity, dementia, or electroencephalogram abnormalities) • Symptomatic (most due to metabolic abnormalities)	Symptomatic treatment may be achieved with benzodiazepine such as clonazepam	
Parkinsonism	Hypokinetic	Various levels of bradykinesia, rigidity, resting tremor, and postural instability	• Idiopathic Parkinson's disease • Drug-induced parkinsonism (occurs with first several days to weeks of antipsychotic initiation, usually more symmetric)	If drug induced: • decrease antipsychotic dosage if possible • consider administering a lower-potency antipsychotic as an alternative[a] • benztropine 1–2 mg PO BID or amantadine 100 mg PO BID (increase to max of 300 mg/TDD)	Drug-induced parkinsonism is very common, almost 50% of outpatients develop signs or symptoms during course of treatments Consider Parkinson-plus syndromes, as neuroleptics may cause extreme extrapyramidal symptoms: • Lewy body dementia (visual hallucinations, fluctuating mental status and parkinsonism)

- Progressive supranuclear palsy
- Multiple system atrophy

Elderly patients are susceptible to cognitive impairments with anticholinergics, antihistamines, and amantadine—use sparingly; taper medication gradually as abrupt discontinuation can exacerbate symptoms

[a]Atypical antipsychotics (serotonin-dopamine antagonists) may represent an alternative medication strategy, because they possess a lower risk for extrapyramidal side effects. Risperidone is most likely to cause EPS at higher doses (>8 mg). Olanzapine has been shown to increase EPS, especially in patients with a history of EPS or Parkinson's disease. Quetiapine has been shown not to have a greater risk of EPS compared with placebo. Meanwhile, clozapine has the dopamine-serotonin affinity profile, which makes it least likely to cause extrapyramidal side effects; and in some cases, it has even been shown to improve tardive dyskinesia and other movement disorders.

Also consider infections (e.g., meningitis), metabolic defects, malignant hyperthermia, heat stroke, myocardial infarction, medication allergies and side effects, drug interactions, and lethal catatonia.

Certain laboratory values may support the diagnosis of NMS. These include elevated level of CK; increased white blood cell count; elevated liver enzyme levels; decreased serum levels of calcium, iron, and magnesium; and abnormal urine findings (proteinuria and myoglobinuria).

NMS often develops within the first few days of treatment with an antipsychotic or after its dosage is increased. It may also occur when suddenly discontinuing levodopa therapy in patients with Parkinson's disease. Risk factors include hypersensitivity to dopaminergic agents, comorbid affective disorders, and physical illness (e.g., dehydration). High-potency antipsychotics, large dosages, rapid dosage increases within a brief span of time, and parenteral administration are also risk factors. There is mounting evidence to suggest that the use of atypical antipsychotics (e.g., clozapine) may lower the risk of developing NMS.

LARYNGEAL DYSTONIA

Acute dystonia is a common movement disorder in patients treated with antipsychotics and is characterized by muscle spasms and contractions that result in a variety of abnormal postures. Laryngopharyngeal spasms are often experienced as a feeling of suffocation, and laryngeal dystonia may cause sudden death. On exam, patients with laryngeal dystonia will often have audible or auscultated stridor.

Patients usually develop drug-induced dystonia within days of beginning treatment with antipsychotics or of having a significant dosage increase. Rule out other possible causes such as metabolic defects, central nervous disorders, tumors, head trauma, and toxins. Nonpsychiatric medications that have been associated with dystonia include antiemetics, toxic levels of phenytoin, levodopa, and antimalarials containing quinine.

Acute Stroke

If acute stroke is suspected as an etiology of a patient's movement disorder, consult neurology immediately.

BEDSIDE

Quick Look Test

Assess the patient for signs and symptoms consistent with either NMS or laryngeal dystonia. In addition to difficulty breathing, the patient may have problems speaking owing to involvement of pharyngeal musculature. Does the patient appear toxic and/or dehydrated? Although very uncomfortable, patients with milder forms of dystonia and drug-induced parkinsonism may continue to follow their daily routines before asking for help. Conversely, patients with suspected NMS are often bedridden and dehydrated and appear quite sick.

Airway and Vital Signs

Most antipsychotic-induced conditions that produce rigidity do not compromise the autonomic system, except for NMS and laryngeal dystonia. In NMS, there usually is a significant elevation in temperature accompanied by tachycardia, tachypnea, and either hypertension or hypotension.

Selective Neurologic Examination

Look for the following signs (which often evolve in this sequence):

1. Mental status changes: be sure to focus on appearance, degree of alertness, level of consciousness, ability to consolidate new information (e.g., recall three words in 5 minutes), affect, perceptual or thought distortions, and any other behavioral abnormality.
2. Rigidity (lead-pipe or cogwheel): check wrists, supination/pronation of arms, rotate ankles, and if no suspicion of cervical trauma, then rotate head for neck rigidity.
3. Tremor: have patient extend both arms out. Feel over extended hands for fine postural tremor. Then have patient point index fingers toward each other to accentuate postural tremor.
4. Motor strength: begin with pronator drift (have patient extend arms with palms facing upward and eyes closed to look for pronation of one arm), then observe finger tapping of index finger and thumb, foot tapping to the floor, and end with confrontation testing of each muscle group.
5. Cerebellar signs: begin with finger to nose testing, then check for dysdiadokinesis (one hand with palm facing up while the other alternates slapping the dorsal and palmar surface over the hand), and then check for heel to shin movements.
6. Dyskinesias: observe lip smacking or licking and tongue protrusions, and note whether or not patient wears dentures (dentures without disease may cause dyskinesias). Have patient open mouth and stick out tongue while opening and closing one hand (for distraction), which may accentuate oral dyskinesias.
7. Gait: always try to test gait if the mental status is intact. Begin with having the patient get out of the seat with arms folded to test for postural stability. Have the patient walk normally then on heels, toes, and end with heels to toes. Observe stooped posture, decrease arm swing, shuffling gait, ability to clear ground,

fenestrating (speeding up without ability to slow down or stop), and balance.

MANAGEMENT

Neuroleptic Malignant Syndrome

The clinical course of NMS is variable but usually progresses rapidly. If NMS is suspected, perform the following steps:

- Discontinue antipsychotic medication
- Order laboratory tests (including CBC, electrolytes, urinalysis, CK, alkaline phosphatase, AST, ALT, and full fever work-up)
- Call a medical consultant—the patient may need to be transferred to a medical unit
- Consider initiating treatment with dantrolene sodium (skeletal muscle relaxant) or bromocriptine (dopaminergic agonist)
  - Dantrolene sodium: available parenterally or orally. Recommended dosage is 1 to 2.5 mg/kg IV QID (TDD 10 mg/kg); oral doses from 50 to 600 mg daily. Hepatotoxicity is associated with higher doses
  - Bromocriptine: treatment of choice for patients who can tolerate oral medications. Start 2.5 mg PO TID, increased dose by 2.5 mg TID q24hr until response (max dose 45 mg/day). Can exacerbate or cause psychosis
  - Length of treatment with dantrolene and/or bromocriptine depends on the form of antipsychotic that caused NMS. For example, for patients taking oral antipsychotics, a course of treatment for 10 days is necessary; however, for depot or long acting injectable antipsychotics, 2 to 3 weeks of treatment may be required

Acute Dystonia

- For laryngeal dystonia, administer benztropine 2 mg IV or IM, repeat dose in 5 to 10 min; can then give lorazepam 1 to 2 mg IV or IM
- For severe but nonlaryngeal dystonic reactions, reassure patient that this is a common and treatable side effect of the antipsychotic. Administer an anticholinergic (benztropine 1 to 2 mg IM or IV)/antihistamine (diphenhydramine 25 to 50 mg IM or IV), repeat twice within 15 min
- Once episode has resolved, be sure to place the patient on standing PO dosages of the previous medications to prevent further repeated complications
  - Typical regimens include Benadryl 25 mg PO BID–QID; trihexyphenidyl 1 to 3 mg PO TID; benztropine 1 to 3 mg PO BID

Always leave a note. Be sure to mention any medications involved or any interventions given.

Suggested Readings

Friedman JH. Atypical antipsychotics in the EPS-vulnerable patient. *Psychoneuroendocrinology.* 2003;28:39–51.

Jankovic J. Movement disorders. In: Goetz C, Pappert E, eds. *Textbook of Clinical Neurology.* 2nd ed. Philadelphia: WB Saunders; 2003:713–740.

J.J. Parkinson disease and other movement disorders. In: Bradley WG, Daroff R, eds. *Bradley's Neurology in Clinical Practice.* Philadelphia: Elsevier Saunders; 2012.

J.J. A.E.L. Diagnosis and assessment of Parkinson disease and other movement disorders. In: Bradley WG, Daroff R, eds. *Bradley's Neurology in Clinical Practice.* Philadelphia: Elsevier Saunders; 2012.

Leucht S, Pitschel-Walz G, Abraham D, Kissling W. Efficacy and extrapyramidal side-effects of the new antipsychotics olanzapine, quetiapine, risperidone, and sertindole compared to conventional antipsychotics and placebo. A meta-analysis of randomized controlled trials. *Schizophr Res.* 1999;35:51–68.

Barriers to Communication: Mutism and Other Problems With Speech and Communication

The on-call evaluation of new, acute changes in speech or communication requires consideration of a broad differential diagnosis. Changes in speech and language may be caused by various psychiatric, medical, and neurologic etiologies. There are a variety of deficits in speech, ranging from dysarthria to complete mutism, that must be differentiated from pathologic changes in cerebral language areas of the brain, as seen in aphasia. The clinician's first role is to make this distinction so that proper evaluation and treatment may be pursued.

PHONE CALL

Questions

1. Are there alterations in vital signs (including oxygen saturation and blood glucose)?
2. How specifically has speech or communication changed? Describe in detail.
3. What is the patient's level of consciousness?
4. What are the patient's psychiatric, medical, and neurologic histories?
5. What is the patient's level of psychomotor activity? Is catatonia suspected?
6. Did the patient recently begin or stop taking any medications (including antipsychotic medications) or undergo any procedures?
7. Is there any suspicion of recent illicit drug use?

Orders

Have the nurse take full vital signs if not already measured (including oxygen saturation and blood glucose).

Inform RN

"Will arrive in … minutes."

Mutism in any suspected case of psychosis, depression, or mania or acute medical illness in a patient unknown to you warrants one-to-one observation pending your arrival.

ELEVATOR THOUGHTS

What causes an acute change in speech or communication?

Mutism is a neuropsychiatric symptom resulting in the cessation of speech. Mutism itself is not a disease. A change in the level of alertness, impaired cerebral language centers, or impaired vocal/oral mechanisms of speech can result from many different psychiatric, neurologic, and medical disorders. See Table 16.1.

The first step in the evaluation of a communication disorder is to distinguish between disorders of speech and disorders of language. Disorders of speech include dysarthria and dysphonia. Dysarthria is a disturbance in articulation. It is caused by problems of the neuromusculature of the mouth, lips, or tongue or of the cerebral or cerebellar structures that coordinate their control. It may appear as

TABLE 16.1	Common Psychiatric and Medical/Neurologic Causes of Mutism

Psychiatric Causes	Medical/Neurologic Causes
Catatonia	Cerebrovascular accidents or other brain lesions
Schizophrenia	Delirium
Mania	Medication/drug intoxication/drug withdrawal (corticosteroids, antipsychotics, anticholinergics, PCP, amphetamines, crystal methamphetamine, cocaine, benzodiazepines, barbiturates, ETOH, etc.)
Depression	Laryngitis
Conversion disorders	Encephalitis, meningitis
Malingering	Seizures
Brief dissociative episodes	Endocrine disorders (myxedema, DKA, hyperparathyroidism, Addison disease)
Selective mutism	Tertiary syphilis
Posttraumatic stress	Neuroleptic malignant syndrome
Autism spectrum disorders	Paraneoplastic syndromes (e.g., anti-NMDA receptor encephalitis)

DKA, Diabetic ketoacidosis; *ETOH,* ethanol; *PCP,* phencyclidine.

slurred speech or as a total inability to speak in extensive cases. It may also be caused by antipsychotic medications and intoxication states. A disorder of phonation, or dysphonia, commonly presents as hoarseness, which stems from pathology of the larynx.

Disorders of cerebral language refer to impairments in symbolic communication, such as an inability to speak, understand, read, write, or repeat. These disorders are called aphasias and can include disturbances in the production of language, the comprehension of language, or both. Aphasias are usually caused by central nervous system (CNS) lesions, such as vascular accidents.

Severely affected patients may present with a near-total inability to produce verbal language, mimicking mutism. Alternatively, an aphasia that impairs language comprehension may sometimes mimic psychotic thought disorders.

Altered language in the context of a confusional state requires a work-up for delirium.

MAJOR THREAT TO LIFE

Inadequate nutrition from catatonia

Disordered language from delirium, particularly with deteriorating vital signs

Mutism in neuroleptic malignant syndrome (NMS)

Aphasia from acutely evolving stroke

Agitation, paranoia, violence, and suicidality in severe sensory aphasia

Violent behavior of psychotic or manic patients coming out of catatonia

Violent or agitated patient with paraneoplastic syndrome (e.g., anti-N-methyl-D-aspartate [NMDA] receptor encephalitis)

Suicide in severely depressed patients coming out of catatonia

BEDSIDE

Quick Look Test

Are there any abnormalities in vital signs?

Unstable vital signs may indicate cerebral infarction, drug (illicit or prescribed) intoxication or withdrawal, NMS, paraneoplastic syndromes (e.g., anti-NMDAR encephalitis), metabolic derangements, epilepsy, anoxia, infection, or other medical etiologies.

Is the patient breathing comfortably?

Irregular (Cheyne-Stokes) respiration may point to a neurologic cause such as cerebral embolism or infarct. The presence of stridor could indicate laryngospasm, particularly if the patient has recently been administered antidopaminergic medications.

These medications would include antipsychotic and antiemetic drugs such as metoclopramide and prochlorperazine.

What is the patient's age?

Older patients with any new, acute communication deficit require evaluation for stroke and delirium. In children, loss of speech is typically from selective mutism, a treatable, nonlife-threatening condition. In young and middle-aged adults, new-onset mutism is more often caused by psychiatric disorders; however, drug and medication toxicity or withdrawal, as well as metabolic disturbances, warrants consideration.

Does the patient have a new unilateral facial droop or other focal neurologic signs?

New-onset changes in speech with a new facial droop point toward ongoing cerebral ischemia or infarct and require immediate neurologic consultation. Sustained abnormal muscle posturing could also represent acute dystonias, which can be observed anywhere in the body but are most commonly seen in the head and neck area. Examples would include torticollis, retrocollis, oculogyric crisis, grimacing, and blepharospasm. They are generally accompanied by anxiety and pain.

What is the patient's level of consciousness?

Impaired arousal or alertness suggests a medical or neurologic etiology. Consider the possibility of a stroke and toxic and metabolic causes of delirium, including NMS. Visible diaphoresis or tremor may suggest delirium tremens from alcohol, benzodiazepine, or barbiturate withdrawal.

What is the level of psychomotor activity?

An alert patient with a "frozen" or bizarre posture may have mutism associated with catatonia (see later). Catatonia may derive from multiple psychiatric and neurologic etiologies.

What is the patient's level of distress?

Patients with mutism from psychiatric causes generally do not appear distressed by their communication deficit. Similarly, patients with amotivational states from frontal lobe pathology are rarely distressed. However, patients with aphasias, particularly motor aphasias (when they have intact comprehension but impaired spontaneous speech), are often quite distressed.

Selective History and Chart Review

Often a full history is not obtainable from the patient. Family members or close friends may provide a history of prior changes in speech. They may also be aware of a history of psychiatric, medical, or neurologic illness; recent changes in medications; or use of illicit drugs. Prior hospital records are also quite useful. In addition, some patients may be able to write information, which will help with the differential diagnosis for the communication problem (see section "Assessment of Speech and Communication").

Has the onset of the change in speech been sudden or gradual?

Gradual loss of verbal communication may often be caused by progressive degenerative brain disease (Alzheimer dementia, frontal-temporal dementia, primary progressive aphasia, and Parkinson disease), neoplasm, or depression. Alternatively, aphasia from stroke typically evolves within hours to days. Traumatic brain injury, delirium, and some psychiatric disorders may also cause more acute changes in communication.

Does the patient have a psychiatric history?

Is there a prior history of mutism or catatonia, and, if so, what diagnosis was made? Is there a prior history of bipolar illness, depression, schizophrenia, malingering, or conversion disorder? Is there a family psychiatric history? Is there a history of prior severe psychological trauma, posttraumatic stress disorder, or dissociative states? Mutism may be the presenting sign of any of these aforementioned psychiatric illnesses.

Have signs of catatonia been witnessed?

Posturing, stereotypy, waxy flexibility, automatic obedience, negativism, extremity rigidity, echolalia, echopraxia, and stupor are all signs of catatonia. Catatonia can be caused by both psychiatric and neurologic or other medical conditions. Some of these etiologies are listed in Table 16.2. Note that catatonia and NMS may have a strong syndromal overlap (rigidity, rigors, mutism); however, NMS presents with characteristic lab abnormalities (elevated creatine kinase - MB [CKMB], leukocytosis), fever, and diaphoresis.

Because true mutism more often occurs with catatonia than without, the absence of catatonic signs should alert the clinician to consider other causes of the communication deficit, such as a metabolic disturbance or aphasia from a cerebral lesion. However, note that mutism from conversion disorder, dissociation, and malingering often presents without catatonia.

TABLE 16.2	Causes of Catatonia
Psychiatric Causes	**Medical/Neurological Causes**
Schizophrenia	Epilepsy (ictal catatonia, postictal psychosis)
Mania	Encephalitis and other CNS infections
Depression	Medications (disulfiram, antipsychotics, maprotiline hydrochloride and aspirin in toxic doses)
	Substance intoxication (PCP) or withdrawal (benzodiazepines), hepatic encephalopathy
	Systemic lupus erythematosus or other rheumatologic disorders

CNS, Central nervous system; *PCP,* phencyclidine.

What medications has the patient taken previously and most recently?

A patient's medication list may highlight medical risk factors. For example, use of insulin, oral hypoglycemics, cholesterol-lowering agents, platelet aggregation inhibitors, anticoagulants, cardiac antiarrhythmics, or antihypertensives can indicate an underlying disease predisposing to stroke. Use of antiepileptic drugs should raise vigilance for absence seizures or postictal mutism. High doses of neuroleptics, along with antiemetics that also block dopamine (e.g., metoclopramide or promethazine) should raise concern for extrapyramidal side effects, from acute dystonic reactions to NMS. Acute dystonias are involuntary contractions of major muscle groups commonly seen in the face, neck, trunk, extremities, and, in life-threatening conditions, the larynx.

Slurred speech accompanied by oversedation and/or ataxia is often seen with medication toxicity. This may be caused by any sedating or anticholinergic medication and is more commonly seen in geriatric patients.

Is there a history of drug abuse?

Severe hypnotic or anxiolytic withdrawal-induced delirium tremens may be mistakenly misdiagnosed as mutism or catatonia. Substance intoxication or withdrawal may also manifest with mutism.

In a child, is the mutism selective to certain situations?

Mutism in children is most commonly selective. It generally occurs between the ages of 3 and 8 years as a failure to speak in school or to adults outside the home. The onset is gradual, and these children have typically been excessively shy, inhibited, or anxious previously.

Behavior not characteristic of selective mutism, such as not talking to immediate family members, abrupt cessation of speech in one environment (e.g., at a particular person's house), or absence of speech in all settings, should raise concerns about other causes of mutism. Mutism in a child who never learned to speak is most likely due to a specific or pervasive developmental disorder (e.g., autism) or deafness. Childhood-onset schizophrenia should also be considered. Petit mal seizures in children may also resemble selective mutism. Anti-NMDAR encephalitis in children has been reported to mimic autistic regression.

Does the patient have risk factors for stroke, including prior stroke, older age, poorly controlled diabetes, hypertension, cigarette smoking, or a family history of stroke?

Aphasias are most often due to embolic infarction of the middle cerebral artery. Aphasias can be divided largely into impaired verbal language output (motor aphasias) and impaired language syntax and comprehension (sensory aphasias).

Has there been a history of recent hypoxia or prolonged hypotension?

Recent hypoxia or prolonged hypotension may result in transcortical motor or sensory aphasias, caused by lesions of the so-called watershed area between the blood supply of the anterior communicating artery and the middle cerebral artery or between the middle and the posterior cerebral arteries.

Is the disordered language due to psychiatric or neurologic pathology?

On rare occasions a sensory aphasia may produce disordered language that needs distinction from a psychotic thought disorder. The sensory aphasias are problems with language reception and comprehension (also called posterior aphasias or Wernicke aphasia). Both Wernicke aphasia and transcortical sensory aphasia present with a normal amount of verbal output (unlike motor aphasia) but with syntactical errors such as paraphasias. Because people with sensory aphasia lack language comprehension, they are initially unaware of the deficit and may even become agitated or paranoid as they are blamed for communication difficulties. On occasion, more severely affected patients may present with incomprehensible language full of jargon that is mistakenly attributed to a psychotic thought disorder. These patients will usually lack the poverty of thought, bizarre thinking, delusions, or hallucinations typical of psychotic disorders.

Assessment of Speech and Communication

Assessment of speech and communication can be made by evaluating the patient's ability to speak spontaneously, repeat, name, write, read, and comprehend. See Table 16.3.

Selective Neurologic Examination

Assessment of every new-onset change in speech or communication should include a neurologic examination. This is particularly critical for older patients and for patients without prior known psychiatric illness, because organic causes of mutism may be overlooked. A neurologic examination can help to determine if the change in speech or communication exists as part of catatonia, aphasia, or dysarthria. Although the on-call psychiatrist should certainly do the initial neurologic examination, mutism in the absence of any known psychiatric history should also trigger a neurology consultation.

General Appearance

On observation, does the patient demonstrate any marked psychomotor abnormalities?

Abnormal posturing or stereotyped movements may point toward catatonia.

TABLE 16.3 Assessment of Speech and Communication

Disorder	Notes	Characteristic Speech	Ability to Repeat	Ability to Name	Comprehension	Ability to Write
Broca	Lesion to posterior inferior frontal lobe	Usually tries to talk, resulting in vocalizations/grunts or short utterances	Decreased	Decrease	Preserved	Poor
Wernicke	Lesion to posterior superior temporal lobe	Spontaneous fluent speech but content is incoherent containing paraphasic errors and neologisms	Decreased	Decreased	Decreased	Physically able to write but content incoherent
Locked-in syndrome	Injury to pons, most often ischemic or hemorrhagic stroke resulting in inability to respond verbally or nonverbally with no alteration in level of consciousness or awareness	None	None	None	Preserved	None
Delirium	Characterized by waxing and waning mental status	Variable	Variable	Variable	Variable	Variable
Catatonia	Characterized by waxy flexibility, posturing, negativism, stereotyped movements	Speech decreased or absent	Variable, echolalia may be present	Decreased	Variable	Decreased

Psychotic depression	May be accompanied by slowed or soft speech, tearfulness, suicidal ideation	Able to speak but may be hesitant	Preserved	Preserved	Preserved	Preserved
Malingering	Associated with secondary gain	Able to speak, but amount of speech variable depending on whether patient thinks he or she is being observed	Preserved	Preserved	Preserved	Preserved
Akinetic abulia	Extensive bilateral anterior frontal disease characterized by impairment of motivation and slowness to initiate actions	Variable	Variable	Variable	Variable	Variable

Face and Eyes

Is the pupillary diameter abnormal? Are pupils reactive to light? Are they equal?

Abnormal pupillary size or reactivity may be seen in drug intoxication or withdrawal states or in brainstem lesions. Asymmetry may point to a focal lesion or event. A psychiatric cause of mutism should be suspected in patients who resist eye opening.

Are there abnormalities in facial musculature?

Focal CNS lesions affecting language production may also cause decreased voluntary control of muscles of facial expression or of oral/vocal regions (as the two functions stem from nearby areas in the brain).

Is tongue protrusion midline?

Remember that the tongue will deviate to the side of the lesion.

Phonation, articulation, and nonspeech movements such as swallowing or coughing should be assessed to rule out failure of the peripheral sensorimotor speech apparatus.

Extremities

Is there bilateral extremity rigidity?

This may be indicative of catatonia, NMS, or severe extrapyramidal symptoms (EPSs) from antipsychotics or from Parkinson disease, all of which may present with mutism.

Is there waxy flexibility of the limbs, as seen in catatonia?

Is there unilateral weakness, spasticity, or exaggerated reflexes?

Patients with impaired speech from motor aphasia will often demonstrate these signs in the contralateral upper extremity and sometimes in the lower extremity.

Are primitive reflexes elicited?

Degeneration or lesions of the frontal lobes can produce the frontal release signs such as snout, suckling, grasp, or rooting reflexes. Similarly, check for the Babinski reflex.

Diagnostic Tests

Neuroimaging

Acute new-onset language disturbance or dysarthria in the geriatric population often requires immediate neuroimaging to rule out a vascular event. For any suspected acute cerebral hemorrhage, an immediate noncontrast head computed tomography scan is indicated. Similarly, for suspected evolving ischemic stroke, a noncontrast head computed tomography scan is generally preferred over magnetic resonance imaging for its ease and rapidity; however, remember that clinical signs may precede the ability to detect an evolving stroke with computed tomography scanning initially. Magnetic resonance imaging, although more expensive and time consuming, is a more sensitive tool to confirm suspicion of the vast majority of CNS lesions of all kinds. Cost aside, it is generally preferred in nonemergent cases.

Laboratory Studies

Impaired speech in the context of a fluctuating level of consciousness may signify a delirium. In this case, appropriate laboratory assessment could include electrolyte panel including calcium and magnesium levels, complete blood count, ammonia, liver enzymes, and toxicologic screenings. If infection is suspected, blood and CSF cultures should be sent. Cerebrospinal fluid (CSF) should also be sent for anti-NMDAR antibodies. If NMS is suspected, creatine kinase (CK) should be checked.

Electroencephalography

Electroencephalography may confirm suspected ongoing epileptic activity or a metabolic encephalopathy causing a change in communication. An electroencephalogram may be acutely indicated if the patient's mutism or other neurologic symptoms are episodic.

Additional Diagnostic Techniques

Lorazepam, parenterally given, will often improve symptoms of catatonia. A typical starting dose is lorazepam 2 mg intramuscularly (IM) or 1 mg intravenously (IV). This may require upward titration of dose and then establishment of the necessary frequency and the total daily dose required. Benzodiazepines will also generally improve delirium that is caused by alcohol, barbiturate, or benzodiazepine withdrawal or from epileptic activity. However, use caution because benzodiazepines will generally worsen most delirium and dementia.

MANAGEMENT

Suspected delirium: proper laboratory and neuroimaging assessment are essential. Medical consultation and management are usually indicated.

Suspected evolving stroke: an immediate noncontrast head computed tomography scan and neurologic consultation are necessary.

Depression: mutism may stem from severe psychomotor retardation. The patient may lack the energy to express thoughts or may have markedly slowed thinking. These patients can usually be urged into speaking. This may not be the case when the patient has a psychotic depression. Psychotic depression generally requires an antipsychotic and an antidepressant.

Schizophrenia: patients with schizophrenia who appear mute will often have associated poverty of thought, energy, or motivation.

They may be too frightened to speak, may be completely pre-occupied by internal stimuli, or may have bizarre beliefs that entail silence. They may be paralyzed by ambivalence. Treatment with an antipsychotic should resolve mutism over time. However, if they have frank catatonia, they will need more acute treatment (see following).

Severe parkinsonism, including acute dystonia: consider giving an anticholinergic such as benztropine 2 mg orally (PO) or IM or diphenhydramine 50 mg PO or IM. Both can also be given IV if more immediate relief is indicated.

NMS: patients with NMS present with extreme rigidity, altered level of consciousness, autonomic instability, fever, and elevated creatinine kinase level. The offending drug (most often a neuroleptic) should be discontinued. If the precipitant was withdrawal of L-dopa or dopamine agonist therapy, it should be reinstated. These patients require admission to an intensive care unit for intensive monitoring and supportive therapy. Benzodiazepines may be used to control agitation if necessary.

Mutism in acute drug-induced psychosis: manage mutism in acute drug-induced psychosis with a benzodiazepine such as lorazepam 1 to 2 mg PO or IM every 4 to 6 hours as needed. Antipsychotics such as haloperidol may be used adjunctively in cases of severe agitation.

Acute dystonia: can be treated with anticholinergic medications, such as benzotropine 1–2 mg IM or diphenhydramine 50 mg IM. Medications should be administered intramuscularly for faster onset of action.

Selective mutism: a common treatment approach to selective mutism in children is behavior modification. General supportive counseling, psychotherapy, speech therapy, and psychopharmacology have all been used as interventions.

General Guidelines for Dealing With Mutism of a Psychiatric Etiology

Frequent brief contacts may be more useful than long interviews.

Simple, concrete questions evoke better responses than do complex, open-ended questions.

Surreptitious observation is important, especially if malingering is suspected.

Nursing and social work staff who spend extensive time with the patient and show empathic concern may gain information more readily.

One-to-one observation may be necessary if dangerousness cannot be assessed.

Additional Considerations in Catatonia

Patients with catatonia may require nutritional support. IV fluid replacement may be indicated initially and ongoing monitoring of oral food intake, fluid intake and output, weight, and electrolytes may be needed.

Unresponsive catatonic patients are awake and alert and should have actions explained to them. Catatonia can be characterized by extreme fluctuations in psychomotor activity. Patients in a catatonic stupor may suddenly and without warning became extremely excited, agitated, and potentially violent. If the level of excitation is dangerous, an antipsychotic such as haloperidol (Haldol) 2 to 5 mg IM or fluphenazine 2 to 5 mg IM can be used, but the patient must be closely observed because dopamine blockers can worsen the stuporous phase of catatonia. Lorazepam 1 to 2 mg IM may be combined with the antipsychotic for additional sedation. In addition to IV or IM lorazepam, electroconvulsive therapy is often an effective treatment for catatonia if pharmacotherapy is not producing an adequate response.

Physical and Sexual Trauma

Victims of trauma may require urgent medical and psychiatric attention. Here, **trauma** is defined as "exposure to actual or threatened death, serious injury, or sexual violence," as defined by criterion A for post-traumatic stress and acute stress disorders in *Diagnostic and Statistical Manual of Mental Disorders,* fifth edition (DSM-V). This chapter is a brief guide for the psychiatric consultant on how to provide psychiatric intervention in the hours after acute trauma. The goals of intervention are to assist emergent medical and forensic evaluation, reduce acute emotional distress, and minimize future psychiatric morbidity. As in previous editions of this book, consideration of the acute management of the victim of rape is here used to illustrate basic principles that can be applied to crisis intervention in general. Special considerations for other populations follow.

Background

Of every 100,000 persons age 12 or older in the United States, 1100 reported to be a victim of rape in 2014, and the majority of incidents of rape were undisclosed. One out of every 10 rape victims is male. Transgender and gender-nonconforming individuals are at higher risk for sexual assault. One in every six women will be a victim of completed or attempted rape at some time in her life.

PHONE CALL

Questions

1. What is the behavior of the patient?
   Symptoms of dissociation and reexperiencing phenomena after trauma may be associated with behavioral agitation and disorganization, which can endanger patient safety and impede evaluation. Suicidal and homicidal comments and violent behavior may follow from feelings of intense fear, anger, shame, and guilt.

2. What is the patient's medical status?

   Rape is a violent act, and victims require immediate medical evaluation. In addition to assessment of physical trauma, including possible head trauma, evidence of alcohol and drug intoxication or withdrawal should be pursued. Abnormal vital signs may be an unrecognized clue that alcohol or substance use is involved.

Orders

1. Agitated patients may require pharmacologic intervention before the psychiatric consultant is able to arrive if the agitation poses acute risk to self or others. One dose of a benzodiazepine (e.g., **lorazepam 1 to 2 mg** or **diazepam 5 to 10 mg orally or parenterally**) may be useful.
2. Especially with patients who display poor behavioral control or express feelings of intense distress, including suicidal or homicidal comments, one-to-one observation is prudent until psychiatric evaluation is completed.
3. Full routine laboratory tests, pregnancy test, and screens for sexually transmitted diseases and indicated radiologic studies should be ordered by the primary team; request urine and blood toxicologic screening, including screening for amnestic "date rape" agents like gamma-hydroxybutyrate (GHB), flunitrazepam (Rohypnol), and ketamine, if it has not been obtained.

Inform RN

"Will arrive in … minutes."

ELEVATOR THOUGHTS

Acute responses to trauma are conceptualized by Osterman and Chemtob as the three "survival mode" functions. Functions of "fight," "flight," and "freeze" generate symptoms of anger, anxiety, and dissociation, respectively. The persistence of these functions and symptoms may contribute to the brief and chronic psychiatric symptomatologies of acute stress and post-traumatic stress disorders. Symptoms of reexperiencing the traumatic event (intrusive thoughts or images, dreams, reliving, distress or physiologic reactivity to external cues), avoidance (of thoughts, activities, memories, relationships, emotions, and expectation of a foreshortened future), hyperarousal (sleep difficulty, irritability, poor concentration, hypervigilance, exaggerated startle), and negative alterations in cognitions and mood (inability to remember totality of trauma, persistent distorted cognitions about cause or consequence of trauma, anhedonia, detachment, persistent negative emotional state) may emerge and persist from 2 to 4 weeks (meeting a diagnosis of acute stress disorder) or greater than 1 month (meeting a diagnosis of post-traumatic stress disorder). These symptoms may also contribute to emerging mood or other anxiety disorders.

MAJOR THREAT TO LIFE

Medical evaluation is the first priority. Disruptions in the patient's level of consciousness and orientation noted on the mental status examination may indicate undiagnosed medical or neurologic problems. Consider the possible role of alcohol or substance use or withdrawal in contributing to a patient's mental status.

Suicidality and homicidality are especially significant concerns because the patient's judgment may be impaired by the psychological shock of the trauma and alcohol or substance intoxication.

BEDSIDE

Quick-Look Test

It is imperative to assess the patient's level of consciousness and orientation.

Airway and Vital Signs

Abnormal vital signs can be a clue to undiagnosed medical or neurologic injury or to alcohol or substance intoxication or withdrawal.

Selective History

For the psychiatric consultant, taking a history from the rape victim can be a therapeutic opportunity as much as a diagnostic one. However, gathering information can proceed only if the patient feels safe and capable of providing it. Part of the trauma of rape is the experience of helplessness during the attack. You can start to restore a patient's feeling of empowerment and physical integrity simply by asking permission prior to beginning the interview and continuing to inquire about the patient's comfort with aspects of the interview, including the questions asked and persons present. It is not the psychiatric consultant's job to determine the accuracy of the patient's story or even catalog the traumatic events, especially because inquiry from law enforcement may already have prompted a detailed account. Furthermore, research shows that single session early debriefing of trauma does not reduce post-traumatic stress disorder (PTSD) symptomatology and may in fact increase the likelihood of a person developing these symptoms. As such, eliciting and responding to the patient's experience of the trauma is the primary goal.

The consultant may think of the therapeutic aims as threefold: to diminish guilt, normalize the trauma response, and assess for safety. Pay special attention to avoid statements that the patient may experience as judgmental because rape victims may already have a sense of shame or even guilt about their experience. History taking may provide opportunities to challenge a patient's feeling of responsibility for the events, an intervention that undercuts "identification with the aggressor" and supports healthier coping strategies and a more realistic understanding of trauma.

Target symptoms for the history include reexperiencing phenomena, hypervigilance, numbing and avoidance, somatic symptoms associated with panic and the specific events of the trauma, intrusive thoughts, distorted or exaggerated cognitions about the cause or consequences of the traumatic event, and intense feelings of anger, dysphoria, helplessness, rage, shame, and guilt. Suicidal or homicidal ideation may be present and should be asked about. These can be especially worrisome if neurologic injury, intoxication, or other acute psychiatric symptoms impair the victim's judgment or impulse control.

As with any patient, preexisting histories of recognized or undiagnosed psychiatric disorders may be present, and preexisting illness predicts increased symptomatology after rape. Screening for a history of psychotic, mood, anxiety, dissociative, personality, and substance use disorders should be preceded by an explanation that the patient's report of trauma-associated symptoms, such as reexperiencing, are not abnormal and that screening questions are not prompted by an impression that the patient is "crazy." Indeed, the elicitation of history may be integrated with psychoeducation about common emotional responses to trauma, including the features of acute stress, post-traumatic stress, adjustment, and depressive disorders, as well as difficulties maintaining intimacy with even long-standing friends and partners. Ultimately, this serves to destigmatize patient experiences, improve patient reporting, heighten the patient's sense of control, and encourage active pursuit of future treatment.

Finally, thorough family and social histories are extremely important in evaluating the rape victim. Because victims know the rapist in one-half of rape cases, the benevolence of family and friends cannot be assumed, and questions about them should be neutral and open ended. All evaluations should include a domestic violence screening such as the one described later (see section "Intimate Partner Violence"). The presence of any children in the patient's household should be determined, the adult providing care during patient evaluation should be identified, and risk of potential harm to the child assessed. After reliable social supports are identified by the patient and consent for their presence and involvement is given, they may be enlisted in the emergent evaluation and outpatient follow-up of the victim. Careful documentation of these issues is paramount, especially because anything you document is potential evidence in a criminal investigation.

Selective Physical Examination

The psychiatric consultant should not be directly involved in the physical examination. The physical examination of a rape victim not only serves the traditional purpose of evaluating the need for medical intervention but also is a primary source of evidence for criminal investigation. Most hospitals have a "rape kit" for this purpose and many have personnel trained in the Sexual Assault Nurse Examiner (SANE) or similar programs. However, because the physical examination can be traumatic and prompt reexperiencing, the psychiatric consultant can play an important role by helping patients prepare for it. Furthermore, when ability to provide informed consent to the examination is questionable, the psychiatric consultant will likely be asked to assess capacity to do so. Orienting the patient to routine procedures for rape victims can help to minimize anticipatory anxiety. In general, forensic evaluations may take up to 6 hours and involve an extensive interview and a comprehensive physical examination including photograph documentation, speculum exam, and sample collection from the patient's mouth, vagina, rectum, fingernails, scalp and pubic hair, and blood. All clothing worn during the time of attack is taken as evidence. Educating the patient that he or she may experience anxiety, flashbacks, intrusive thoughts, and somatic symptoms (e.g., palpitations, dyspnea, and sensations recalled from the rape) during the examination helps to normalize the experience and tolerate associated distress.

For patients who are unsure if they wish to proceed with the forensic exam, it may be helpful to educate them on their right to revoke consent at any time during the examination process. Careful inquiry about patient preferences—including the desire to have family members or friends present or absent—offers the patient a feeling of control and may prove relevant as law enforcement seeks to identify possible suspects. In general, it is helpful to remove as many people from the examination room as possible. Patients should be asked about their preference for the gender of examining clinician, and this request should be honored when possible.

MANAGEMENT

For the patient who can participate in a psychiatric interview, acute intervention is aimed at assisting emergent medical and forensic evaluation, reducing acute emotional distress, and minimizing future psychiatric morbidity. Interventions described previously include cultivating the patient's feeling of safety in the hospital, supporting an open discussion of traumatic events while allowing the patient discretion about the duration and detail of discussion, challenging self-blame, preparing the patient for physical evaluation and possible responses to it, educating the patient about the possible symptomatic sequelae of trauma, and including safe and requested social supports. Additional education about the likely course of medical treatment, including human immunodeficiency virus (HIV) postexposure prophylaxis, possible prophylactic treatment for other sexually transmitted diseases, and possible postcoital pregnancy prophylaxis may be useful. Throughout the emergent evaluation and continued treatment, the psychiatric consultant may be in a privileged position to help incorporate new information, assist the decision-making process, and supportively counteract emerging distress.

There is currently no medication indicated for the treatment of acute psychological trauma. Despite early promising open-label studies and a theoretical basis for its use, propranolol has not been shown to be effective in reducing the prevalence of PTSD symptoms when used immediately after trauma. Use of benzodiazepines in the acute period post-trauma should be cautioned against because there is some limited evidence that it may increase long-term PTSD symptoms. However, in the case of acute agitation posing a danger to self or others, use may be warranted of a low-dose benzodiazepine (e.g., lorazepam 1 to 2 mg PO or IV).

Finally, the psychiatric consultant must judge how safe it is for the rape or trauma victim to leave the hospital. This judgment is based on the relative significance of psychiatric symptoms, including suicidality and homicidality, alcohol or substance intoxication, medical or neurologic injury, the availability of social supports including family and friends, and a safe physical environment. All patients should be referred for follow-up care through crisis intervention or outpatient clinical programs and along with available social supports should be instructed on how to obtain emergency services if intense distress or dangerous behaviors emerge.

SPECIAL CONSIDERATIONS FOR OTHER POPULATIONS

Child Abuse

Child abuse is highly prevalent, yet rarely the chief complaint or identified problem when a child is brought in for evaluation. There are close to 1 million substantiated cases of child abuse in the United States per year, and in 2015 an estimated 1670 children died from abuse and neglect. Pediatricians and all physicians must be alert to unexplained physical findings, behavioral abnormalities, and child-caregiver interactions that raise any suspicion that a child is being neglected or abused. All states require physicians to report suspicion of child neglect or abuse.

Intimate Partner Violence

Intimate partner violence (IPV) includes physical violence, sexual violence, threats of physical or sexual violence, stalking, and psychological aggression by a current or former intimate partner. One million women and 150,000 men are victims of physical abuse or sexual assault by their partner each year. This type of violence can occur among heterosexual or same-sex couples; in fact, according to 2010 Centers for Disease Control and Prevention (CDC) data, bisexual women experienced significantly higher lifetime prevalence of rape, physical violence, and/or stalking by an intimate partner when compared with lesbian and heterosexual women. Other factors that elevate risk include young age, substance abuse, marital difficulties, pregnancy (for women), and economic hardships.

Victims often do not present with a complaint of abuse and may indeed be accompanied in hospital by the perpetrator of their abuse. Because potential indicators of abuse (including inconsistent explanation of injuries, frequent medical or emergency room visits, unexplained or vague medical complaints, inconsistent compliance with treatment) are nonspecific, the American Congress of Obstetrics and Gynecologists (ACOG) and the US Preventive Services Task Force (USPTF) both recommend universal screening for all women for IPV. Several screening instruments may be used and are available on the Centers for Disease Control and Prevention, National Center for Injury Prevention and Control website.

On examination, injuries can be present anywhere on the body but are often in the breast, abdomen, genital, and buttock areas.

Interventions for domestic violence include providing the patient with support and consultation with a social worker and calling the National Domestic Violence Hotline (1-800-799-7233) or providing a referral for counseling. If a child is suspected to suffer as a result of abuse or is a witness to the spousal abuse, concerns should be documented and reporting to Child Protective Services may be required. Please see separate chapter on Child Abuse.

Elder Abuse

Please see separate chapter on Elder Abuse.

For survivors of disasters, feeling helpless in the face of calamity is an especially significant experience. You can help to start the process of restoring a sense of control to survivors by attending to concrete needs and issues such as physical safety, food, and shelter and using supportive interventions such as consoling and comforting. Disaster survivors often experience survivor guilt based on the randomness of who has survived. The root of survivor guilt is a cognitive distortion that the psychiatric consultant can target by challenging the feelings of responsibility that many survivors have. Delivering psychiatric intervention to a group of survivors is often beneficial because members of the group can provide support for each other and help the psychiatric consultant challenge cognitive distortions.

Suggested Readings

American Psychiatric Association. *Diagnostic and Statistical Manual of Mental Disorders.* 4th ed Washington, DC: American Psychiatric Association; 2000. text revision.

Argolo FC, Cavalcanti-Ribeiro P, Netto LR, Quarantini LC. Prevention of posttraumatic stress disorder with propranolol: a meta-analytic review. *J Psychosom Res.* 2015;79(2):89–93.

Basile KC, Hertz MF, Back SE. *Intimate Partner Violence and Sexual Violence Victimization Assessment Instruments for Use in Healthcare Settings: Version 1.* Atlanta (GA): Centers for Disease Control and Prevention, National Center for Injury Prevention and Control; 2007.

Bureau of Justice Statistics, National Crime Victimization Survey, 1993–2014.

Calhoun KS, Resick PA. Post-traumatic stress disorder. In: Barlow DH, ed. *Clinical Handbook of Psychological Disorders.* 2nd ed. New York: Guilford Press; 1993:48–98.

Case B, Varma C. Physical and sexual trauma. In: Bernstein CA, Levin Z, Poag M, Rubinstein M, eds. *On Call Psychiatry.* Philadelphia: Elsevier; 2006.

Gelpin E, Bonne O, Peri T, Brandes D, Shalev AY. Treatment of recent trauma survivors with benzodiazepines: a prospective study. *J Clin Psychiatry.* 1996;57:390–394.

Hoge EA, Worthington JJ, Nagurney JT, et al. Effect of acute posttrauma propranolol on PTSD outcome and physiological responses during script-driven imagery. *CNS Neurosci Ther.* 2012;18(1):21–27.

Kaplan HI, Sadock BJ, eds. *Pocket Handbook of Emergency Psychiatric Medicine.* Baltimore: Williams & Wilkins; 1993.

Osterman JE, Barbiaz J, Johnson P. Emergency psychiatry: emergency interventions for rape victims. *Psychiatr Serv.* 2001;52:733–740.

Osterman JE, Chemtob CM. Emergency intervention for acute traumatic stress. *Psychiatr Serv.* 1999;50:739–740.

U.S. Administration for Children and Families. *Child Maltreatment 2015.* Washington, DC: U.S. Department of Health and Human Services; 2015.

Van der Kolk BA, McFarlane AC, Weisaeth L, eds. *Traumatic Stress.* New York: Guilford Press; 1996.

Walters ML, Chen J, Breiding MJ. *The National Intimate Partner and Sexual Violence Survey (NISVS): 2010 Findings on Victimization by Sexual Orientation.* Atlanta, GA: National Center for Injury Prevention and Control, Centers for Disease Control and Prevention; 2013.

The Pregnant Patient

The psychiatrist on call may be asked to assess and manage the pregnant patient. In managing a peripartum patient, providers must be cognizant that treatment decisions affect both mother and the developing fetus. The on-call psychiatrist must carefully weigh the risks of treatment with psychiatric medications in pregnancy and lactation against the risks of untreated symptoms, which may include agitation, psychosis, mania, severe depression, functional impairments, and suicidal or violent ideation. The appropriate knowledge of the risks and benefits of psychotropic medications and other treatment options for the pregnant patient will allow the psychiatrist on call to handle these complicated issues sensitively and thoughtfully.

As the literature is continuing to grow regarding safety profiles and long-term sequelae of psychiatric medication during pregnancy, the psychiatrist on call should refer to the listed resources, which are kept up to date and can be accessed while on call.

PHONE CALL

Questions

In addition to questions regarding the presenting consult question, the following may be useful during the initial screening phase:

1. How many weeks pregnant is the patient?
2. Have there been any complications in the pregnancy?
3. Does the patient have other medical problems? Does the patient take any medications?
4. What was the reason for admission or presentation?
5. What was the previous mental status and level of functioning? Is there a change in patient's mental status?
6. Is the patient actively using cigarettes, drugs, or alcohol?

Chart Review

The following questions should be answered by a chart review and selective history:

Past Medical History (PMH):

Does the patient have any medical problems?

What is the patient's obstetrical history (including prior pregnancies, duration, type of delivery, complications in mother and/or infant, abortions)?

Is the patient engaged in prenatal care (including taking prenatal vitamin, attending obstetrical appointments)?

Past Psychiatric History (PPH):

Does the patient have any preexisting psychiatric diagnoses, including onset in prior peripartum periods?

Is the patient currently in psychiatric care?

Does the patient have any prior history of drug or alcohol use?

In Utero Exposures:

Has the patient taken or is she currently taking any medications (including psychotropics) at any point during this pregnancy?

Has the patient or is she currently using cigarettes, alcohol, or illicit drugs at any point during this pregnancy?

It may be helpful to document the prior items as a complete list of in utero exposures to consider as part of the assessment.

Social History (SH):

What is the patient's support network? Does the patient have a partner or family who are involved?

Does the patient have other children? If so, who is caring for them while the patient is in the hospital?

Does the patient have any prior involvement with child protective services?

Any historical or current intimate partner violence?

Was the pregnancy planned?

Does the patient have a family history of psychiatric problems (including onset in peripartum periods)?

Orders

Close observation may be necessary until the psychiatrist arrives. If patient is extremely agitated, violent, or suicidal, 1:1 observation should be ordered immediately.

Inform Consulting Staff

"Will arrive in … minutes." As with all patients, if the pregnant patient is acutely agitated, psychotic, or suicidal, she must be seen more urgently and prioritized.

ELEVATOR THOUGHTS

Liaison: Dealing With Heightened Anxiety in Team Members

Patients with serious mental illness are at increased risk of receiving poor prenatal care and may also experience difficulties communicating their needs effectively. By acting as a liaison between medical caregivers and patients, the psychiatrist can maximize the patient's ability to engage productively with their medical caregivers and improve outcomes.

In particular, these patients may be unable to effectively verbalize physical pain associated with labor or obstetric complications. The psychiatrist can play an important role in advocating for these patients with the obstetrics team. Many of the breathing techniques involved in the management of labor pain are designed to reduce hyperventilation and can prevent anxiety and panic. Working effectively with the labor and delivery staff, who can coach the patient to breathe slowly through pain, can be an effective adjunct or alternative to medication.

In the face of anxiety about harming the fetus, neonate, or mother, staff may be tempted to undermedicate the patient or to abruptly discontinue existing psychiatric medications. Part of a psychiatrist's role is to educate the primary team and contain some of this anxiety.

Causes of Delirium/Agitation in Pregnancy

In a pregnant patient with any change in mental status, one must evaluate the patient for delirium, which should include a full medical work-up. Possible medical etiologies include:

- Preeclampsia/eclampsia
- Stroke—rare in pregnant/postpartum, but increased risk compared with age-matched controls
- Posterior reversible encephalopathy syndrome—may present with headache, seizures, and altered mental status
- Wernicke's encephalopathy—can be a rare consequence of hyperemesis gravidarum
- Pituitary apoplexy (vs. Sheehan syndrome)

BEDSIDE

Quick Look Test

When evaluating a psychiatric emergency in a pregnant patient, it is important to immediately assess the acuity of the situation. If there is an acute risk of physical dangerousness resulting from suicidal/homicidal threats or gestures, agitation, psychosis, or delirium, emergency medication and/or restraints may be necessary to maintain safety for both the patient and the providers.

MAJOR THREAT TO LIFE

The major threats to the life of the peripartum patient and her fetus include:

- Suicide
- Aggression/violence
- Infanticide (in postpartum period)
- Postpartum psychosis
- Alcohol withdrawal

Suicide

Suicide accounts for 3% to 13% of maternal deaths in high-income countries. Risk factors for suicide among peripartum women include history of prior suicide attempts, teenage pregnancy, history of intimate partner violence, and obstetric or neonatal complications. In a UK study of suicide in women, pregnant women were more likely than nonpregnant counterparts to have a recent diagnosis of mental illness, were more likely to have a diagnosis of depression, and were less likely to be receiving pharmacologic or psychological treatments at the time of suicide. It was also observed that pregnant and postpartum women who committed suicide frequently used violent or high-lethality methods, suggesting a high degree of suicidal intent.

Women may be at higher risk of suicide in the earliest phase of pregnancy. In a Hungarian study of pregnant women who attempted suicide via intentional poison ingestion, approximately 61% of these women attempted suicide before the third month of gestation. The study suggested that there was a peak in suicidal behavior around the time of initial discovery of pregnancy and in the context of the associated psychosocial and interpersonal stressors.

A suicidal mother will likely need close observation with an individual staff member and should also be screened carefully for infanticidal ideation (discussed later).

Violence/Aggression Due to Psychosis, Lack of Behavioral Control

A delirious, agitated pregnant woman should be treated urgently. Verbal de-escalation is preferred, if possible, though the on-call psychiatrist should consider medications if there is acute danger. In each case, psychotropics that have effectively addressed agitation in the patient in the past should be considered first.

Notably, there are no efficacy or safety studies comparing the risks and benefits of different pharmacologic interventions for agitation in pregnancy, and the latest Clinical Consensus Guidelines to address this topic were issued in 2001. At this time, expert consensus (76%) recommended a high-potency antipsychotic as a first-line treatment. The experts were unable to reach a consensus on second-line treatments; among the experts, 44% recommended adjunctive benzodiazepines, 33% recommended risperdal alone, and 29% recommended a combination of benzodiazepine and antipsychotic.

If the pregnant patient must be physically restrained for any reason, she should be placed on her left lateral side only. A supine position is contraindicated, particularly in the second and third trimesters, because the enlarged uterus can obstruct the vena cava and lead to vasovagal symptoms, including dizziness, pallor, sweating, and nausea. In very rare cases, vena cava compression can lead to maternal cardiovascular instability or compromise and fetal distress or demise.

Infanticide

Infanticide, homicide of an infant, is among the leading causes of infant death, with infants at particularly high risk during the first year of life. Many of these deaths can be attributed to an incident of extreme abuse. Maternal risk factors for infanticide include young age, low educational attainment, history of exposure to domestic violence, and late initiation of prenatal care. Women who commit neonaticide, or who kill an infant in the first 24 hours of life, may have concealed their pregnancy or exhibited denial of the pregnancy. Risk factors of infants that place them at higher risk of infanticide include low gestational age, low birthweight, low Apgar score, and male sex.

In formulating a risk assessment with specific attention to risk of harm to baby, the psychiatrist should consider a woman's past history of violence or child abuse, history of psychosis, and collateral information from family, friends, and outpatient psychiatrists. In addition, the consulting psychiatrist should directly ask about past or current thoughts of harming or killing the baby. If a mother has infanticidal thoughts, close observation of the mother by staff, separation of the mother and baby, and psychotropic medication may be necessary.

Postpartum Psychosis

Postpartum psychosis impacts approximately 1 to 2 of every 1000 deliveries. Risk factors include prior diagnosis of bipolar disorder, family history of bipolar disorder, primiparity, marital problems, and sleep deprivation. Women who stop mood-stabilizing treatment during pregnancy are more likely to experience postpartum psychosis than women who continue mood-stabilizing medications. Postpartum psychosis typically occurs within the first 4 weeks after delivery and exhibits a sudden onset. Patients present with delusions and/or hallucinations, acute irritation, hyperactivity, decreased need for sleep, and significant mood changes with poor decision-making. As symptoms may be waxing and waning, multiple points of evaluation may be necessary for accurate diagnosis.

Postpartum psychosis is associated with a suicide rate of 5% and an infanticide rate of 4%. It constitutes an acute psychiatric emergency and typically necessitates inpatient hospitalization. Treatment of acute postpartum psychosis may include lithium, an atypical antipsychotic, or electroconvulsive therapy (ECT).

Alcohol Withdrawal in Pregnancy

Alcohol use disorders have a lower prevalence in pregnant women than in nonpregnant women, and pregnant women may be more inclined to limit or eliminate alcohol use. Nonetheless, it is essential to diagnose and treat alcohol withdrawal in pregnancy where appropriate. Risks of alcohol withdrawal to the pregnant woman include seizures, hemodynamic instability, and delirium tremens. Risks to the fetus include risk of preterm delivery, placental abruption, and fetal distress.

In the United States, benzodiazepines are the first-line treatment for acute alcohol withdrawal. Our understanding of fetal risks of benzodiazepine use in the first trimester remains inconclusive. While an early study demonstrated an association between first-trimester benzodiazepine use and congenital abnormalities, more recent studies have not substantiated this risk. Infants exposed to benzodiazepines in the third trimester or close to delivery are at increased risk of floppy infant syndrome, which can include hypotonia, lethargy, hypothermia, and breathing difficulties. Infants are also at risk of neonatal benzodiazepine withdrawal, which can include irritability, hyperreflexia, hypertonia, movement abnormalities, breathing difficulties, and growth retardation.

In a pregnant woman suffering from alcohol withdrawal, the benefits of treatment with a benzodiazepine for both mother and fetus outweigh the risks of fetal exposure. In general, consider limiting polypharmacy and fetal exposures by choosing only one benzodiazepine to treat alcohol withdrawal. Lorazepam may be a preferred choice for a benzodiazepine taper because it has no active metabolite, but it is long-acting enough to cover withdrawal in the mother. As alcohol metabolism can change in pregnancy, Clinical Institute Withdrawal Assessment for Alcohol scale (CIWA) can be useful in monitoring patient symptoms.

MANAGEMENT

Because of ethical concerns, there are limited randomized controlled trials of medication effects during pregnancy. Therefore the scientific information regarding medications in pregnancy is limited to case reports, and cohort and case-control studies, largely retrospective rather than prospective. It is difficult to account for all confounding variables in these studies, such as maternal diagnoses, illness severity (of which medication use may be a marker), smoking, substance use, medical comorbidities, or other medication exposures—all of which can impact maternal, fetal, and infant outcomes. The on-call psychiatrist's decision-making should integrate patient preferences, take into account the available data (including safety and efficacy in pregnancy and lactation), and include clinical assessment of the individual situation. General treatment principles include using nonpharmaceutical or behavioral treatments for mild to moderate symptoms, limiting polypharmacy, preference for medications that have historically been beneficial for the patient, and using the lowest effective dose of medication.

While there used to be letter categories assigned by the US Food and Drug Administration (FDA) regarding a medication's published effects in pregnancy, on December 13, 2014, the FDA published the Pregnancy and Lactation Labeling Final Rule, which changed the labeling requirements for the pregnancy and lactation sections for prescription drugs. This removed the pregnancy letter categories, which many felt were confusing and oversimplified important risk/benefit treatment guidelines. In their place, the FDA created descriptive subsections for pregnancy exposure and risk, lactation, and effects to reproductive potential for females and males. These changes began June 30, 2015. All new submissions have already begun to use the new labeling guidelines; previously approved drugs will switch to the new labeling gradually.

In managing the pregnant patient with an acute psychiatric issue, it is important to consider (1) teratogenicity, (2) adverse reproductive outcomes, (3) neonatal complications, and (4) long-term neurobehavioral effects. Depending on the stage of pregnancy, these effects will be more or less relevant to your decision-making.

First Trimester

The first 3 months represent the time of organogenesis, so the choice and dosage of medication must be weighed against the known risk of teratogenicity. In any pregnancy, there is a risk of congenital malformation; this baseline risk is estimated to be between 2% and 5%. Attempt to manage symptoms behaviorally first, with methods such as creating a quiet space, practicing breathing techniques, and providing distraction.

Second Trimester

In the second trimester, although organogenesis has been largely completed, attention must still be paid to the choice of medication because of risk of withdrawal in the newborn and to honor the wishes of the mother for lactation. In the case of agitation, suicidality, violence, and psychosis, high-potency neuroleptics such as haloperidol along with diphenhydramine can be used. In the case of panic and anxiety not responsive to behavioral techniques, lorazepam is preferred.

Third Trimester and Labor

During the third trimester, pregnant patients require close monitoring of symptoms, as expanding blood volume and changes in metabolism can decrease serum levels across pregnancy. Dose increases may be needed to maintain stability. Similarly, once prepregnancy drug metabolism is restored postpartum, the patient's medication dose may need to be decreased.

Increasing levels of progesterone during pregnancy can induce hyperventilation, and the increasing uterine size can compress the diaphragm, both of which can worsen anxiety and panic. Effective use of breathing techniques can work to ameliorate anxiety during late pregnancy and labor. Reducing the patient's sense of isolation by including family members can also be effective in the management of anxiety. Make attempts to reduce stress and overstimulation inside the labor and delivery room, if at all possible.

Prior to labor, optimization of outcomes for the patient and neonate will require coordination with peds and the obstetrics (OB) team to ensure all providers involved are aware of the patient's medications and the infant's in utero exposures. It is often useful to discuss postpartum planning with the patient and her supports, if available. Discussing plans for breastfeeding, available supports to help with infant care, partner involvement, plans for caring for the infant overnight, and optimizing the patient's sleep will all help ensure a smooth postpartum transition.

Close psychiatric and pediatric follow-up is necessary to fully explore the risks and benefits of lactation with psychiatric medication. In new mothers with serious mental illness or with unstable home situations, close postpartum follow-up with social services is warranted.

Medications in Pregnancy

If bipolar disorder or major depression is suspected in a pregnant patient, a full risk assessment should be performed prior to discontinuing medications. In cases in which risk of relapse, severity of symptoms, and resulting functional impairments or dangerousness are high, discontinuation of medication may not be preferred, and close monitoring of the fetus may be preferable.

Neuroleptics

- In the case of severe agitation or psychosis resulting from schizophrenia, delirium, intoxication, or mood disorders, high-potency traditional neuroleptics such as haloperidol and perphenazine have not clearly shown any increased teratogenic effects on the fetus.
- First-generation medications are often used in psychiatric emergencies during pregnancy—most often haloperidol. Of the second-generation antipsychotics, olanzapine and quetiapine have the lowest documented placental transfer ratios—5% to 14% and 3.7%, respectively.
- In 2011, the FDA updated the pregnancy section of the labels for all antipsychotic drugs to highlight the risk of neonatal complications following exposure in the third trimester, including extrapyramidal signs (abnormal involuntary muscle movements), sedation, breathing and feeding difficulties, agitation, tremor, and abnormally increased or decreased muscle tone.
- Diphenhydramine can be used to manage insomnia or extrapyramidal symptoms and has more reassuring safety data in pregnancy than benztropine.

Mood Stabilizers

- Valproic acid is a known teratogen and is generally avoided in pregnancy.
- Lithium carries increased risk of congenital heart malformation (Ebstein anomaly), but absolute risk remains low and women may be maintained on lithium during pregnancy with very close monitoring and coordination between the psychiatrist and obstetrician (including a fetal echocardiogram in the second trimester).
- There are increasing safety data on lamotrigine, and supplementation with folic acid 4–5 mg daily is recommended for all women of childbearing age taking antiepileptic drugs.
- There are limited data on other antiepileptic drugs used as mood stabilizers.

Antidepressants

- Selective serotonin reuptake inhibitors (SSRIs) are being used with increasing frequency during pregnancy.
- With the exception of paroxetine, SSRIs are not associated with increased risk of congenital malformation.
- There is some concern that maternal SSRI use may be associated with increased risk of persistent pulmonary hypertension of the newborn, but the absolute risk remains very low.

- Use of SSRIs in the third trimester close to delivery may be associated with transient neonatal distress syndromes that typically self-resolve without treatment or intervention.

Anxiolytics

- If acute anxiety cannot be managed behaviorally, then lorazepam is the preferred as-needed medication.
- Though earlier studies suggested an association with cleft lip and palate (with absolute risk being very low), several prospective studies have not shown an association between benzodiazepines and congenital malformations.
- Because of the concern for active metabolites, clonazepam and diazepam are usually avoided during pregnancy.
- Administration near delivery might cause sedation or decreased tone in the infant.

For up-to-date information regarding medications in pregnancy and lactation, we recommend the following resources:

- Mother to Baby: For fact sheets on medications in pregnancy and lactation in English and Spanish, https://mothertobaby.org
- MGH Center for Women's Mental Health: https://womensmentalhealth.org/
- Lactmed: NIH database with medication levels in breast milk, as well as known evidence regarding infant exposures, https://toxnet.nlm.nih.gov/newtoxnet/lactmed.htm
- Postpartum Support International: Listing of referral resources by state for woman with postpartum depression and anxiety, www.postpartum.net
- Reprotox: A subscription information system on environmental hazards to human pregnancy, reproduction, and development, with free subscription access for trainees, https://reprotox.org

Suggested Readings

Bhat A, Hadley A. The management of alcohol withdrawal in pregnancy—case report, literature review, and preliminary recommendations. *General Hospital Psychiatry.* 2015;37(3):273e1–273e3.

Czeizel AE, Timar L, Susanszky E. Timing of suicide attempts by self-poisoning during pregnancy and pregnancy outcomes. *International Journal of Gynecology and Obstetrics.* 1999;65(1):39–45.

De-Giorgio F, Grassi VM, Vetrugno E, d'Aloja E, Pascali VL, Arena V. Supine hypotensive syndrome as the probable cause of both maternal and fetal death. *Journal of Forensic Sciences.* 2012;57(6):1646–1649.

DeVido J, Bogunovic O, Weiss RD. Alcohol use disorders in pregnancy. *Harv Rev Psychiatry.* 2015;23(2):112–121.

Friedman SH, Horowitz SM, Resnick PJ. Child murder by mothers: a critical analysis of the current state of knowledge and a research agenda. *Am J Psychiatry.* 2005;162(9):1578–1587.

Khalifeh H, Hunt IH, Appleby K, Howard LM. Suicide in perinatal and non-perinatal women in contact with psychiatric services: 15 year findings from a UK national inquiry. *Lancet Psychiatry*. 2016;3 (3):233–242.

Ladavac AS, Dubin WR, Ning A, Stuckeman PA. Emergency management of agitation in pregnancy. *General Hospital Psychiatry*. 2007;29 (1):39–41.

Overpeck MD, Brenner RA, Trumble AC, Triflietti LB, Berendes HW. Risk factors for infant homicide in the United States. *N Engl J Med*. 1998;339 (17):1211–1216.

Rahi M, Heikkinen T, Hartter S, et al. Placental transfer of quetiapine in relation to P-glycoprotein activity. *J Psychopharmacol*. 2007;21: 751–756.

Schenker S, Yang Y, Mattiuz E, Tatum D, Lee M. Olanzapine transfer by human placenta. *Clin Exp Pharmacol Physiol*. 1999;26:691–697.

Sit D, Rothschild AJ, Wisner KL. A review of postpartum psychosis. *J Women's Health (2002)*. 2006;15(4):352–368. https://doi.org/10.1089/jwh.2006.15.352.

Wyszynski A, Lusskin S. The pregnant patient. In: Wyszynski A, Wyszynski B, eds. *A Manual of Psychiatric Care for the Medically Ill*. Arlington, VA: American Psychiatric Publishing Inc.; 2005. Chapter 7.

Intoxication

Substance abuse evaluation is an important component of a thorough psychiatric interview. Our understanding of the neurobiologic mechanisms of addiction has progressed rapidly. Although we now have a more complex understanding of the intricacies of substance use and substance-induced disorders, evaluating and treating an intoxicated patient remain the most challenging situations to the psychiatrist on call. Often intoxicated patients are behaviorally difficult and may present with potentially life-threatening conditions; hence they require immediate attention. Although these patients may appear to have a primary psychiatric disorder, intoxication must clear before other diagnoses can be considered.

This chapter should serve as a guide to recognizing and managing intoxication syndromes. Obtaining a thorough history is key to providing care quickly and effectively.

PHONE CALL

Questions

1. What is the level of consciousness?
2. What are the vital signs?
3. What were the substances used?
4. How much was used?
5. How long ago was the last use?
6. What is the behavior?

Orders

Measure blood alcohol level and obtain urine toxicology results immediately.

Inform RN

"Will arrive in … minutes."

ELEVATOR THOUGHTS

What substances has the person been using?

First, consider the category of drug ingested. These most commonly include alcohol, hallucinogens, inhalants, marijuana, opiates, psychostimulants, and sedative-hypnotics. More recently, synthetics such as bath salts, synthetic cannabinoid receptor agonists (SCRAs), and "club drugs" such as methylenedioxymethamphetamine (MDMA), ketamine, and gamma-hydroxybutyrate (GHB) have increased in popularity. Often more than one substance will be involved. Street drugs have the added complication of not being pure, often containing additives and mixtures of drugs. Be aware of a mixed withdrawal and intoxication state. In general, intoxicated patients can be divided into two categories: lethargic or obtunded patients and agitated or restless patients.

If the patient appears lethargic or is in a coma, suspect intoxication from the following:

1. Opiates: meperidine (Demerol), morphine, heroin, opium, methadone, narcotic analgesics (OxyContin, Vicodin, fentanyl)
2. Sedative-hypnotics: benzodiazepines, barbiturates, zolpidem (Ambien), zaleplon (Sonata), eszopiclone (Lunesta), GHB, meprobamate (Equanil, Miltown)
3. Alcohol

If the patient is described as restless or agitated, suspect intoxication from the following:

1. Alcohol
2. Psychostimulants: cocaine, amphetamines, "bath salts," or other mephedrone derivatives
3. Hallucinogens: phencyclidine hydrochloride (PCP), lysergic acid diethylamide (LSD), ketamine, psilocybin ("mushrooms"), ayahuasca
4. Methylenedioxymethamphetamine (MDMA, "ecstasy")
5. Marijuana, synthetic cannabinoid receptor agonists ("K2/Spice")

BEDSIDE

Quick Look Test

What is the patient's appearance and level of activity?

What is the patient's level of consciousness?

What is the patient's history (enlist friends and relatives if necessary)?

Vital Signs

What are the patient's vital signs?

Selective History

What substances were inhaled, ingested, or injected?
How much was used?
How long ago was the last use?
Does the patient habitually use the substance? If so, how much and how often?
Does the patient use over-the-counter remedies?

Selective Physical Examination

1. Pupils
2. Tremors
3. Mental status examination
4. Neurologic examination

SUBSTANCE-SPECIFIC INTOXICATION SYNDROMES

Alcohol

Signs and symptoms include the following:
1. Slurred speech
2. Ataxia
3. Disinhibition
4. Aggression
5. Tachycardia
6. Hypothermia
7. Nystagmus
8. Respiratory depression
9. Coma
   General management involves the following:
1. Evaluate the patient in a quiet area.
2. Monitor vital signs.
3. Be aware of potential agitation and violence. It is reasonable, if the substance causing the behavioral disturbance is unknown, to start with benzodiazepines, such as lorazepam 1 to 2 mg orally (PO) or intramuscularly (IM) every 4 hours as needed, to treat agitation, especially if a component of alcohol withdrawal is suspected. However, if alcohol intoxication or sedative use is suspected, use caution with parenteral (IM or intravenous [IV]) benzdiazepines, as they can precipitate respiratory depression. Using an IM antipsychotic such as Haldol or an atypical may be safer in those cases.
4. Patients suspected of using excessive alcohol should be given thiamine (100 mg IM then PO for 6 days) to prevent the onset

of Wernicke encephalopathy. If a patient is exhibiting symptoms of thiamine deficiency (including ataxia, hypothermia and hypotension, confusion, ophthalmoplegia or nystagmus, memory disturbances, coma or unconsciousness), consider high-dose thiamine replacement (thiamine 500 mg IV q8 hours for 3 days, then 100 mg IV daily 1 to 3 days, then 100 mg PO daily indefinitely). Folate 1 mg PO should be given for 7 days. Patients with other vitamin B deficiencies should be given supplements appropriately.

5. Treat unconscious patients supportively, starting with IV fluids and glucose (give thiamine prior to giving glucose to avoid acute cerebral damage); maintain airway; and monitor vital signs.

Serious Alcohol Intoxication

A person with a blood alcohol level of 0.08 mg/dL or greater is considered legally intoxicated. A level of 0.3 to 0.4 mg/dL can cause coma and respiratory suppression. Patients who are alcohol-dependent often can tolerate higher levels.

Management involves the following:

1. IV fluids
2. Thiamine 500 mg IV every 8 hours for prophylaxis against Wernicke encephalopathy
3. Fifty milliliters of 50% glucose to prevent hypoglycemia
4. Intensive care unit monitoring
5. Monitoring for withdrawal symptoms

Psychostimulants (Cocaine, Amphetamines)

Signs and symptoms include the following:

1. Restlessness, agitation (most common presentation), anxiety, irritability, panic attacks
2. Euphoria, increased energy and alertness, insomnia
3. Psychosis, hallucinations, paranoia
4. Decreased appetite—may lead to hypovolemia or hypotension
5. Increased respiratory rate
6. Dilated, reactive pupils
7. Cardiac arrhythmias, tachycardia, hypertension, chest pain, palpitations, myocardial infarction
8. Fever/hyperthermia
9. Seizures
10. Neurologic signs secondary to stroke
11. Coma

Chronic high-dose cocaine users may exhibit paranoia that can mimic schizophrenia. A patient who has used extremely high doses may exhibit autonomic instability and hyperthermia, which may progress to seizures, strokes, and death. Chronic methamphetamine users can also have psychotic symptoms and mood changes.

General management involves the following:

1. Evaluate in a quiet area.
2. Urine drug screen may help delineate diagnoses of substance-induced versus primary psychotic or mood disorder; screens for cocaine are positive for 1 to 2 days after use. However, mephedrone derivatives are typically not detected in urine drug screens.
3. Benzodiazepines can be used for acute agitation and anxiety. Use lorazepam (Ativan) 1 to 2 mg as often as every 1 to 2 hours (generally not to exceed 8 mg in a 24-hour period) until the patient has calmed down.
4. Severely paranoid or agitated patients can also receive antipsychotic medications. Consider the use of olanzapine, risperidone, or quetiapine. As cocaine lowers the threshold for seizures, avoid Haldol, chlorpromazine, and clozapine. Monitor for effects every 30 minutes to 1 hour and continue administration until the patient is appropriately sedated. As symptoms are often self-limiting, antipsychotic use beyond 72 hours is often unnecessary and is not encouraged.
5. Be aware of medical complications, such as myocardial infarction, stroke, and intracranial hemorrhage.
6. Any temperature greater than 102°F is a medical emergency, could indicate comorbid infection, and should be treated aggressively with a cooling blanket and intravenous fluids.
7. Seizures should be treated as any other seizure with IV diazepam (Valium) 5 to 20 mg or lorazepam 2 to 4 mg, and repeated at 15-minute intervals as necessary. Seizures indicate the need for a monitored setting and potentially ICU-level care.
8. If paranoia persists for longer than 12 hours, hospitalization should be considered. Otherwise, discharge to a responsible person may be appropriate. An immediate follow-up appointment may be considered to verify that symptoms have resolved.

Marijuana (Cannabis) and Synthetic Cannabinoid Receptor Agonists (K2 and Spice)

Signs and symptoms include the following:

1. Euphoria, silliness, feeling of well-being
2. Altered perceptions
3. Lack of coordination
4. Increased appetite, thirst
5. Tachycardia
6. Injected conjunctivae
7. Increased anxiety, paranoia

SCRAs are generally more toxic than marijuana. Originally designed to act at the cannabinoid receptor, they now comprise a vast array of synthetic substances that have a wide range of effects that vary by batch, origin, and content and may contain toxins such as acetone. Due to the variety of compounds, standard urine drug screening does not detect SCRAs, though specific testing for these compounds is available at some institutions or by special request; suspect if symptoms are suggestive of drug use but drug screening is negative. Other compounds to consider if standard screening is negative include bath salts, mephedrone, and flakka. Marijuana smoking tends to produce relatively mild side effects in most users, with heavy intoxication potentially causing protracted vomiting, hallucinations, or paranoia. The following more serious adverse effects are more common with SCRAs:

1. Hypertension, tachycardia, temperature fluctuations, syncope
2. Agitation, aggressiveness, and other behavioral issues
3. Gastrointestinal symptoms, such as hyperemesis, nausea, and vomiting (often conspicuous features)
4. Hallucinations, psychosis, and panic attacks
5. Seizures and death

Management involves the following:

1. Reassure the patient that the effects will subside.
2. Treat acute anxiety with benzodiazepines such as lorazepam 1 to 2 mg PO every 4 hours as needed. (Do not exceed 8 mg in a 24-hour period.)
3. Especially with synthetic cannabinoids, treat psychotic symptoms with antipsychotic medications, such as haloperidol (Haldol) 5 mg PO or IM every 30 minutes until the patient has calmed down (up to ~20 mg in a 24-hour period).
4. For synthetic cannabinoids, consider hospitalization when the reaction lasts longer than 24 hours despite vigorous intervention.

Opioids

Opioids include opium, morphine, heroin, methadone, oxycodone, hydrocodone, fentanyl, and so on.

Signs and symptoms include the following:

1. Pinpoint pupils unresponsive to light, except with meperidine, which may produce dilated pupils
2. Depressed respiration and level of consciousness
3. Bradycardia
4. Hypothermia
5. Pulmonary edema
6. Coma, death

Overdose is a medical emergency because of pulmonary edema and respiratory depression, and requires treatment in the intensive care unit.

Management involves the following:

1. Support the airway.
2. Treat with naloxone 0.4 to 2.0 mg IV every 2 to 3 minutes until respirations are stable. After 10 mg, consider other causes for symptomatology.
3. The half-life of naloxone is much shorter than that of most opioids (approximately 1 hour), so observe closely for the reemergence of symptoms (e.g., coma) and retreat with naloxone; failure to do so may result in patient death after release from the emergency room. Overdose with long-acting opiates may require naloxone drip.
4. Monitor for withdrawal symptoms.

Hallucinogens

Hallucinogens include LSD, psilocybin (mushrooms), ayahuasca, mescaline (peyote), diethyltryptamine (DET), and dimethyltryptamine (DMT).

Signs and symptoms include the following:

1. Labile affect
2. Cyclic reactions with alternating periods of lucidity and hallucinations
3. Perceptual distortions, including hallucinations, and synesthesia, in which, for example, sound is perceived as color
4. Dilated pupils
5. Tachycardia, palpitations
6. Diaphoresis
7. Tremor, incoordination
8. Hypertension
9. Hyperthermia
10. Piloerection

The effects mostly occur over 6 to 12 hours but may last up to several days. One common emergency room presentation is that of a patient having a "bad trip," which is an adverse drug reaction following the use of hallucinogenic drugs. Manifestations may vary from an acute panic reaction to a temporary psychotic state. The patient may report feelings of helplessness, fear of losing control, fear of going crazy, and suspiciousness that can reach proportions of frank paranoia. Patients may also complain of intense anxiety, depression, and hallucinations, predominantly visual.

Flashbacks are another unique presentation that may occur with chronic LSD use. A flashback is a spontaneous recurrence of the original LSD trip. It usually occurs suddenly and lasts from several minutes to several hours.

Management involves the following:

1. Reassurance is the most important therapeutic intervention.
2. Maintain close observation to monitor for dangerous behavior.

3. Treat with lorazepam 1 to 2 mg PO or IM every 1 to 2 hours until the patient has calmed down.
4. Consider hospitalization when the reaction lasts longer than 24 hours despite vigorous intervention.

Phencyclidine and Ketamine

PCP can have hallucinogenic, stimulant, or central nervous system depressant effects, depending on the dose taken. Ketamine is a dissociative anesthetic used in human and veterinary medicine. Its effects are similar to those of PCP, but it is much less potent and shorter-acting. Of note, ketamine is odorless and tasteless, and is often given to victims unknowingly; hence it is sometimes referred to as a "date rape" drug.

Signs and symptoms include the following:
1. Nystagmus, ataxia, dysarthria
2. Hyperreflexia, numbness
3. Disorientation, memory impairment
4. Hallucinations, synesthesia
5. Agitation, combativeness
6. Decreased sensitivity to pain
7. Rigidity, muscle contractions
8. Hypertension
9. Tachycardia
10. Stupor
11. Seizures
12. Coma, death

Management involves the following:
1. Monitor vitals and cardiopulmonary functioning; supportive treatment when necessary.
2. Consider hospitalization, because overdose can be fatal.
3. Minimize sensory stimulation. Attempts to reassure the patient may aggravate the situation.
4. Treat anxiety or agitation initially with lorazepam 1 to 2 mg PO or IM; can repeat every 30 to 60 minutes until patient is calm, while watching for respiratory suppression.
5. Can treat psychosis with antipsychotics (i.e., Haldol 5 mg PO or IM, max. 20 mg/24 hours, olanzapine 5 to 10 mg PO or IM, max. 20 mg/24 hours), but use caution as this may lower the seizure threshold.

Sedative-Hypnotics

Sedative-hypnotics include benzodiazepines, barbiturates (phenobarbital, secobarbital), zolpidem, zaleplon, and eszopiclone.

Signs and symptoms include the following:
1. Ataxia
2. Slurred speech

3. Nystagmus
4. Confusion
5. Depressed respiration and level of consciousness
6. Hypotension
7. Coma, death

Overdose with benzodiazepines alone is rarely fatal. Mixture with other sedatives, however (particularly alcohol), can cause fatal respiratory depression.

Management involves the following:

1. Sluggishness, altered mental status, or coma represents a life-threatening emergency.
2. Monitor vital signs and support the airway as needed.
3. Activated charcoal to reduce further absorption if the drug was taken in the last 30 minutes.
4. Flumazenil (Romazicon) is a benzodiazepine antagonist that may be used to reverse the effects of an overdose. However, severe adverse events have been recently reported, including cardiotoxicity (arrhythmias) and seizures (avoid in patients with benzodiazepine dependency or concomitant tricyclic antidepressant overdose). Avoid in patients with increased intracranial pressure (e.g., head trauma), as flumazenil adversely affects cerebral hemodynamics. Would only consider use with guidance from toxicology, as supportive treatment can be provided until substances are metabolized.
5. Monitor for withdrawal symptoms.
6. Ineffective treatments: gastric lavage, elimination enhancement by forced diuresis.

Inhalants

Signs and symptoms include the following:

1. Altered states of consciousness ranging from euphoria to clouding of consciousness
2. Dizziness, syncope, ataxia, slurred speech
3. Psychosis
4. Nausea, vomiting, epigastric distress
5. Chest pain
6. Tachycardia, ventricular fibrillation
7. Organ damage (brain, liver, kidney, heart)
8. Chemical-like odor on the breath, residue on clothing/hands
9. Oral/nasal ulcerations, Huffer rash (perioral/nasal dermatitis), rhinitis, epistaxis
10. Death—can occur from anoxia, cardiac dysfunction, allergic reaction, injury to lungs, CNS depression

Acute intoxication can last from 15 to 45 minutes. Drowsiness and stupor may last for hours.

Management involves the following:

1. Monitor vitals and apply "ABCs" of life support.
2. Decontamination of skin and clothing to prevent burns and further harm.
3. Attempt to identify the solvent. Leaded gasoline may require the use of a chelating agent.
4. Restoration of oxygenation should resolve symptoms within minutes.
5. Treat acute psychosis with haloperidol 2 to 5 mg PO or IM. For agitation, use benzodiazepines.

Club Drugs: Methylenedioxymethamphetamine, Gamma Hydroxybutyrate, Ketamine

"Club drugs," including MDMA ("ecstasy, "molly"), GHB, and ketamine ("special K"; see previous) are increasingly popular among young adults at nightclubs, parties, and raves. They are not detectable on routine urine toxicology screens.

Methylenedioxymethamphetamine/"Ecstasy"

MDMA ("ecstasy," "E," "X," "molly") has become a very popular drug among young adults and adolescents, particularly in the "club/rave" and "electronic dance music" (EDM) scene. It has both stimulant and hallucinogenic effects. MDMA can exert a range of psychiatric effects, including confusion, depression, memory impairment, and anxiety. These symptoms can occur for weeks following chronic use. Although the risk of death from MDMA remains low, MDMA overdose can lead to hyperthermia and dehydration, especially when users have been awake for long periods of time with decreased fluid intake (e.g., dancing for extended periods in hot, enclosed places). In rare cases, MDMA overdose can produce a syndrome similar to neuroleptic malignant syndrome, characterized by rigidity, hyperthermia, dehydration, mental status changes, and rhabdomyolysis, leading to renal failure, convulsions, and autonomic dysregulation. There have been reports of disseminated intravascular coagulation resulting from extreme hyperthermia related to MDMA overdose.

If MDMA overdose is suspected, the condition should be treated promptly. Management involves the following:

1. Rehydration is imperative to prevent renal failure.
2. Electrolytes should be monitored closely.
3. Hyperthermia should be corrected (cooling blankets).

Gamma-Hydroxybutyrate

GHB is a central nervous system depressant used for its sedative and euphoric effects. It is known as one of the date rape drugs (along with ketamine and flunitrazepam [Rohypnol], a benzodiazepine). GHB precursors are available in nutritional supplements and are used by bodybuilders for their anabolic properties.

GHB overdose can be lethal via respiratory depression or seizures. Effects are synergistic when combined with alcohol or other sedative-hypnotics, making these combinations especially dangerous.

Signs and symptoms include the following:

1. Sedation
2. Nystagmus, ataxia
3. Nausea, vomiting
4. Bradycardia, hypothermia
5. Depressed respiration and level of consciousness
6. Seizures (especially in combination with cocaine/stimulants)
7. Coma, death
8. Often, combativeness and myoclonus on recovery of consciousness

Management involves the following:

1. Observation, monitoring, and supportive treatment
2. Atropine for symptomatic and persistent bradycardia
3. Hospitalization if symptoms are severe or persist more than 6 hours; admit to intensive care unit if breathing is labored.

Anticholinergic Drugs

These include diphenhydramine, benztropine, atropine, and belladonna. Note that many psychotropic medications have anticholinergic effects, and overdose may have an element of anticholinergic toxicity.

Signs and symptoms are related to the anticholinergic effects (e.g., "red as a beet, dry as a bone, mad as a hatter"):

1. Hot, flushed skin
2. Dry mouth, thirst
3. Blurred vision
4. Confusion, delirium
5. Dilated pupils
6. Tachycardia, arrhythmias
7. Hypertension
8. Urinary retention

Management involves the following:

1. Provide supportive medical management.
2. Discontinue the offending agent.
3. Reassure the patient.
4. Treat agitation with lorazepam 1 to 2 mg PO or IM every hour until the patient is calm.
5. For severe medical symptoms or uncontrolled agitation, can be used to reverse the anticholinergic effects. Use with caution in patients with concomitant medical illness.

Selective Serotonin Reuptake Inhibitors

Serotonin syndrome may occur in the setting of a selective serotonin reuptake inhibitor overdose, or with combinations of medications including selective serotonin reuptake inhibitors, serotonin norepinephrine reuptake inhibitors, tricyclic antidepressants, and synthetic opioids (e.g., meperidine), triptans, antiemetics (e.g., ondansetron), antibiotics (linezolid), dextromorphan, levodopa, St. John's wort, and drugs of abuse (MDMA, cocaine, methamphetamines, LSD).

Signs and symptoms of the serotonin syndrome include the following:

1. Classic triad: Mental status changes (e.g., delirium, anxiety, irritability, confusion), neuromuscular irritability (primarily rigidity and clonus, but also ataxia, tremor, hyperreflexia), and autonomic instability (e.g., hypotension or hypertension, tachycardia, diaphoresis, sialorrhea, mydriasis, tachypnea)
2. Gastrointestinal disturbance
3. Hyperthermia (can be $>41°C$)
4. Severe cases can be life-threatening. Other complications include seizures, renal failure, and disseminated intravascular coagulopathy (DIC).

Management involves the following:

1. The syndrome is self-limited and often resolves after discontinuation of the offending agent. In severe cases, supportive measures and intravenous hydration (crystalloids) may be necessary.
2. For rigidity, dantrolene can be used though benefit is unclear; dose is 1.0 to 2.5 mg/kg IV and then 1 mg/kg q6 hours until 10 mg/kg reached.
3. If supportive therapy fails, can use cyproheptadine, a 5-ht2a antagonist, though its benefit is unclear and use for serotonin syndrome is not FDA approved. Starting dose is 12 mg followed by 2 mg every 2 hours until effective.
4. Atypical antipsychotic (olanzapine, risperidone) use is controversial; while some studies report that these drugs treat serotonin syndrome, others report these drugs can induce serotonin syndrome.

Serotonin syndrome and neuroleptic malignant syndrome may present with some similar features. A careful history of current medications is therefore essential.

Caffeine

Signs and symptoms mimic those caused by stimulants. Lethal dose is 10 g (150 to 200 mg/kg); for reference, coffee contains 50 to 200 mg of caffeine, tea 40 to 100 mg, and energy drinks 40 to 300 mg per serving. Manage the patient symptomatically: provide support and anxiolytic medication if necessary.

Suggested Readings

Alusik S, Kalatova D, Paluch Z. Serotonin syndrome. *Neuro Endocrinol Lett.* 2014;35(4):265–273.

Benowitz NL. Caffeine. Chapter 39, In: Olson KR, ed. *Poisoning & Drug Overdose.* 6th ed. New York, NY: McGraw-Hill; 2012.

Cooper ZD. Adverse effects of synthetic cannabinoids: management of acute toxicity and withdrawal. *Curr Psychiatry Rep.* 2016;18(5):52.

Katus LE, Frucht SJ. Management of serotonin syndrome and neuroleptic malignant syndrome. *Curr Treat Options Neurol.* 2016;18(9):39.

Nguyen J, O'Brien C, Schapp S. Adolescent inhalant use and prevention, assessment, and treatment: a literature synthesis. *Int J Drug Policy.* 2016;31:15–24.

Quan D. Benzodiazepines. In: Tintinalli JE, Stapcyzynski J, Ma O, Yealy DM, Meckler GD, Cline DM, eds. *Tintinalli's Emergency Medicine: A Comprehensive Study Guide.* 8th ed. New York, NY: McGraw-Hill; 2016.

Substance-Related and Addictive Disorders. *American Psychiatric Association: Diagnostic and Statistical Manual of Mental Disorders.* 5th ed. Arlington, VA: American Psychiatric Association; 2013.

Tang Y, Martin NL, Cotes RO. Cocaine-induced psychotic disorders: presentation, mechanism, and management. *J Dual Diagn.* 2014;10 (2):98–105.

Toxicological Findings of Synthetic Cannabinoids in Recreational Users. Kronstrand R et al. doi:10.1093/jat/bkt068.

Tsutaoka B. Benzodiazepines. Chapter 31, In: Olson KR, ed. *Poisoning & Drug Overdose.* 6th ed. New York, NY: McGraw-Hill; 2012.

Substance Withdrawal

Substance withdrawal is commonly encountered in both psychiatric and medical patients. The psychiatrist on call is asked to evaluate and treat patients who are behaviorally difficult, have comorbid psychiatric diagnoses, suffer clinical stigmata of withdrawal, and/or complain of various subjective discomforts related to the substance(s) from which they are withdrawing.

Primary concerns for substance withdrawal include medical and psychiatric stability, and identification of the specific substance(s) and most recent use. Although many symptoms (e.g., distress, irritability, dysphoria) are mild and self-limited, others may progress to life-threatening situations, such as delirium tremens (DTs) and seizures. When the patient is stable, a complete history will include usage patterns including query of prescription monitoring database (if available), prior withdrawal symptoms, comorbid medical conditions, and other data specific to the substance(s), outlined as follows. As substance use disorders are chronic and relapsing in nature, complete care for withdrawal should ideally include referral to appropriate aftercare.

PHONE CALL

Questions

1. What are the patient's vital signs?
2. What is the patient's level of consciousness (e.g., comatose, obtunded but responsive, disoriented with clouded sensorium)?
3. Does the patient appear dangerous to himself or herself, or to others?
4. Are there obvious signs concerning for withdrawal (e.g., autonomic arousal, piloerection, lacrimation, vomiting, diarrhea, dilated or pinpoint pupils)?
5. Is there a history of drug use or evidence of drug use (e.g., alcohol on breath, needle tracks)?

6. If the patient admits to drug use or abuse, what substances were used, when was the last use, how much was used, and by what route was it administered?
7. What medications is the patient taking?

Orders

If the patient is severely agitated, violent, or suicidal, one-to-one observation should be started immediately.

Inform RN

"Will arrive in … minutes."

1. If any of the above information is lacking (e.g., vital signs), ask the nurse to obtain it while you are on your way.
2. If indicated, ask the nurse to prepare intramuscular (IM) medications—for example, lorazepam (Ativan) 2 mg and/or haloperidol (Haldol) 5 mg.

ELEVATOR THOUGHTS

What causes substance withdrawal?

Prolonged and repeated exposure to drugs of abuse is associated with receptor downregulation in the central nervous system (CNS), and substance dependence is defined physiologically by the presence of craving and withdrawal as a result of these changes. Withdrawal syndromes result from the discontinuation or decrease of the substances (or their analogues) responsible for this habituation. The signs and symptoms of withdrawal are often opposite those of intoxication, and the severity of withdrawal is directly proportional to the severity of dependence. In severely dependent patients, withdrawal may occur when intoxicants are still detected, but at a relatively lower level than those at which the patient has been habituated.

Substance-Specific Syndromes

1. Alcohol withdrawal, including withdrawal delirium (DTs)[a]
2. Sedative, hypnotic, or anxiolytic withdrawal[a]
3. Opioid withdrawal
4. CNS stimulant (cocaine and amphetamine) withdrawal
5. Nicotine withdrawal
6. Antidepressant withdrawal
7. Anticholinergic withdrawal
8. Marijuana withdrawal
9. Synthetic cannabinoid receptor agonist (SCRA) withdrawal[a]

---

[a]Indicates a potentially lethal withdrawal syndrome.

In addition to these syndromes, be alert for:

1. Multiple concurrent intoxication and withdrawal syndromes
2. The presence of withdrawal symptoms despite concurrent evidence of intoxication (e.g., alcohol on breath)
2. Medical sequelae of substance use, including trauma associated with altered states, endocarditis, septic shock, or hepatitis C virus/human immunodeficiency virus (HCV/HIV) associated with intravenous (IV) drug use
3. Malnutrition
4. Malingering for secondary gain of substance treatment (e.g., methadone), food, shelter, or avoidance of court appearances

INITIAL ASSESSMENT

Level of consciousness, airway, and vital signs: Is the patient stable and able to protect his or her airway in the event of emesis? Is he or she agitated or distressed?

Mental status exam (MSE): While you may choose to defer a complete MSE until the patient is stable and withdrawal is being managed, use the initial assessment to look for evidence of substance use (e.g., track marks, alcohol on breath, jaundice), evidence of trauma (e.g., head trauma that might be the result of sudden loss of consciousness), evidence of acute physical pain, evidence of withdrawal (e.g., diaphoresis, dilated pupils, tremor), evidence of recent seizure (e.g., incontinence, tongue lacerations), psychosis (e.g., internal preoccupations, disorganized thought), suicidal ideation, and homicidal ideation; perform a basic cognitive assessment if possible.

Physical exam: Likewise, a complete physical exam may be deferred at this time. However, a targeted exam can yield important information. In addition to the general observations included in the MSE, perform a focused neurologic exam with special attention to pupil size, extraocular movements, tendon reflexes, cerebellar function, and gait. If there is suspicion of alcohol use history, look for stigmata of liver failure. If there is suspicion of IV drug use, look for evidence of infective endocarditis, liver injury (HCV), and opportunistic infections associated with AIDS.

History/Chart Review

1. Is there a history of substance abuse? What have the most recent patterns of use been (amounts, routes)? Has the patient ever had withdrawal symptoms, including DTs, seizures, or prior hospitalizations for withdrawal? Is there any history of IV drug use?
2. Has the patient been enrolled in detoxification or rehabilitation programs or methadone clinics? If the patient is enrolled in a methadone maintenance program, contact the program and obtain the daily maintenance dosage and date of last dose administered.

3. Is there a psychiatric history of a mood or psychotic disorder? Has the patient been hospitalized or taken psychotropic medications? Has the patient followed up with treatment?
4. Is there a history of suicide attempts or violence?
5. Is there a family history of substance abuse or other psychiatric illness?
6. Is the patient in pain? Ask about the localization and quality of pain. Has the patient been prescribed pain medication (e.g., opiates), and for what duration?

Labs: The patient needs a careful medical evaluation to rule out a possible life-threatening condition. The autonomic instability and delirium of severe alcohol withdrawal can mimic an infectious process, and confusion and agitation could be due to CNS injury. A medical evaluation may include some or all of the following, depending on what pathology is suspected: complete blood count, blood chemistry and possibly fingerstick glucose, liver function tests, thyroid function tests, rapid plasma reagin, vitamin B12, folate, hepatitis panel, HIV test, blood cultures, chest x-ray, electrocardiogram, lumbar puncture, and head computed tomography scan.

Confirm or rule out suspected substances of abuse by obtaining urine toxicology and blood alcohol levels, if they have not already been obtained. Some emergency rooms are equipped with dipstick urine toxicology kits. However, note that not all substances of abuse are detected by these screens (i.e., synthetic opiates such as buprenorphine, short-acting benzodiazepines such as alprazolam).

SPECIFIC WITHDRAWAL CONDITIONS

Alcohol Withdrawal
Signs and Symptoms

1. Autonomic hyperactivity (e.g., sweating or pulse rate greater than 100 bpm, elevated blood pressure)
2. Increased hand tremor
3. Insomnia
4. Nausea or vomiting
5. Transient visual, tactile, or auditory hallucinations or illusions
6. Psychomotor agitation
7. Anxiety
8. Generalized tonic-clonic seizures

See the following for discussion of withdrawal seizures, DTs, and Wernicke encephalopathy.

Time course: Tremors usually begin within 5 to 10 hours after alcohol use has been stopped or reduced. They are related to a hyperadrenergic state. Symptoms peak in intensity during the second day of abstinence and usually remit by the third to fifth day in uncomplicated withdrawal. Alcohol withdrawal seizures usually occur within the first 24 to 48 hours of withdrawal, and DTs may occur within 3 to 5 days.

N.b.: If the patient has a history of concomitant cocaine dependence or is taking beta blockers, vital sign elevation may not be a reliable indication of withdrawal, because large amounts of cocaine may result in adrenergic depletion, and beta blockers may suppress adrenergic response. In this case, alterations in mental status may be the best indication of withdrawal, and presumptive prophylaxis should be initiated.

Immediate Steps

Consider admission if the patient presents with fever, autonomic instability, seizures, protracted nausea, vomiting, diarrhea, or signs of Wernicke encephalopathy.

1. Assess and treat withdrawal symptoms. Evidence of autonomic arousal by vital signs (increasing heart rate or blood pressure) or CIWA (Clinical Institute Withdrawal Assessment) score >8 indicates the need for treatment. The CIWA scale asks the patient or the treating clinician to assign a rating from 0 to 15, with 15 being more severe, to the patient's agitation, anxiety, auditory disturbances, clouding of sensorium, headache, nausea/vomiting, paroxysmal diaphoresis, tactile disturbances, tremor, and visual disturbances. CIWA >15 has been shown to have a relative risk of 3.72 for severe alcohol withdrawal.

   Benzodiazepines relieve the withdrawal symptoms by serving as an alcohol substitute at GABA receptors; they also raise the seizure threshold and provide sedation. Specific benzodiazepines and benzodiazepine administration protocols may vary, but evidence shows that treating symptoms as they arise ("symptom-triggered therapy") results in shorter duration of treatment and less overall drugs administered than scheduled or tapered-dose therapy. If you suspect the patient may suffer from liver failure, use lorazepam, oxazepam, or temazepam, which are not hepatically metabolized. Suggested symptom-triggered therapy using lorazepam is 2 mg PO for CIWA greater than 8 or vitals indicating withdrawal, or 2 mg IV q2h if vomiting is present. For withdrawal seizures and DTs, see the later discussion. Note that in the absence of other evidence of DTs, hallucinations themselves do not require treatment with benzodiazepines.

2. Ensure hydration. Encourage fluid intake by mouth (PO) if patient is able to protect his or her airway and not suffering from nausea, vomiting, or diarrhea. In such cases, consider IV fluids. Patients who drink heavily may become volume

depleted due to poor PO intake apart from alcohol, which can lead to tachycardia and nausea independent of withdrawal.

3. Give vitamins and minerals. All patients suspected of chronic alcohol use should receive IV or IM thiamine 100 mg before glucose, as well as 1 mg folate, and 1 tablet vitamin B complex. Mg, Ca, K, and glucose should be corrected if necessary. Continue to replete thiamine, folate, and vitamin B PO daily for the next week if the patient remains hospitalized.

4. Continue to monitor while treating and repleting. Monitor vitals, level of consciousness, and CIWA regularly, and retreat with benzodiazepines as needed. Remember that heavy drinkers may begin withdrawing while their blood alcohol level remains elevated.

Management of Seizures

Seizures occur in 5% to 15% of patients, are typically tonic-clonic, and are one or two in number. They usually develop within 24 to 48 hours but can also occur as late as 7 days following the cessation of alcohol use. About 30% of patients who have seizures will develop withdrawal delirium. Treat withdrawal seizures with lorazepam 2 mg IV. Diazepam 5 mg IV can also be used, although it is longer-acting and has active metabolites. Call a neurology consultation for all seizures.

Management of Withdrawal Delirium

Withdrawal delirium (DTs) is a medical emergency. It occurs in less than 5% of individuals and usually begins 48 to 96 hours (or rarely 1 week) after cessation or decrease in alcohol intake. It typically occurs in individuals who have been drinking heavily for 5 to 15 years. If seizures also occur, they almost always precede the development of delirium. Withdrawal delirium may last 1 to 5 days. If untreated, mortality may be as high as 20%.

This potentially life-threatening condition includes disturbances in consciousness and cognition (e.g., disorientation, memory impairment), visual, tactile, or auditory hallucinations; agitation; and marked autonomic hyperactivity (e.g., tremulousness, tachycardia, hyperthermia, diaphoresis). It may lead to circulatory collapse, coma, and death. When alcohol withdrawal delirium develops, it is likely that a clinically related general medical condition may be present (e.g., liver failure, pneumonia, gastrointestinal bleeding, sequelae of head trauma, hypoglycemia, pancreatitis, an electrolyte imbalance, or postoperative status).

In addition to the preceding guidelines for the management of uncomplicated withdrawal:

1. Secure an IV access.

2. Lorazepam 1 to 4 mg IV q5–15 minutes. Doses should be repeated until symptoms clear. Patients should be calm and

lightly sedated. Severely dependent individuals may have high benzodiazepine requirements. If symptoms are not adequately controlled, escalation to barbiturates or propofol may be indicated, which would require ICU-level care.

3. Haloperidol 2 to 5 mg, IM or IV, every 2 to 4 hours may be used to control severe cases of agitation or psychosis. It should be used with caution, however, because it may lower the seizure threshold and is metabolized hepatically.

4. Avoid physical restraints, if possible, because the patient may fight them and cause injury. Be alert to the possibility of sharp elevations in creatine phosphokinase level. Adequate sedation with benzodiazepines should be used to avoid the need for restraint.

5. Observe the patient closely for the development of focal neurologic signs.

6. Put the patient on a high-calorie, high-carbohydrate diet.

Other Complications

Other complications encountered during alcohol withdrawal include the Wernicke-Korsakoff syndrome and alcohol hallucinosis. Although they are not believed to be caused directly by alcohol withdrawal, they may complicate the clinical picture.

Wernicke encephalopathy is an acute, potentially reversible neurologic disorder thought to be caused by thiamine deficiency. It is characterized by disturbances of consciousness (ranging from mild confusion to coma), ophthalmoplegia (sixth cranial nerve palsy), nystagmus, broad-based ataxia, peripheral neuropathy, hypothermia, and hypotension. It is usually seen in individuals with chronic heavy alcohol abuse and nutritional deficiencies. This disorder has a high mortality rate if untreated and can also progress to a more chronic condition known as Korsakoff psychosis. Korsakoff psychosis usually presents as a disturbance of short-term memory, inability to learn new information, and compensatory confabulation. See the previous discussion for thiamine repletion guidelines; it is important to give thiamine to all patients suspected of chronic alcohol use.

Alcoholic hallucinosis is characterized by vivid and persistent illusions and hallucinations (auditory or tactile). This disorder may last several weeks or months. Antipsychotics may relieve agitation and hallucinations in those patients who do not improve spontaneously. Haloperidol 2 to 5 mg PO or IM every 6 to 8 hours (if the patient is acutely dangerous and refusing PO medication) **may be used.**

Sedative/Hypnotic/Anxiolytic Withdrawal

Agents in this category include benzodiazepines, phenobarbital, pentobarbital, secobarbital, meprobamate, ethchlorvynol, glutethimide, chloral hydrate, and methaqualone. Withdrawal syndromes are likely to occur after chronic use of 40 to 60 mg/day of diazepam, 400 to 600 mg/day of pentobarbital, and 3200 to 6400 mg/day of meprobamate, or their equivalents. Signs and symptoms may resemble those of alcohol withdrawal, including the potential lethality. Collectively signs and symptoms are more diverse than those of alcohol withdrawal, given the diversity of sedatives, hypnotics, and anxiolytics:

1. Autonomic hyperactivity (e.g., sweating or pulse rate >100 bpm)
2. Hand tremor
3. Insomnia
4. Nausea or vomiting
5. Transient visual, tactile, or auditory hallucinations or illusions
6. Psychomotor agitation
7. Anxiety
8. Grand mal seizures

Time course: Variable, according to the half-lives of substances abused. Symptoms can occur as quickly as within hours of decreased use or take up to days to appear, and may persist for days to weeks.

Immediate Steps

1. Assess for withdrawal as outlined for alcohol.
2. For uncomplicated withdrawal, quantify the patient's use before onset of withdrawal, and convert to benzodiazepine equivalency using the benzodiazepine available on formulary at your institution. See bibliography or use resources available at your institution for benzodiazepine/barbiturate equivalency tables. Chlordiazepoxide has a relatively long half-life, is moderately sedating, and is a reasonable choice. A suggested chlordiazepoxide regimen is to give 80% of the known used amount in chlordiazepoxide equivalents, or as much as is needed to control withdrawal symptoms over the first 24 hours. Then reduce the dose daily, giving 50% of the first dose on each of the first 2 days, and tapering off chlordiazepoxide over the next 7 to 10 days. In some cases, detoxification with "high-potency" benzodiazepines such as alprazolam may require taper of a long-acting high potency agent such as clonazepam to fully address withdrawal. Patients with hepatic impairment may require lorazepam or oxazepam, due to an inability to metabolize chlordiazepoxide.
3. For complicated withdrawal (seizures, delirium), manage as outlined for alcohol.

4. Rule out metabolic, infectious, hepatic, and structural abnormalities. Hypoglycemia and Wernicke encephalopathy must always be considered.

Opiate Withdrawal

Opioid withdrawal is uncomfortable but not life-threatening. The objective in treating withdrawal is to reduce, rather than suppress, symptoms. Patients should be told to expect some discomfort but be reassured that they will not be allowed to suffer or experience pain.

Signs and Symptoms

In approximate order of appearance, the signs and symptoms of opiate withdrawal are as follows:
1. Anxiety, irritability, and craving
2. Dysphoric mood
3. Lacrimation and rhinorrhea
4. Insomnia
5. Yawning
6. Increased sensitivity to pain
7. Muscle, bone, and joint aches
8. Fever (usually low grade) and hot and cold flashes
9. Pupillary dilation, piloerection ("cold turkey"), and sweating
10. Nausea, vomiting, and diarrhea
11. Hyperadrenergic state: increased blood pressure, pulse, and respiratory rate
12. Muscle twitching and kicking ("kicking the habit")

Time course: In most individuals who are dependent on short-acting drugs, such as heroin or morphine, withdrawal symptoms occur within 6 to 24 hours after the last dose. They peak at 48 to 72 hours and last 7 to 10 days. Symptoms may take 36 to 72 hours to emerge in the case of longer-acting drugs, such as methadone or l-α-acetyl-methadol (LAAM).

Warning: In adults, the presence of high-grade fever, altered mental status, and seizures is inconsistent with opioid withdrawal and should alert the clinician to the possibility of another withdrawal syndrome (e.g., alcohol or sedative withdrawal), CNS infection, trauma, or sepsis.

Immediate Steps

1. Assess the severity of withdrawal. The physician relies on objective findings (e.g., piloerection, sweating, rhinorrhea, pupillary changes, tachycardia, hypertension) to determine whether withdrawal is present; subjective complaints are less reliable as to the severity of the withdrawal, and motivated and savvy patients may malinger symptoms of withdrawal in order to

obtain medications. The Clinical Opioid Withdrawal Scale (COWS) is a freely available clinician-administered tool to quantify the severity of withdrawal symptoms and overall withdrawal syndrome.

2. If the patient is enrolled in a methadone maintenance program, that program should be contacted to verify the daily dosage and date last administered. Once verified, the patient may be given his or her maintenance dose daily during hospitalization (if not being detoxified this admission). See the following "Medications" section.

Medications

The main principle of treatment is replacement of the opioid agent. Methadone has become the replacement of choice in most cases because of its long half-life and ease of oral administration. If the patient's daily dosage can be verified through a methadone maintenance program, it can be safely given to the patient. If not, most patients in significant opioid withdrawal will have symptomatic relief with 5 to 10 mg of methadone initially, regardless of the patient's daily intake of heroin or methadone. The advantage of such a dosage is that it can be given safely, even to individuals who have never taken opioids, without the risk of respiratory arrest. Consider IM administration because of its predictable absorption and efficacy, given the nausea, vomiting, and diarrhea commonly associated with opioid withdrawal, which may interfere with methadone absorption.

The methadone dose should be repeated every 4 to 6 hours until withdrawal symptoms disappear. Total methadone intake during the first 24 hours should not exceed 30 mg in most cases. The amount given the first day should be divided into two daily doses on the second day and then tapered at a rate of 10% to 20% per day. Institutions vary as to their policies regarding use of methadone tapers versus symptom-triggered stat dosing. Symptom-triggered therapy is safest, as it avoids oversedation. If patients are on a taper, specify to nursing that doses should be held if the patient is sedated.

Other opioid agents can be used in agonist substitution therapy:

1. Clonidine (Catapres) is an alpha-2-agonist antihypertensive agent that appears to be effective in alleviating insomnia, restlessness, nausea, vomiting, diarrhea, muscle aches, and craving associated with opioid withdrawal. As an adjunct to methadone treatment, it can help attenuate withdrawal and reduce its duration and cost. Clonidine can also be used in lieu of methadone in patients for whom methadone is contraindicated (e.g., documented allergy). Clonidine can be administered at 0.1 to 0.3 mg PO 3 or 4 times a day for 2 weeks. Do not exceed 0.8 mg a day. The principal side effects are hypotension and sedation, and the dosage should be carefully individualized. Do not administer if

the systolic blood pressure is less than 90 mm Hg or the diastolic blood pressure is less than 60 mm Hg. Clonidine should be tapered on discontinuation because of the possibility of rebound hypertension.

2. Buprenorphine is a partial opiate agonist that may be given instead of methadone and/or clonidine. As a partial agonist, buprenorphine does not carry associated risks of sedation or drug-drug interaction, yet still relieves symptoms of withdrawal within 20 minutes. Patients must be abstinent from opiates for at least 24 hours prior to administration and should be in withdrawal, as administration of buprenorphine results in displacement of full agonists with associated dysphoria and subjective complaints. Note that buprenorphine requires a US Drug Enforcement Administration (DEA) act waiver, addiction psychiatry certification, or completion of federal buprenorphine training to prescribe.

Other Complications

Commonly used medications can treat symptoms associated with withdrawal, among them loperamide for diarrhea, antacids for nausea, and nonsteroidal anti-inflammatory drugs (NSAIDs) for headache and muscle cramps.

IV drug abusers may suffer from other medical complications of their habit. Be alert to possible signs of endocarditis, trauma, intoxication with other substances, and malnutrition. The possibility of HIV and hepatitis C infection should also be considered.

Central Nervous System Stimulants (Cocaine and Amphetamines)

Withdrawal signs and symptoms include the following: Dysphoria, fatigue, psychomotor retardation or agitation, sleep changes, and increased appetite. Withdrawal is not life-threatening. In general there is a less precise syndrome for withdrawal from stimulants, compared with alcohol, sedative/hypnotics, and opioids, and "symptoms" may be caused by lack of sleep and nourishment secondary to intoxication, rather than physiological withdrawal.

1. Fatigue
2. Vivid, unpleasant dreams
3. Insomnia or hypersomnia
4. Increased appetite
5. Psychomotor retardation or agitation
6. Anhedonia

Time course: A triphasic pattern of behavior is described for cocaine withdrawal:

1. Crash phase (9 hours to 4 days after the last binge): This phase begins with agitation, depression, anorexia, and high drug craving. These are followed by a decrease in drug craving and by

fatigue, depression, and a desire for sleep. The patient's sensorium is intact when awakened.

2. Withdrawal phase (1 to 10 weeks after the last binge): This phase begins with normalization of sleep and mood patterns, only to be followed again several days later by anhedonia, anergia, and anxiety, with high cocaine craving.

3. Extinction phase (may last for years): This phase represents a period of extended vulnerability to relapse, especially to conditioned cues.

Immediate Steps

It is important to assess for suicidality during the crash phase of withdrawal, because patients may experience intense dysphoria and be at risk for impulsive suicide attempts, but may also malinger suicidality for secondary gain of shelter, food, or medications. Suicidal patients may require admission to the hospital.

Patients should be encouraged to attend a detoxification or rehabilitation program and be referred to a support group, such as Narcotics Anonymous. Family or group therapy can also be helpful.

Medication

No medications are indicated for treatment of withdrawal syndromes. However, for agitated patients, lorazepam 1 to 2 mg, PO or IM, may be given; if paranoid ideation is present to a significant extent, antipsychotics, such as haloperidol (Haldol) 5 to 10 mg PO or IM (if leading to acutely dangerous behavior), or its equivalent, may be added.

Club Drugs: Methylenedioxymethamphetamine ("Ecstasy") and Gamma-Hydroxybutyrate

Methylenedioxymethamphetamine Withdrawal

Methylenedioxymethamphetamine (MDMA) causes an increase in the release of multiple neurotransmitters in the brain, most notably serotonin. Hence, patients may experience symptoms associated with a relative deficiency of serotonin for several days following use of the drug.

SIGNS AND SYMPTOMS

1. Dysphoria, irritability
2. Anorexia
3. Concentration difficulties
4. Fatigue

Antidepressant medications may be used for treatment. There have also been case reports of long-term psychotic symptoms following discontinuation of MDMA. Treat symptomatically.

Gamma-Hydroxybutyrate Withdrawal

Gamma-hydroxybutyrate (GHB) has a very short half-life, and withdrawal from GHB is similar to that of other GABA-potentiating substances, including alcohol and sedatives. A withdrawal syndrome typically occurs after prolonged use of the drug.

SIGNS AND SYMPTOMS

1. Anxiety
2. Tremor
3. Insomnia
4. Autonomic instability—tachycardia, elevated blood pressure, diaphoresis
5. Disorientation, delirium
6. Psychosis—paranoia, auditory and visual hallucinations
   Management involves the following:
1. Symptomatic and supportive treatment
2. Benzodiazepines (often very high doses may be necessary)
3. Barbiturates (if treatment refractory to benzodiazepines)
4. May require ICU-level monitoring if delirium is present

Nicotine Withdrawal

Signs and Symptoms

Nicotine withdrawal is commonly encountered during hospitalization in a nonsmoking facility. The withdrawal syndrome includes four or more of the following:

1. Irritability, frustration, or anger
2. Anxiety
3. Difficulty concentrating
4. Increased appetite
5. Restlessness
6. Depressed mood
7. Insomnia

Time course: Typically the sense of craving begins within 24 hours of decreased use, peaks around 48 to 72 hours, and then declines gradually over a period of 2 to 3 weeks. As with cocaine and other drugs, craving can be powerfully evoked by cues previously associated with smoking or tobacco use.

Medication

Nicotine replacement therapy (NRT), which provides nicotine to prevent withdraw but dissociates its physiological effects from the act of smoking, doubles long-term abstinence rates (from 4% to 8%). When combined with behavioral therapy, success rates of up to 40% have been reported. It is important to ensure that the patient does not smoke while undergoing replacement therapy, because nicotine overdose can occur. NRT is available as a transdermal patch, which may be combined with other forms of NRT including gum, lozenge, inhaler, and nasal spray. The patch should be dosed 21 mg q24h for patients who smoke ≥10 cigarettes/day, and 14 mg for those who smoke less. Patch application sites should be rotated daily. Gum should be dosed 4 mg for patients who smoke ≥25 cigarettes/day, and 2 mg for those who smoke less, both ordered q2h prn. Lozenges should be dosed 4 mg for patients who smoke within 30 minutes of waking, and 2 mg for those who smoke less both ordered q2h prn. The inhaler and nasal spray are prescription-only medications, while the others are available over the counter.

Clonidine (Catapres) has also been effective in alleviating withdrawal symptoms. However, it is not FDA approved for this indication and appears to be less effective than transdermal nicotine.

Compliance with long-term smoking cessation can be supported with the initiation of bupropion (Zyban) or varenicline (Chantix). Bupropion should be initiated only with patients who do not have seizure disorders. Dosing of 150 to 300 mg/day for 7 to 12 weeks is recommended. Varenicline should be uptitrated over 1 week to 1 mg BID, for 12 weeks, with a quit date 1 to 4 weeks after starting. Both drugs have FDA Black Box Warnings regarding "hostility, agitation, depressed mood, and suicidal thoughts or actions," which should be discussed as part of your risks/benefits/alternatives conversation with patients.

Marijuana Withdrawal

Marijuana withdrawal is not life-threatening, but like all withdrawal syndromes is uncomfortable for patients, and as with all substance-dependent presentations, cointoxicants should be suspected. Prolonged marijuana use is associated with the rare occurrence of cannabis hyperemesis syndrome; be alert for metabolic derangements if patients complain of recent nausea/vomiting or abdominal pain, which usually resolves with cessation of marijuana use.

Signs and Symptoms

1. Irritability, anger, or aggression
2. Nervousness or anxiety
3. Sleep difficulty (e.g., insomnia, disturbing dreams)
4. Decreased appetite or weight loss
5. Restlessness
6. Depressed mood
7. At least one of the following physical symptoms causing significant discomfort: abdominal pain, shakiness/tremors, sweating, fever, chills, or headache

Time course: Symptoms usually develop within 24 to 72 hours of decreased use. They are worst during the first 7 days and can last for weeks. Sleep disturbances in particular may last for months.

Treatment: There is no THC or cannabinoid replacement therapy; symptoms should be treated with prn sleep agents, loperamide, NSAIDs, and so on as indicated.

Synthetic Cannabinoid Receptor Agonist (K2, Spice, etc.) Withdrawal

SCRA withdrawal has yet to be systematically characterized, likely because of the relative recent emergence and popularity of the substance; however, there is some literature addressing its withdrawal toxidrome. Given the increasing prevalence in use, especially among young people, SCRA withdrawal should be considered in those patients reporting daily use multiple times per day, as serious withdrawal symptoms have been reported in these patients. However, the same symptoms have also been reported to be due to acute intoxication, and severe reactions are limited to single case reports in the literature at this time.

Signs and Symptoms

1. Behavioral: Anxiety, mood swings, irritability, agitation, insomnia
2. Somatic: Nausea, vomiting, loss of appetite, headache, chest pain, palpitations, dyspnea
3. Rare: Tachycardia, hypertension; 1 case report of seizure

Time course: Onset and severity of withdrawal symptoms seem to correspond with the amount of daily SCRA use. Based on the current available literature, anxiety, mood swings, nausea, and loss of appetite typically are the first withdrawal symptoms to appear, and often can occur within 1 to 2 hours of last use. Withdrawal symptoms seem to peak on day 2 (following discontinuation), remain present at a similar level for up to a weak, and then slowly begin to subside.

Treatment: In one study, inpatient admission for medically supervised withdrawal was recommended to greater than 50% of patients with problematic daily synthetic cannabinoid use ($n = 47$); however, only 20 enrolled and were followed in the study, limiting the generalizability of their recommendations. In that study, diazepam and quetiapine were used as needed to treat withdrawal symptoms in those patients admitted to the inpatient detoxification, with patients reporting that quetiapine was more effective in alleviating symptoms. In other case studies, phenobarbital has been used for seizure prophylaxis; clonidine as well as other medications for symptomatic treatment have also been used. Given the limitations of available literature and experience, symptomatic and supportive treatment is the most reasonable course.

Selective Serotonin Reuptake Inhibitor Discontinuation Syndrome

Discontinuation of a selective serotonin reuptake inhibitor (SSRI) with a short half-life (e.g., paroxetine) is more likely to precipitate withdrawal than an agent with a longer half-life (e.g., fluoxetine).

Signs and Symptoms

1. Nausea, vomiting, diarrhea, and abdominal pain
2. Malaise
3. Myalgias
4. Fatigue
5. Hot flashes and diaphoresis
6. Anxiety
7. Insomnia
8. Shocklike sensations
9. Vivid dreams

Less common symptoms may include movement disorders, such as akathisia and parkinsonism, or psychiatric symptoms, such as hypomania, mania, and panic attacks.

Immediate Steps

The treatment of antidepressant withdrawal, if severe, is to reinstitute the antidepressant and then taper the drug gradually. Fluoxetine may be used for a patient withdrawing from a short–half-life SSRI, because it will self-taper. Minor symptoms usually abate spontaneously.

Anticholinergic Drug Withdrawal
Signs and Symptoms

Withdrawal symptoms usually resemble those of influenza. Anticholinergic drugs may occasionally produce depressed mood, maniclike symptoms, or seizures when withdrawn abruptly. Reinstitution of the medication and gradual tapering are the mainstays of treatment.

Suggested Readings

American Psychiatric Association. Substance-related and addictive disorders. In: *Diagnostic and Statistical Manual of Mental Disorders.* 5th ed. Washington, DC: American Psychiatric Association; 2013.

Bernstein E, Bernstein JA, Weiner SG, D'Onofrio G. Substance use disorders. In: Tintinalli JE, Stapczynski J, Ma O, Yealy DM, Meckler GD, Cline DM, eds. *Tintinalli's Emergency Medicine: A Comprehensive*

Study Guide. 8th ed. New York, NY: McGraw-Hill; 2016. http://accessmedicine.mhmedical.com/content.aspx?bookid=1658&Sectionid=109448503. Accessed October 11, 2016.

Cooper ZD. Adverse effects of synthetic cannabinoids: management of acute toxicity and withdrawal. *Curr Psychiatry Rep.* 2016;18(5):52. https://doi.org/10.1007/s11920-016-0694-1.

Eisendrath SJ, Cole SA, Christensen JF, Gutnick D, Cole M, Feldman MD. Depression. In: Feldman MD, Christensen JF, Satterfield JM, eds. *Behavioral Medicine: A Guide for Clinical Practice.* 4th ed. New York, NY: McGraw-Hill; 2014. http://accessmedicine.mhmedical.com/content.aspx?bookid=1116&Sectionid=62688871. Accessed October 19, 2016.

Foy A, March S, Drinkwater V. Use of an objective clinical scale in the assessment and management of alcohol withdrawal in a large general hospital. *Alcohol Clin Exp Res.* 1988;12(3):360–364.

Kasper DL, Fauci AS, Hauser SL, Longo DL, Jameson J, Loscalzo J. Alcohol use disorder. In: Kasper DL, Fauci AS, Hauser SL, Longo DL, Jameson J, Loscalzo J, eds. *Harrison's Manual of Medicine.* 19th ed. New York, NY: McGraw-Hill; 2016. http://accessmedicine.mhmedical.com/content.aspx?bookid=1820&Sectionid=127560547. Accessed October 11, 2016.

Macfarlane V, Christie G. Synthetic cannabinoid withdrawal: a new demand on detoxification services. *Drug Alcohol Rev.* 2015;34:147–153.

Martin PR. Substance-related disorders. Chapter 15. In: Ebert MH, Loosen PT, Nurcombe B, Leckman JF, eds. *CURRENT Diagnosis & Treatment: Psychiatry.* 2nd ed. New York, NY: McGraw-Hill; 2008. http://accessmedicine.mhmedical.com/content.aspx?bookid=336&Sectionid=39717887. Accessed October 10, 2016.

Nacca N, Vatti D, Sullivan R, Sud P, Su M, Marraffa J. The synthetic cannabinoid withdrawal syndrome. *J Addict Med.* 2013;7:296–298.

Rigotti NA. Tobacco use. In: Feldman MD, Christensen JF, Satterfield JM, eds. *Behavioral Medicine: A Guide for Clinical Practice.* 4th ed. New York, NY: McGraw-Hill; 2014. http://accessmedicine.mhmedical.com/content.aspx?bookid=1116&Sectionid=62688534. Accessed October 17, 2016.

Rodgman CJ, Verrico CD, Worthy RB, Lewis EE. Inpatient detoxification from a synthetic cannabinoid and control of postdetoxification cravings with naltrexone. *Prim Care Companion CNS.* 2014;16:4.

Rustin T. Substance abuse. In: Lipsom Glick R, et al. eds. *Emergency Psychiatry: Principles and Practice.* Philadelphia, PA: Lippincott Williams and Wilkins; 2008.

Sampson CS, Bedy SM, Carlisle T. Withdrawal seizures seen in the setting of synthetic cannabinoid abuse. *Am J Emerg Med.* 2015;33:1712.e3.

Sullivan JT, Sykora K, Schneiderman J, Naranjo CA, Sellers EM. Assessment of alcohol withdrawal: the revised clinical institute withdrawal assessment for alcohol scale (CIWA-Ar). *Br J Addict.* 1989;84(11):1353–1357.

Sullivan S. Cannabinoid hyperemesis. *Can J Gastroenterol.* 2010;24(5):284–285.

Wesson DR, Ling W. The clinical opiate withdrawal scale (COWS). *J Psychoactive Drugs.* 2003;35(2):253–259.

Insomnia

Insomnia is often a symptom of another disorder. The key to treating insomnia is to search for the underlying cause. As with any consultation, each patient deserves a complete evaluation and appropriate treatment. It is tempting to quickly prescribe sedating medications for patients complaining of sleeplessness, especially if you are fatigued. Beware of medicating patients for insomnia, however, without first assessing them. This will avoid inappropriate treatment for those with hidden medical, psychiatric, or more serious sleep disorders.

Insomnia is the complaint of insufficient sleep associated with adverse daytime consequences such as anergy, malaise, cognitive slowness, and irritability. Insomnia is best understood as a symptom with numerous potential underlying causes. Mild transient sleep disturbance secondary to anxiety or physical discomfort is very common in hospitalized patients. If the patient has no compromise in daytime functioning, it is acceptable to monitor the insomnia and defer treatment with hypnotics.

PHONE CALL

Questions

1. Who is requesting help—the patient or the staff?
2. What is the patient's admission diagnosis, and when was he or she admitted to the hospital?
3. Is the patient also anxious, agitated, or acting strangely? Remember that a patient who is sleepless and agitated or acting bizarrely requires prompt evaluation to rule out an acute psychiatric illness or delirium.
4. Has the patient had complaints of insomnia previous to this hospitalization or this consultation? If so, what forms of treatment were suggested? Were these beneficial to the patient?
5. Has there been any recent change in the patient's clinical status or medications?

Orders

When the patient is well known to the staff, has no symptoms of acute medical or psychiatric distress, or has an established history of difficulty initiating or maintaining sleep and responded well to medication in the past, it is acceptable to consider renewing sleep medications over the phone. However, if this is a patient with a new complaint, an in-person assessment is important.

Inform RN

"Will arrive in … minutes."

REMEMBER

A patient who is sleepless and agitated or acting bizarrely requires prompt evaluation.

ELEVATOR THOUGHTS

What causes insomnia?

The etiology will often be readily identified by assessing the onset, duration, and nature of the patient's sleep complaint.

1. Environmental and behavioral factors
   a. Unpleasant or noisy sleep environment
   b. Situational anxiety
   c. Preoccupation with falling asleep
   d. Disrupted circadian rhythm (e.g., shift work or jet lag)
2. Psychiatric and neurologic disorders
   a. Affective disorders (e.g., depression or mania)
   b. Anxiety disorders (e.g., generalized anxiety disorder, obsessive-compulsive disorder, panic attacks, posttraumatic stress disorder, adjustment disorder with anxiety)
   c. Psychosis (e.g., intrusive hallucinations or paranoia)
   d. Akathisia
   e. Dementia
   f. Neurodegenerative disorders (e.g., Parkinson disease, Alzheimer disease)
3. Substance abuse and withdrawal symptoms
   a. Stimulant intoxication (including caffeine)
   b. Alcohol or sedative withdrawal
   c. Nicotine withdrawal
4. Medications (Box 21.1)
5. Related medical problems (Box 21.2)

BOX 21.1	Possible Iatrogenic Causes of Insomnia

Antiasthmatics: β2-agonists, theophylline
Anticonvulsants: Phenytoin, carbamazepine, valproic acid
Antidepressants: Phenelzine, tranylcypromine, protriptyline, desipramine, imip-ramine, amoxapine, selective serotonin reuptake inhibitors, tricyclic with-drawal, venlafaxine, bupropion
Antihypertensives: Beta blockers, methyldopa, diuretics, reserpine, clonidine
Antipsychotics: Phenothiazines, butyrophenones
Cimetidine
Decongestants: Pseudoephedrine, phenylephrine
Levodopa, baclofen, methysergide
Sedative-hypnotics (rebound insomnia), barbiturates, benzodiazepines, narcotics
Stimulants: amphetamines, methylphenidate, pemoline
Tetracycline
Thyroxine, steroids, birth control pills

BOX 21.2	Common Medical Causes of Insomnia

Neurologic Disorders
1. Stroke
   a. Increased incidence of obstructive sleep apnea, central sleep apnea, or periodic limb movement disorder
   b. Increased incidence of depression after stroke
2. Alzheimer disease—In later stages is associated with circadian rhythm disorder
3. Parkinson disease—Associated with parasomnias (e.g., rapid eye move-ment [REM] behavior disorder) and insomnia
4. Chronic pain—Produces difficulty in initiating and maintaining sleep

Cardiovascular Disease
1. Nocturnal angina pectoris
2. Congestive heart failure (CHF)
   a. Supine posture redistributes blood to the central circulatory system, worsening paroxysmal nocturnal dyspnea.
   b. CHF is accompanied by Cheyne-Stokes respiration, leading to repeated awakenings.
3. Hypertension—Insomnia may be caused by uncontrolled hypertension or may be secondary to use of antihypertensive medications.

Pulmonary Disease[a]
1. Chronic obstructive pulmonary disease (COPD)—Note: Nasal canula O_2 reduces sleep-onset latency, increases the duration of uninterrupted sleep, and improves nocturnal oxygen saturation in this population.
2. Obstructive sleep apnea (OSA)—Insomnia may be related to awakenings due to obstructed airway, or poor tolerance of or discomfort with continuous positive airway pressure (CPAP) treatment.
3. Asthma

Continued

| BOX 21.2 | Common Medical Causes of Insomnia—cont'd |

Gastrointestinal Disorders
1. Gastroesophageal reflux disease (GERD)—Symptoms can occur only during sleep or can significantly worsen during sleep.

Endocrine Disorders
1. Thyroid disorders
2. Diabetes mellitus—May be related to hyperglycemia, hypoglycemia, nocturia, or pain from peripheral neuropathy.
3. Perimenopause—Insomnia may respond to hormone replacement therapy.
4. Obesity

ª Drug therapies for COPD and asthma, including methylxanthines, oral beta-agonists, and oral glucocorticoids, can also cause insomnia.

MAJOR THREATS TO LIFE

Overmedication or inappropriate medication with sedatives
Unrecognized medical problem manifesting as insomnia
Undiagnosed obstructive or central sleep apnea syndrome

BEDSIDE

Remember that the primary task is to distinguish symptoms of benign sleeplessness from other conditions that require further evaluation and for which a sedating medication may be contraindicated (Box 21.3).

Quick Look Test

Is the patient in bed or wandering?
Does the patient look uncomfortable or anxious?
Does the patient seem manipulative or demanding?
Does the patient have tachycardia, hypertension, or fever?
Is there a trend in the patient's vital signs that would suggest another clinical concern (e.g., uncontrolled hypertension or withdrawal states)?

| BOX 21.3 | Contraindications to Sedative-Hypnotic Medications |

Concomitant use of alcohol or narcotics (potentiation)
Hepatic or respiratory failure
Delirium or confusion
Sleep apnea
Myasthenia gravis

Selective Chart Review

1. When and why was the patient admitted?

   Recently admitted patients may have difficulty sleeping owing to the new environment or to new medications. Alternatively, the patient may have an underlying chronic, unrecognized sleep disturbance.

   Patients who have been hospitalized for a while may develop disturbed circadian rhythms secondary to frequent daytime naps and disruptions from nighttime sleep (e.g., for vital sign measurements or blood work, or because of neighboring patients).

2. Is there a history of substance abuse?

   Sleep disturbance may be one of the first signs of intoxication with various substances (e.g., caffeine, cocaine, herbaceuticals) or, more importantly, acute withdrawal states from alcohol, benzodiazepines, or narcotics. Withdrawal states can become life-threatening.

   Recovering substance abusers may sleep poorly for months to years after cessation of drinking or illicit drug use. Heavy nicotine dependence often leads to a nighttime withdrawal syndrome of frequent awakenings to smoke cigarettes.

3. What are the patient's age, gender, and current medical/psychiatric status?

   Pay special attention to medical problems that may make the patient uncomfortable, especially those with associated pain. Elderly patients have a greater incidence of occult primary sleep disorders and a greater likelihood to have disturbed sleep secondary to multiple medications and other medical and psychiatric disorders.

4. Have there been sleep complaints in the past or were sleep disorders observed previously? If so, which treatments were attempted and which were successful?

Selective History

The sleep history should include a general characterization of the severity, duration, variability, and daytime consequences of sleep deprivation.

Common questions to ask include the following:

1. When did your insomnia begin?
2. Do you have difficulty in falling asleep, staying asleep, waking too early, or a combination? How long are you typically awake before falling asleep again?
3. It is also very important to look at the nursing record and speak with nursing staff about their observations of the patient at night. Many patients have the perception that they have not slept all night, despite being witnessed asleep for many hours.

| BOX 21.4 | Cognitive/Behavioral Approaches to Insomnia |

1. Limit electronic device usage 1–2 h prior to bedtime. Consider using "blue light" filters as a risk reduction strategy if patient refuses to limit electronics use.
2. Minimize interruptions and offer eye masks and/or earplugs if available.
3. Lie in bed only when attempting to sleep—this may be difficult to do in the hospital.
4. If unable to sleep, get out of bed and try sitting up and reading.
5. Use relaxation techniques to decrease anxiety:
   a. Progressive muscle relaxation
   b. Visualization
   c. Correct negative thoughts (e.g., "I didn't sleep last night, so I won't be able to sleep tonight.")
   d. Avoid catastrophic thoughts (e.g., "I'll die if I don't get a good night's sleep.")
   e. Insert positive thoughts

Behavioral interventions are often most appropriate in this case (Box 21.4).

Alternatively, anxiety, environmental noise, or physical discomfort (especially pain) can make it difficult to fall asleep. A variety of intrinsic sleep and psychiatric disorders can lead to problems in maintaining sleep at night. Remember to ask the patient what he or she perceives as the cause of the multiple awakenings. Also, ask about nightmares with early awakenings, restlessness, leg "kicking" or cramping in the limbs, and loud snoring with gasping or choking on awakening (collateral sources of information can be helpful with these questions).

4. Are you sleepy during the day? Do you nap?
   Remember that a diagnosis of insomnia includes daytime sleepiness and decreased perception of sleep at night. Does the patient complain of fatigue, difficulty in completing tasks, mood symptoms, irritability, or concentration problems?
5. Do you drink caffeine or alcohol? Do you use benzodiazepines or narcotics? Do you smoke cigarettes?
6. Do you have any other symptoms of psychiatric illness (e.g., depression, anxiety, obsessive-compulsive disorder, psychosis, dementia, or delirium)?

COMMON CAUSES OF INSOMNIA

Medical Problems

Some common medical problems that cause insomnia are listed in Boxes 21.2 and 21.3. Chronic insomnia may be a symptom of a

BOX 21.5	Psychiatric Causes of Insomnia

Anxiety disorders
Affective disorders
Dementia
Psychosis (neuroleptic-induced akathisia or night-day reversal in paranoid schizophrenics)
Substance intoxication (caffeine, stimulants, amphetamines, cocaine, "ecstasy")
Substance withdrawal (caffeine, alcohol, nicotine, benzodiazepines)

disease in virtually any organ or a side effect of medication. It is preferable to relieve the insomnia associated with a chronic medical condition by treating the underlying medical illness. Only when there is no accepted treatment for the primary medical condition or when treatment of the medical condition fails to alleviate the insomnia should the consultant treat the sleep symptom by itself.

Psychiatric Disorders

Psychiatric disorders are the leading cause of chronic insomnia (Box 21.5). Insomnia is a symptom of major depression, dysthymia, mania, and anxiety, but can also be a component of psychosis, dementia, and substance abuse or withdrawal.

Primary Sleep Disorders

Restless legs syndrome occurs during wakefulness and is a sensation of unpleasant pulling or drawing deep in the muscles of the lower extremities that worsens in the evening hours. Symptoms decrease with dopamine agonists (e.g., levodopa/carbidopa, pergolide) or bedtime doses of clonazepam.

Periodic limb movement disorder occurs during sleep and is movement of limbs that may be accompanied by electroencephalographic arousal, disturbing the continuity of sleep. Treatment is the same as for restless legs syndrome.

Obstructive sleep apnea involves repetitive closure of the upper airway during sleep, resulting in increased labor of breathing accompanied by multiple arousals from sleep. Loud snoring with choking or gasping occurs. Treatment is continuous positive airway pressure, use of a dental appliance, or upper airway surgery. Obstructive sleep apnea requires evaluation in a sleep laboratory or by an ear, nose, and throat specialist.

Central sleep apnea is characterized by a repetitive loss of respiratory drive, leading to a cyclic fluctuation in respiratory effort, electroencephalographic arousal, and disturbance of sleep continuity. Consultation should be assisted by a pulmonary specialist.

Poor Sleep Hygiene

Poor sleep hygiene insomnia results from sleep-incompatible behaviors just before or throughout bedtime. Such behaviors include exercising or eating close to bedtime, not allowing for "winding down" time before bedtime, and failing to protect the sleeping environment from adverse temperatures and avoidable sources of noise. In particular, electronic devices such as mobile phones, televisions, and tablets are known to interfere with sleep. As many hospitals permit access to these devices, a careful assessment of the patient's electronic usage can be extremely helpful in the assessment of insomnia.

MANAGEMENT

Successful treatment of insomnia requires alleviating nighttime complaints without compromising daytime functioning. Medication treatment of secondary insomnia should be evaluated on a case-by-case basis. Use of hypnotic agents should be recommended only after the primary cause has been evaluated. The ideal hypnotic would be completely absorbed, have minimal first-pass hepatic metabolism, be rapidly transferred from blood to brain, be completely metabolized by the end of sleep time, and be associated with minimal tolerance and dependence.

1. Evaluate, address, and treat the underlying causes of insomnia.
2. Evaluate and recommend changes in sleep hygiene (Box 21.6).
3. Recommend cognitive/behavioral approaches (see Box 21.4).
4. Evaluate the need for adjunct sedative-hypnotic medication (Box 21.7). Select a medicine that also treats the underlying axis I or II disorder.

BOX 21.6   Important Elements of Good Sleep Hygiene

Quiet, comfortable environment
No electronic devices 2 h prior to bedtime
No stimulants, alcohol, heavy meals, or vigorous exercise within 3–4 h before bedtime
Moderate exercise earlier than 4 h before bedtime
No daytime naps
Regular wake time
For hospital: out of bed when possible during daytime hours
Reinforce waking hours with exposure to light early in the day and physical activity if possible
Address life stressors and any obsessive concerns regarding ability to sleep

BOX 21.7   Adjunct Medication to Treat Insomnia

Benzodiazepines[a] (should be used at their lowest effective dose and only for acute complaints of insomnia)

Alprazolam (Xanax) 0.25–0.5 mg PO QHS ($t_{1/2} = 12$ h)

Lorazepam (Ativan) 0.5–2 mg PO QHS ($t_{1/2} = 10$–20 h)

Temazepam (Restoril) 7.5–30 mg PO QHS ($t_{1/2} = 8$–25 h)

Novel Benzodiazepine-Receptor Agonists[b]

Zolpidem tartrate (Ambien) 5–10 mg PO QHS ($t_{1/2} = 2.5$ h); women generally require lower doses.

Zaleplon (Sonata) 5–10 mg PO QHS ($t_{1/2} = 1$ h)

Sedating Antidepressants (indicated for depressed/anxious patients)

Trazodone (Desyrel) 25–150 mg PO QHS

Doxepin (Sinequan) 25–50 mg PO QHS

Mirtazapine (Remeron) 15–30 mg PO QHS; 15 mg is more sedating

Antihistamines[c]

Diphenhydramine hydrochloride (Benadryl) 25–50 mg PO QHS

Hydroxyzine hydrochloride (Atarax/Vistaril) 25–100 mg PO QHS

Sedating Antipsychotics[d] (indicated for patients with psychosis, mania, or cognitive impairment/sundowning)

Quetiapine (Seroquel) 25–50 mg PO QHS

Thioridazine (Mellaril) 10–50 mg PO QHS

Haloperidol (Haldol) 2–5 mg PO QHS (0.5–2 mg for sundowning)

Others

Gabapentin (Neurontin) 100 mg PO QHS

Melatonin 1 mg PO 2 h prior to bedtime

[a]Potential for recreational abuse, increased risk of falls, delayed reaction time, increased risk of machinery accidents, residual morning sedation, rebound insomnia, anterograde amnesia, tolerance, and dependence.

[b]Tolerance, dependence, and withdrawal syndromes unclear.

[c]Potential for morning sedation, dry mucous membranes, risk of anticholinergic delirium.

[d]Potential for inducing akathisia.

$t_{1/2} =$ half-life.

Headache

Headaches are a common complaint on a psychiatric service and may be a symptom of a serious medical condition or a manifestation of a psychiatric disorder such as anxiety or depression. Primarily, headaches have been classified into two categories depending upon the etiology: (1) primary headaches that are recurrent and chronic in nature, and (2) secondary headaches that result from a known central nervous system (CNS) pathology. The on-call resident should be able to evaluate the character of the headache, determine the seriousness of the patient's complaints, and institute appropriate neurologic consultation and timely treatment.

PHONE CALL

Questions

1. How severe is the headache?

    The severity of headache on a scale of 1 to 10 should be noted. Alternatively, the severity can also be judged from functional disabilities that the headaches might cause.

2. Was the onset sudden or gradual?

    In general, sudden onset headaches raise serious concerns, while gradual onset headaches are usually more benign in nature. A sudden onset headache reaching maximum intensity in less than 1 minute is considered to be a thunderclap headache and is a neurologic emergency that needs an urgent neurology consultation.

3. What are the current vital signs relative to the patient's baseline?

    Fever in the setting of headache is an ominous sign and may represent a CNS infection (e.g., meningitis, encephalitis, brain abscess), while significantly elevated blood pressure may indicate a vascular crisis (e.g., hypertensive emergency, stroke, intracranial hemorrhage).

4. Does the patient look sick, has there been a change in the level of consciousness, and are there concerning symptoms such as visual changes, nausea, or vomiting?

Altered mental status in the setting of a headache may point to ischemic/hemorrhagic stroke, hypertensive emergency, or subarachnoid hemorrhage (SAH). A migraine headache can present with visual auras and nausea; vomiting associated with a cluster headache, though lasting less than 3 hours, can be extremely painful and distressing.

5. Does the patient have a history of chronic or recurrent headaches?

It is important to ask for a history of prior headaches, as presentation with similar features can be diagnostic and could point to the fact that the symptoms are more benign. Alternatively, abrupt onset of new headache symptoms may warrant an urgent evaluation.

6. What is the patient's medical history?

The reason for hospitalization as well as the patient's medical comorbidities should be ascertained, as they may point to a probable cause for the patient's complaints. The presence of vascular risk factors can suggest stroke or hemorrhage, whereas a history of malingering or conversion disorder in the absence of objective findings may decrease suspicion of an acute process requiring urgent medical intervention.

7. What medications is the patient taking?

Certain medications (e.g., nitrates) and drug withdrawal syndromes (e.g., alcohol, nicotine) are known to cause headaches.

Orders

1. Ask the nurse for vital signs (e.g., blood pressure, heart rate, temperature) if they have not been recorded in the last 30 minutes.

2. If the headache is mild and you are confident that it represents recurrence of a previously diagnosed problem, it may be appropriate to prescribe a nonnarcotic analgesic (e.g., acetaminophen or ibuprofen). If you cannot see the patient immediately because of other emergencies, ask the nurse to call back in 1 to 2 hours if the headache has not been relieved by medication.

Inform RN

"Will arrive in…minutes."

If the patient's headache is associated with fever, vomiting, visual changes, or an altered mental status, or if he or she has a severe headache with an acute onset, you should see the patient immediately. An assessment at the bedside is also necessary if the headache is more severe than usual for the patient or if the character of the pain is different from usual.

ELEVATOR THOUGHTS

See Table 22.1.

TABLE 22.1	Headache Classification

Primary Headache Disorders

Common Causes	Less Common	Secondary/Symptomatic Headaches

1. Migraine
2. Tension HA
3. Cluster HA
	• Paroxysmal hemicrania
	• Hemicrania continua
	• Benign exertional HA
	• Benign cough HA
	• Headache associated with sexual activity
	• Short-lasting unilateral neuralgiform headaches syndrome
		1. Infections
		  a. Meningitis
		  b. Encephalitis
		  c. Sinusitis
		2. Posttraumatic
		  a. Concussion
		  b. Cerebral contusion
		  c. Subdural or epidural hematoma
		3. Vascular
		  a. Subarachnoid hemorrhage
		  b. Intraparenchymal hemorrhage
		  c. Cerebral infarction
		  d. Carotid or vertebral artery dissection
		4. Increased intracranial pressure
		  a. Space-occupying lesions
		  b. Malignant hypertension (hypertensive crisis)
		  c. Benign intracranial hypertension
		5. Decreased intracranial pressure
		  a. Spontaneous intracranial hypotension
		  b. Postlumbar puncture headache
		6. Drug exposure or withdrawal
		  a. Nitrates
		  b. Calcium channel blockers
		  c. Acquired immunodeficiency syndrome (AIDS) medications
		  d. Caffeine, nicotine, alcohol, or illicit drug withdrawal
		7. Local causes
		  a. Temporal arteritis
		  b. Acute angle-closure glaucoma
		  c. Referred pain from ear, eyes, jaw, and teeth

HA, Headache.

MAJOR THREAT TO LIFE

1. Subarachnoid hemorrhage is associated with a very high mortality rate if left untreated.
2. Bacterial meningitis must be recognized early if antibiotic therapy is to be successful.

3. Herniation (transtentorial, cerebellar, central) may occur as a result of a tumor, a subdural or epidural hematoma, or any other mass lesion.
4. Hypertensive crisis may result from sympathomimetic drugs or the interaction of monoamine oxidase inhibitors (MAOIs) and tyramine-containing foods, and requires immediate control of blood pressure (BP) to prevent serious consequences.

It is imperative to be cognizant of these conditions and order appropriate tests and neurologic and/or neurosurgical consultation. A noncontrast computed tomography (CT) scan of the head is the first important step in evaluation of these conditions. (Further evaluation and management is discussed under the "Management" section.)

BEDSIDE

Quick Look Test

Does the patient look well (comfortable), sick (uncomfortable), or critical?

- Most patients with chronic headache appear well. Those with severe migraines, subarachnoid hemorrhage, meningitis, or hypertensive crisis appear sick. Patients presenting with cluster headaches are restless and prefer to pace around rather than rest in bed.

Vital Signs

1. What is the patient's temperature?

    When a fever is associated with a headache, you must decide whether a lumbar puncture should be performed to rule out meningitis.
2. What is the patient's BP?

    A sudden and dramatic increase in BP associated with a severe occipital headache, stiff neck, sweating, nausea, and vomiting in a patient taking MAOIs signifies a hypertensive crisis. Malignant hypertension (hypertension with papilledema) is usually associated with a systolic BP > 190 mm Hg and a diastolic BP > 120 mm Hg. Headache usually does not occur as a symptom of hypertension unless there has been a recent increase in pressure. In this setting, hypertension may reflect subarachnoid hemorrhage, acute stroke, or increased intracranial pressure from an intracranial mass lesion.
3. What is the patient's heart rate?

    Hypertension association with bradycardia may be a manifestation of increasing intracranial pressure.

Selective History and Chart Review

1. Onset

    The abrupt onset of a severe headache suggests a vascular cause, the most serious being subarachnoid or intracerebral hemorrhage.

2. Severity

    Most tension (muscle contraction) headaches are not incapacitating. However, migraine headaches are associated with severe pain, and the patient might look quite sick. As previously discussed, thunderclap headaches require the utmost attention. Most common causes of a thunderclap headache are subarachnoid hemorrhage and reversible cerebral vasoconstriction syndrome.

3. Duration and progression

    Migraines and tension headaches can last days, whereas cluster headaches typically only last for a maximum of 3 hours. Primary headaches tend to be stable and recurrent in nature, whereas recent onset with progressive worsening could point to a secondary cause of headache such as subdural hematoma, subarachnoid hemorrhage, brain abscess, or tumor.

4. Diurnal variation

    Certain headaches such as cluster headaches, hypnic headaches, brain tumors, and occasionally migraines can wake the patient from sleep.

5. Position

    Most tension headaches are improved by lying down. Headaches that are worse in the supine position suggest increased intracranial pressure, and an intracranial mass should be considered. Orthostatic headaches that occur only in sitting/standing position and are relieved in supine positions occur in spontaneous intracranial hypotension from various different causes.

6. History of recent trauma

    An epidural hematoma may occur after even a relatively minor head injury, particularly in teenagers or young adults. Subdural hematomas can appear insidiously (6 to 8 weeks) after seemingly mild head trauma and are not uncommonly seen in the alcoholic patient.

7. History of procedures

    A lumbar puncture is often followed by a headache appearing several hours to 1 day after the procedure. The incidence is higher when a large-bore needle is used or if several punctures are performed. This type of headache is usually bifrontal or generalized and is worse when the patient sits upright. It is believed to be caused by intracranial hypotension resulting from cerebrospinal fluid loss, which results in displacement of pain-sensitive structures when the patient is upright. The patient may experience relief when lying flat (prone or supine).

8. Visual changes

Acute angle-closure glaucoma can be precipitated by pupillary dilatation. The patient commonly complains of a severe unilateral headache located over the brow, which may be accompanied by nausea, vomiting, and abdominal pain.

9. Prodromal symptoms

Nausea and vomiting are associated with increased intracranial pressure, but may also occur with migraines or angle-closure glaucoma. Photophobia and neck stiffness are associated with meningitis. Typical prodromal symptoms of a migraine include nausea, vomiting, photophobia, visual scotomata, geometric visual phenomena, and unilateral paresthesias; presence of these may be helpful in making the diagnosis.

10. MAOIs

Headache accompanied by a stiff neck, sweating, nausea, or vomiting in a patient taking MAOIs may signify a hypertensive crisis, secondary to the ingestion of tyramine-containing foods or various over-the-counter medications, and is a medical emergency requiring immediate pharmacologic intervention.

11. Other medications

Drugs such as nitrates, calcium channel blockers, and nonsteroidal antiinflammatory drugs can cause headaches.

12. History of caffeine, nicotine, alcohol, or other drug use

Acute withdrawal from any of these substances can cause headaches. Be aware of the heavy smoker who is placed in the hospital and acutely stops smoking.

13. Temporomandibular joint dysfunction

Patients who experience any clicking or popping when using or closing the jaw, grind their teeth at night, or wake with mandibular tension may be suffering from temporomandibular joint dysfunction. These patients may report pain predominantly in the ear or face.

14. Joint disease in the neck or upper back

Tension headaches in the elderly are often caused by cervical osteoarthritis. These headaches characteristically start in the neck and radiate to the temple or forehead.

15. History of chronic (recurrent) headaches

Migraine and tension headaches follow a pattern. It is important to ask the patient if this headache is the same as a "usual" headache.

16. Psychiatric diagnosis

Headaches and psychiatric disorders often coexist, so any patient with a primary headache disorder should be screened for psychiatric conditions. Several comorbidity studies have shown that underlying psychiatric conditions lead to worsening of severity, frequency, and treatment efficacy of migraine and tension headaches. Conversely, headaches can present as a part of underlying psychiatric syndromes such as somatoform and psychotic disorders (classified as "Headaches attributed to psychiatric disorder" in *The International Classification of Headache Disorders*, 3rd edition). Nonetheless, nonpsychiatric medical causes must always be ruled out before a psychiatric diagnosis can be made. For patients with a somatoform disorder, the complaint of headache should always be taken seriously, and your approach should be a supportive one.

Selective Physical Examination

1. Head, eyes, ears, nose, and throat
   a. Nuchal rigidity (meningitis or subarachnoid hemorrhage)
   b. Papilledema (increased intracranial pressure)
   c. Red eye (acute angle-closure glaucoma)
   d. Hemotympanum, or blood in the ear canal (basal skull fracture)
   e. Tender, enlarged temporal arteries (temporal arteritis)
   f. Retinal hemorrhages (hypertension)
   g. Lid ptosis, dilated pupil, eye deviated down and out (posterior communicating cerebral artery aneurysm)
   h. Tenderness on palpation, or failure of transillumination of the frontal and maxillary sinuses (sinusitis or subdural hematoma)
   i. Inability to fully open the jaw (temporomandibular joint dysfunction)
2. Neurologic
   a. Mental status changes and altered level of consciousness may accompany meningitis, intracranial hemorrhage, electrolyte and metabolic disturbances, or complicated alcohol withdrawal
   b. Drowsiness, yawning, and inattentiveness associated with a headache all are ominous signs and may be the only signs evident in a patient with a small subarachnoid hemorrhage
   c. Asymmetric pupils associated with rapidly decreasing level of consciousness can represent a life-threatening situation. Call for a neurosurgical consult immediately to assess for uncal herniation
   d. Asymmetry of pupils, visual fields, eye movements, limbs, tone, reflexes, or plantar responses suggests structural brain

disease. If this is a new finding, a computed tomographic scan or magnetic resonance imaging of the head is necessary.
   e. Kernig sign: passive flexion of the hip and knee, followed by pain or resistance on passive knee extension, indicates possible meningitis
   f. Brudzinski sign: pain with flexion of the hips or knees in response to passive neck flexion is present in both meningitis and subarachnoid hemorrhage; note that both Kernig and Brudzinski signs have very low sensitivity (5%), but high specificity, and therefore can be used to rule in meningitis as the correct diagnosis.
3. Musculoskeletal
   a. Palpate the skull and face looking for fractures, hematomas, and lacerations. Evidence of recent head trauma suggests the possibility of a subdural or epidural hematoma.

MANAGEMENT

Serious Conditions

1. Bacterial meningitis

   Meningitis should be suspected if there is a headache accompanied by fever, nuchal rigidity, Kernig or Brudzinski sign, and/or signs of cerebral dysfunction (confusion, delirium, or decreasing level of consciousness, ranging from lethargy to coma). Rigors/chills, profuse sweating, photophobia, weakness, nausea, vomiting, anorexia, and myalgias are also common findings. An immediate noncontrast CT scan and lumbar puncture are indicated. Consult the medicine service regarding antibiotics and further management of meningitis. Signs of increased intracranial pressure can develop later in the disease course and carry a grave prognosis. A subdural empyema or a brain abscess may cause nuchal rigidity and increased intracranial pressure. If there is any sign of increased intracranial pressure (papilledema, focal neurologic signs, or obtundation), a lumbar puncture is contraindicated because of the risk of brain herniation.

2. Space-occupying lesions and hemorrhages

   When a lumbar puncture is contraindicated, a CT scan will help identify an intracranial mass or any obstruction to cerebrospinal fluid outflow. Neurosurgery should be consulted immediately for any patients with a subdural, epidural, or subarachnoid hemorrhage or space-occupying lesion (brain abscess, tumor), causing raised intracranial pressure.

3. Hypertensive crisis/malignant hypertension

   Hypertensive crisis requires immediate reduction in BP by the administration of IV labetalol given as a 20 to 40 mg push, which may be repeated after 10 minutes. Alternatively, if the patient is awake and able to protect his airway, oral medications such as captopril 25 mg, labetalol 200 mg, or clonidine 0.1 mg can be used. Call for a medical consultation immediately, and consider transferring the patient to a medical service.

4. Glaucoma

A patient with acute angle-closure glaucoma should be referred to an ophthalmologist immediately.

Less Serious Conditions

1. Tension (muscle contraction) headaches

Chronic tension headaches may be symptomatically treated with nonnarcotic analgesics. This is the most common type of headache you will see in the hospital. Psychiatric patients are particularly susceptible to them, as they can be brought on by emotional stress and often occur in the context of anxiety and depressive disorders. A long-term treatment plan, if not already established, should be discussed with the treatment team.

2. Migraine headaches

Mild migraines can be treated adequately with aspirin or acetaminophen. More severe migraines will respond best if treatment is initiated during the prodromal stage; however, it is unlikely that you will be called until the headache is well established. Ask the patient what he or she usually takes for migraine headaches, because this will probably be the most effective agent for that patient. Common abortive therapies include sumatriptan 25 mg orally (repeated every 2 hours as needed, maximum 200 mg daily dose) or ergotamine/caffeine 1/100 mg 1 to 2 tablets at onset (repeated every 30 minutes as needed for maximum 6 mg/day, 10 mg/week). Refractory migraines, especially those accompanied by nausea and vomiting, may require intravenous hydration and antiemetics; consult the neurologic service as appropriate.

3. Cluster headaches

Cluster headaches are difficult to treat. Most resolve spontaneously within 45 minutes, and oral treatment has minimal effect. Many patients gain partial relief when administered oxygen by nasal canula or nonrebreather mask (100% FiO_2 at a flow rate of 12 to 15 L/min). If a severe cluster headache develops in the hospital, first-line therapy consists of subcutaneous or intranasal triptan (subcutaneous sumatriptan 6 mg, repeat at least 1 hour after first dose if needed), as long as triptans are not contraindicated (ischemic heart disease, peripheral vascular disease, uncontrolled hypertension, stroke). Intranasal lidocaine applied with a cotton swab can also be helpful, but is less well studied. When bridging patients to a preventive therapy such as verapamil, a steroid taper or dihydroergotamine 1 mg intravenously now and repeated in 1 hour may be effective for short-term relief.

4. Postconcussion headaches

Postconcussion headaches (provided that subdural and epidural hemorrhages have been ruled out) should be treated with an analgesic agent that is unlikely to cause sedation (e.g., acetaminophen, codeine). Aspirin or nonsteroidal antiinflammatory drugs are contraindicated for the posttrauma patient, because the inhibition of platelet aggregation may predispose the patient to bleeding complications.

5. Benign intracranial hypertension

Benign intracranial hypertension (pseudotumor cerebri) is a syndrome of unknown etiology, with increased intracranial pressure (headache and papilledema) and no evidence of a mass lesion or hydrocephalus. Refer the patient to a neurologist for further evaluation.

Suggested Readings

Cohen AS, Burns B, Goadsby PJ. High-flow oxygen for treatment of cluster headache: a randomized trial. *JAMA*. 2009;302(22):2451.

Law S, Derry S, Moore RA. Triptans for acute cluster headache. *Cochrane Database Syst Rev*. 2013;(7):CD008042.

Robbins MS, Starling AJ, Pringsheim TM, Becker WJ, Schwedt TJ. Treatment of Cluster Headache: The American Headache Society Evidence-Based Guidelines. *Headache*. 2016;56(7):1093–1106.

The International Classification of Headache Disorders, 3rd edition (beta version). Headache Classification Committee of the International Headache Society (IHS). *Cephalalgia*. 2013;33(9):629–808.

Chest Pain

Questions

1. What are the patient's vital signs? Have they changed?
2. Is the patient dyspneic, diaphoretic, or tachypneic?
3. When did the pain begin? How does the patient describe it? How does it relate to eating or position?
4. Does the patient have a history of cardiovascular disease (myocardial infarction [MI], coronary artery disease, angina), cardiac risk factors (e.g., hypertension, hyperlipidemia, smoker), gastroesophageal reflux, or peptic ulcer disease?
5. Has the patient had any recent surgery or procedures?
6. Has the patient used recreational drugs? Which drugs?

Orders

Assume that a serious medical condition (e.g., myocardial ischemia, MI, pulmonary embolism, aortic dissection) is the cause of the pain until proven otherwise. A good first rule is that all patients with chest pain should have an immediate electrocardiogram (EKG).

This creates a permanent record of cardiac activity at the time of pain that is useful for the following:

1. Assessing the heart's electrophysiologic status for ST segment, Q wave, and T wave changes and rhythm disturbances
2. Comparing with a prior EKG and assessing for change from baseline
3. Consulting with other physicians (e.g., a cardiologist) who might be called in later

A nurse or EKG tech should be asked to do an EKG while you are on your way to the ward. If no one is available, ask to have the machine set up and ready for your arrival to begin the assessment rapidly.

It is usually best to evaluate the patient personally before ordering medications. A patient with a known history of angina or other cardiac disease or who has been treated with nitroglycerin in the past may be given 0.4 mg sublingual nitroglycerin every 5 minutes up to three times before your arrival (hold for systolic blood pressure <90 mm Hg). With the goal of preventing further possible coronary artery thrombus formation, you may consider having the patient chew and swallow one 325 mg aspirin tablet.

If the patient is reported as dyspneic or has had recent chest surgery, trauma, or invasive procedure (chest tube, pleural tap), consider ordering a stat portable chest x-ray (CXR) to check for pneumothorax, mediastinal widening (occasionally seen in ruptured aortic aneurysm), or other pathology.

If a patient is febrile, the CXR may show signs of pneumonia.

Inform RN

"Will arrive in … minutes."

Get to the patient as quickly as possible! Try to have the EKG started or at least set up for your arrival; it will save valuable time in the event of a true medical emergency. Remember that complaints of chest pain need to be evaluated without delay. Although patients on psychiatric wards are typically more stable medically, some also have comorbid medical illnesses that might be missed.

ELEVATOR THOUGHTS
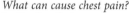

What can cause chest pain?
1. Cardiac factors
    a. Angina
    b. MI
    c. Aortic dissection
    d. Pericarditis
2. Pulmonary factors
    a. Pulmonary embolism
    b. Pneumothorax
    c. Pneumonia with pleuritis
3. Gastrointestinal factors
    a. Gastroesophageal reflux or esophageal spasm
    b. Peptic ulcer disease
    c. Cholelithiasis, cholecystitis
4. Musculoskeletal factors
    a. Costochondritis
    b. Rib fracture
    c. Muscle spasm
5. Skin factors
    a. Herpes zoster

6. Psychiatric factors
   a. Anxiety disorders
   b. Somatoform disorders
   c. Factitious disorder
   d. Substance-related disorders (e.g., amphetamine or cocaine intoxication/withdrawal)

LIFE-THREATENING CAUSES

MI or myocardial ischemia
Aortic dissection
Pulmonary embolus
Pneumothorax

Each of these represents a major threat to life and must be diagnosed and managed quickly. In general, psychiatric wards are not ideally suited to manage or monitor medical emergencies. Although you may feel confident in your abilities to manage medical issues, these situations can get out of hand quickly and should be managed by those with more experience who will be caring for the patient should he or she need to be transferred off the psychiatric ward.

If the situation appears likely to be one of those listed, get the medical consultant, cardiology consultant, or cardiac care unit team involved right away. They will usually appreciate being involved early in the management and can be very helpful in facilitating transfer to the appropriate setting. Always evaluate the patient personally before calling the consultants. You will be better able to report the details of the situation that they will want to know.

BEDSIDE

Quick Look Test

Does the patient look: well (comfortable, resting), sick (uncomfortable or distressed), or critically ill (about to die)?

The overall appearance of the patient can usually provide important clues to the severity of a problem. Calm, conversant, and relatively comfortable-appearing patients are less likely to have a life-threatening cause of their chest pain. Patients with chest pain resulting from myocardial ischemia or MI usually appear pale, anxious, and diaphoretic. However, the ultimate assessment can only be made after a thorough history and physical examination. A patient in the midst of a panic attack can appear just as ill as one suffering from an acute infarction. On the other end of the spectrum, a patient with autonomic sensory neuropathy—that is, someone with advanced diabetes—might report vague or even no pain during a severe MI. There is no substitute for getting a thorough history from the patient and an EKG.

Airway and Vital Signs

What is the patient's blood pressure?

Most patients who complain of chest pain will be normotensive. Hypotension can occur with MI, cardiogenic shock, pulmonary embolism, and tension pneumothorax. Hypertension may occur in the anxious patient with chest pain and in the patient with cocaine/amphetamine intoxication. Severe hypertension (systolic blood pressure >180 mm Hg, diastolic blood pressure >110 mm Hg) should be treated, because it can worsen myocardial ischemia and aortic dissection.

What is the patient's heart rate?

Sinus tachycardia can occur with chest pain of any origin. If the heart rate is greater than 100 beats per minute, life-endangering tachydysrhythmias, such as ventricular tachycardia or atrial fibrillation, should be considered as medical emergencies. Immediate intervention, such as cardioversion, may be required.

Does the patient have bradycardia?

Although bradycardia can indicate myocardial ischemia or MI, in particular an inferior wall MI, unless it is dangerously slow, it often may not require immediate treatment but should be monitored closely.

What is the patient's breathing pattern and quality?

A rapid respiratory rate can occur with any type of chest pain. It is important to remember that tachypnea may be a result of hypoxemia, which may result from myocardial ischemia or MI. Tachypnea also commonly accompanies panic attacks.

Painful breathing (dyspnea) most often indicates a pleural or musculoskeletal cause (pleuritis, pneumothorax, costochondritis, rib fracture).

Mental Status Examination

Does the patient have signs of depression or anxiety?

You should perform an abbreviated mental status examination to identify conditions that should be treated urgently. An anxious patient may appear extremely agitated and frightened and have other somatic complaints besides chest pain. A patient having a panic attack will probably respond to a fast-acting benzodiazepine. Similarly, a patient with somatic complaints may be very depressed. A depressed patient with somatic complaints may often describe a depressed mood, have a constricted range of affect, and admit to suicidal ideation, possibly requiring one-to-one observation.

One useful mnemonic for exploring the causes of chest pain is "PQRST":

P—What is the position/location of the pain?

Q—What is the quality of the pain (sharp, dull, ripping, tearing, pressing, squeezing, other)?

R—Does the pain radiate to other locations (left arm, jaw, back, other)?

S—How does the patient rate the severity of the pain (on a scale of 1 to 10)?

T—What is the time course of the pain (sudden onset, intermittent, constant, other)?

1. *How does the patient describe the quality of the pain? Has the patient experienced the same kind of pain before?*
   Crushing, squeezing, viselike pain or pressure is how MI is typically described. Severe tearing or ripping pain may indicate aortic dissection. Often patients who have had prior cardiac incidents will be able to tell you how this pain compares to their previous episode.

2. *Does the pain radiate?*
   Radiation to the back may indicate peptic ulcer disease or aortic dissection. MI typically radiates to the jaw, neck, and internal aspect of the left arm. Localized pain is often seen with rib fracture, costochondritis, or trauma. A dermatomic distribution is classic for herpes zoster. Diffuse pain is nonspecific and could be an indication of somatization disorder or panic.

3. *Does the pain change with deep breathing or coughing?*
   Pain that changes may be pleuritic and suggests pleuritis, fracture, costochondritis, pneumonia, pericarditis, pulmonary embolism, or pneumothorax.

1. Vital signs
   a. Repeat
2. Respiratory
   a. Crackles (pneumonia; congestive heart failure, which may be secondary to MI; pulmonary embolism)
   b. Decreased breath sounds (consolidation, pleural effusion)
   c. Absence of breath sounds (pneumothorax)
3. Cardiovascular
   a. Murmurs, gallops, rubs (MI, pericarditis, congestive heart failure)
   b. Jugular venous distension (tension pneumothorax, congestive heart failure with right-sided heart failure, pulmonary embolus with right-sided strain/overload, pericardial effusion)

4. Abdominal
   a. Tenderness, guarding, or rebound (peptic ulcer disease with or without perforation, cholecystitis)
5. Skin
   a. Rash in dermatomic distribution (herpes zoster)
6. Musculoskeletal
   a. Tenderness reproducible on palpation (costochondritis, rib fracture, trauma)

MANAGEMENT

For suspected myocardial ischemia or infarction: The patient should be given 325 mg aspirin to chew and sublingual nitroglycerin 0.4 mg separated by 5 minutes up to three times, making sure not to cause a drop in systolic blood pressure below 90 mm Hg. Call the medical consultant, cardiology consultant, or cardiac care unit team right away to get them involved early so that the patient can be transferred to and managed in the appropriate setting. You are responsible for the care of the patient until the transfer of care is complete. You should attempt to stabilize the patient and start the appropriate medical work-up while awaiting transfer or arrival of the medical team.

Stabilizing the patient for transfer should include the following:
1. Monitoring vital signs
2. Performing serial EKGs
3. Obtaining routine laboratory tests (complete blood count, blood chemistries, troponin, creatine kinase with MB fraction, prothrombin, and partial thromboplastin times)
4. Getting a CXR
5. Gaining IV access with the largest-gauge needle possible
6. Starting oxygen at 2 to 4 L/min or as recommended by the medical consult
7. Pain control: You may consider intravenous morphine sulfate 2 mg intravenous every 5 to 10 minutes until pain subsides or side effects occur (nausea, respiratory depression, hypotension) to calm the patient and decrease the stress on the heart.

Pulmonary embolism: Include portable CXR film and measure arterial blood gas while awaiting transfer to medicine.

Pneumonia: Include portable CXR film and send sputum and blood for culture and sensitivity tests. If the patient is in respiratory distress, administer oxygen after getting recommendations on rate of delivery from the medical consult.

Gastroesophageal reflux disease: If you feel confident that gastroesophageal reflux disease is the correct diagnosis, the patient can be managed on the psychiatric unit without urgent medical attention and may be treated initially with an antacid such as aluminum hydroxide 30 mL orally. Elevation of the head may be helpful. Suggest a gastrointestinal consultation for the next day. Perform an EKG. It will not harm the patient and may show unexpected results.

Peptic ulcer disease: Antacids may be given, but they might not offer the patient much relief. Suggest a gastrointestinal consultation for the next day.

Costochondritis: Costochondritis can be treated with nonsteroidal antiinflammatory drugs such as ibuprofen 600 mg orally (maximum of 3200 mg per day) every 6 to 8 hours, if not contraindicated secondary to other medical conditions (e.g., in a patient who is taking an anticoagulant or has peptic ulcer disease).

Herpes zoster: Initially the patient with herpes zoster may require pain treatment with nonsteroidal antiinflammatory drugs or even narcotics, if not contraindicated. Suggest an infectious disease consult for the next day.

Psychiatric: For any suspected psychiatric etiology, the first step is always a thorough psychiatric interview. Simple reassurance and support are often helpful for patients with panic attack, somatization disorders, or depression. If the patient remains anxious, treatment with a fast-acting benzodiazepine such as lorazepam 1 to 2 mg by mouth or intramuscularly may be initiated. It may be repeated every 2 hours with a maximum dose of 10 mg in 24 hours.

Cocaine or amphetamine intoxication: The patient with chest pain secondary to substance intoxication could be experiencing myocardial ischemia or even MI. Cocaine and amphetamines can cause life-threatening arrhythmias, and an urgent medical consultation is indicated. Proceed with cardiac work-up and management.

Suggested Readings

Boie ET. Initial evaluation of chest pain. *Emerg Med Clin North Am.* 2005;23:937–957.

Huffman JC, Pollack MH, Stern TA. Panic disorder and chest pain: mechanisms, morbidity, and management. *Prim Care Companion J Clin Psychiatry.* 2002;4(2):54–62.

Ringstrom E, Freedman J. Approach to undifferentiated chest pain in the emergency department: a review of recent medical literature and published practice guidelines. *Mt Sinai J Med.* 2006;73(2):499–505.

Nausea and Vomiting

Background

Nausea is a subjective sensation of gastric discomfort resulting in aversion to oral intake. This is associated with the behavioral drive to remove the noxious ingestant by vomiting. These two related symptoms are relatively nonspecific and can arise from a variety of causes, including primary gastrointestinal disease, central nervous system disorders, endocrine and metabolic disorders, systemic illness, disorders of the thorax, as well as adverse reactions to medications (e.g., theophylline, digoxin, valproic acid, selective serotonin reuptake inhibitors, opiates, dopamine agonists). Pregnancy should always be ruled out in premenopausal women.

PHYSIOLOGY

Diverse central and peripheral inputs converge downstream on the act of vomiting. The solitary nucleus (located in the midbrain's tegmentum) integrates afferent impulses arising in the gastrointestinal (GI) tract, vagal and sympathetic pathways, the diencephalon/limbic system (emotional stimuli), and the vestibular system. The solitary nucleus also interacts with the chemoreceptor trigger zone of the area postrema, which is located in the floor of the fourth ventricle. The area postrema is a circumventricular organ characterized by absence of the blood–brain barrier, permitting direct communication with humoral factors. Hence it is affected by many drugs, as well as metabolic abnormalities such as acidosis and uremia. The vomiting center, which is composed of several motor nuclei located in the lateral reticular formation of the medulla, generates stereotyped efferent impulses in response to these stimuli.

Vomiting is usually preceded by nausea. Nausea is associated with reduced gastric tone and increased duodenal tone, allowing backward movement of duodenal contents into the stomach. Retching follows the sensation of nausea, during which deep inspiratory movements against a closed glottis decreases thoracic pressure and raises abdominal pressure, creating a favorable pressure gradient for retrograde movement of gastric contents into the esophagus. The final act of vomiting results from sustained contractions of the muscles of the abdominal wall, retrograde contractions of the stomach and duodenum, and simultaneous relaxation of the lower esophageal sphincter.

It is important to distinguish between vomiting and regurgitation, which is unaccompanied by nausea, retching, or straining; usually occurs within minutes of eating; and tastes like the food eaten. Rumination syndrome is distinguished by daily effortless regurgitation and is most common in cognitively impaired children, although it has been identified in normal adults.

PRESENTATION AND DIFFERENTIAL DIAGNOSIS

Nausea and vomiting are usually associated with other phenomena; taking note of the overall clinical context helps one identify the underlying disease process. Tachycardia is common, often caused by volume depletion (particularly if diarrhea and/or GI bleeding are also present) and poor oral intake, as well as emotional distress and discomfort. Hypersalivation and diarrhea may also occur (the control centers in the medulla for these phenomena are near the vomiting center). Certain characteristics of vomiting—its amount, duration, content, and relationship to meals—are helpful in suggesting its cause and differentiating it from regurgitation.

Abrupt onset of symptoms can point toward obstruction, an infectious process, medication/drug effects, food poisoning, or a new intracranial process, whereas gradual onset or a pattern of recurrence suggests subacute/chronic diagnoses such as gastroesophageal reflux disease (GERD), gastroparesis, migraine headache, or worsening toxic metabolic state. Vomiting of psychogenic origin (as in anorexia nervosa, bulimia, or certain psychotic or delusional states) occurs often just after or during meals and is characteristic in that the patient usually manages to avoid vomiting in a public place. Early morning vomiting is a feature of anxiety states but can also occur in pregnancy, alcoholism, and uremia. Intestinal obstruction induces copious vomiting with bile present; the vomitus may also have a fecal odor. Vomiting of undigested food eaten several hours up to a day earlier suggests delayed gastric emptying. This could be the result of gastric outlet obstruction or motor disturbance of the stomach, such as that which occurs in diabetes, scleroderma, or hypokalemia. Acute onset of vomiting associated with fever, myalgias, arthralgias, fatigue, diarrhea, or other features of viral illness suggests a viral gastroenteritis or, if symptoms have become chronic, viral gastroparesis.

Certain intoxication and withdrawal syndromes can present with nausea and vomiting. Acute alcohol/opioid intoxication and withdrawal, marijuana withdrawal, stimulant (amphetamine/cocaine) intoxication, sedative/hypnotic withdrawal, and caffeine withdrawal are known to variably cause these symptoms.

The nature of the vomitus can provide information about the cause. In obstructive vomiting, the presence of bile indicates that obstruction is distal to the pylorus. Blood in the vomitus occurs only in esophageal, gastric, or duodenal disease and may represent an inflammatory or malignant process. In patients with alcohol abuse or dependence, bleeding from esophageal varices should be considered the cause of bloody vomitus until it can be ruled out by endoscopy. Prolonged vomiting of any cause may produce a tear in the lower esophageal or gastric fundal mucosa, which may bleed profusely (Mallory-Weiss syndrome).

Major categories of disorders associated with vomiting are outlined in Box 24.1.

Of these clinical entities, intracranial processes, acute intraabdominal processes, severe systemic infections, and toxic metabolic disorders demand immediate attention.

BOX 24.1   Disorders Associated With Vomiting

Gastrointestinal/Intraabdominal
- Acute gastroenteritis
- Gastroparesis
- Gastric outlet obstruction
- Small/large bowel obstruction
- Gastroesophageal reflux disease
- Gastritis/peptic ulcer disease
- Cholecystitis/cholangitis
- Acute pancreatitis
- Spontaneous bacterial peritonitis
- Mesenteric ischemia

Toxic or Metabolic Disorders
- Toxin/drug-induced or withdrawal states (e.g., alcohol, narcotics, digitalis glycosides, food-borne toxins)
- Uremia
- Acidosis/ketosis
- Electrolyte abnormalities (e.g., hypercalcemia)
- Pregnancy (estrogens)
- Adrenal/thyroid/parathyroid disorders

Infectious
- Viral infections
- Sepsis
- Pyelonephritis

Psychogenic
- Anorexia nervosa/bulimia

Continued

BOX 24.1	Disorders Associated With Vomiting—cont'd

- Anxiety
- Conversion disorder

Neurologic
- Increased intracranial pressure (trauma, stroke, meningitis, malignant hypertension, mass lesion)
- Vertigo/motion sickness
- Seizure disorders
- Migraine

Renal
- Renal colic

Cardiopulmonary
- Myocardial infarction
- Posttussive vomiting

Cyclic Vomiting of Childhood
Acute Glaucoma

Adapted from Table 84.1, Clinical Methods: The History, Physical, and Laboratory Examinations 3rd Ed; Table 1, Scorza et al.

PHONE CALL

Questions

1. When was the patient admitted?
2. When did the nausea and vomiting start? Did nausea precede the vomiting?
3. What is the nature of the emesis (e.g., hematemesis or bright red blood, darker blood with clots, brown "coffee grounds" emesis, bilious, feculent odor, undigested food)?
4. What is the amount of emesis (volume and frequency)?
5. What are the associated vital signs (e.g., fever, tachycardia, hypotension)?
6. What are the associated signs and symptoms (e.g., abdominal, chest, back, pelvic, or rectal pain; diarrhea; constipation; fever; myalgias/arthralgias; relation to nausea)?
7. What are the patient's diagnoses and comorbid conditions (history of abdominal or pelvic surgery, cardiac disease)?
8. Which medications is the patient taking?
9. Is there any history of substance abuse or toxic ingestion?
10. How does the patient look now (e.g., moribund, distressed, resting quietly)?

Orders

If the patient is hypotensive and/or has signs of end-organ dysfunction (e.g., altered mental status, decreased urine output, elevated serum troponin, or ischemic changes on electrocardiogram [EKG]), have an intravenous unit set up with a large-bore short catheter (at least 18 G or 16 G) ready for insertion. Give a bolus of isotonic 0.9% normal saline or lactated Ringer's solution, adjusting the volume for the patient's comorbidities.

If the emesis is bloody or large volume, order an 18 French nasogastric tube, as well as an intermittent suction device (e.g., Gomco machine) and irrigation set to the bedside if these are not installed in the patient's room. Tell the nurse to save the vomitus for your inspection.

Inform RN

"Will arrive in … minutes."

Significant alterations in vital signs, pain, or large amounts of hematemesis necessitate seeing the patient as soon as possible.

ELEVATOR THOUGHTS

1. Is the patient vomiting? If so, how much?
2. What is the content of the vomitus? Does it contain blood?
3. Is there an association with eating?
4. Is the patient pregnant?
5. What are the potential causes of vomiting?
   a. GI disease
   b. Central nervous system (CNS) disorders
   c. Endocrine and metabolic disorders
   d. Systemic illness
   e. Side effect of medications

MANAGEMENT

Serious intraabdominal processes that may present with vomiting include the following:
- Gastric outlet obstruction
- Intestinal obstruction
- GI inflammation
- Perforation of a viscus
- Peritonitis
- Pancreatitis
- Intraabdominal or pelvic abscess

Almost all of these disorders will present with nausea, vomiting, and associated signs and symptoms. Most ominous are peritoneal signs (e.g., lack of bowel sounds, abdominal distension, diffuse tenderness, abdominal wall rigidity with involuntary guarding), which indicate that a surgical consultation should be obtained emergently.

Emergent intracranial processes that are associated with vomiting generally do so by causing increased intracranial pressure.

These include closed head injuries, acute bleeding, cerebral edema (e.g., acute hyponatremia, tumor or infection with vasogenic edema, large ischemic stroke with cytotoxic edema), hydrocephalus, and meningitis. The patient should be evaluated for change in mental status or evolving neurologic deficits. Any change in neurologic status will require neurologic consultation.

In many instances, however, nausea and vomiting are drug-induced. In psychiatric patients, nausea and vomiting may be the result of pharmacotherapy or toxicity. For example, lithium toxicity and selective serotonin reuptake inhibitor pharmacotherapy (as well as therapy with other psychotropic drugs) can cause nausea and vomiting. Anticholinergic agents may cause vomiting by inhibiting motor activity and causing partial gastric outlet obstruction. See Table 24.1 for rates of nausea and vomiting associated with common psychotropic medications. If there is concern for toxicity with an unknown medication or substance, order

TABLE 24.1	Average Rates of Side Effect Nausea and Vomiting in Commonly Prescribed Psychotropic Medications[a]		
Drug Class	Medication	Rate of Nausea Up to ( ) %	Rate of Vomiting Up to ( )%	Dose-Dependent Relationship?
Antidepressants	Mirtazapine	1.5	—	—
	Bupropion SR	18	4	√
	Bupropion XL	18	4	√
	Venlafaxine	58	6	√
	Duloxetine	23	3	—
	Desvenlafaxine	41	9	√
	Levomilnacipran	17	5	—
	Vortioxetine	32	6	—
SSRIs	Escitalopram	15	—	—
	Sertraline	25	4	—
	Citalopram	21	4	—
	Paroxetine CR	22	2	√
	Fluoxetine	29	3	—
Mood stabilizers	Lamotrigine	19	9	√
	Valproate	22	12	—
Atypical antipsychotics	Olanzapine	9	—	At doses >15 mg
	Ziprasidone	12	—	√
	Aripiprazole	15	11	—

SSRIs, Selective serotonin reuptake inhibitors.
[a]Information summarized from package inserts, accessed at www.accessdata.fda.gov, April 4, 2017.

serum osmolality and levels of common offending agents and known home medications, obtain an EKG, and consult with toxicology, emergency medicine, and critical care as needed for direction on medical stabilization, GI decontamination, and antidote administration.

For any patient who has prolonged or severe vomiting, the initial management should include intravenous hydration, intermittent nasogastric suction, determination of baseline laboratory values including complete blood count, electrolytes, liver function tests, arterial blood gases, serum drug levels (for patients taking lithium, valproic acid, or digoxin), glucose, and lactate, and initiation of a search for etiology. These management protocols are outside the scope of psychiatry and require the appropriate medical, surgical, or neurologic consultation.

A note of caution regarding the pharmacotherapy of vomiting is warranted. The use of prokinetic, antiemetic, or antinausea agents, such as metoclopramide, hydroxyzine, or prochlorperazine, should be avoided until the etiology of the vomiting is determined. Abdominal pain should not be aggressively treated with narcotics or nonsteroidal antiinflammatory drugs until medical evaluation and appropriate consultations have been completed, as pain may be an important marker of the progression of many serious intraabdominal processes; moreover, inappropriate use of pain medication can worsen underlying disease (e.g., narcotics in ileus, nonsteroidal anti-inflammatory drugs [NSAIDs] in upper GI bleed).

Suggested Readings

American Gastroenterological Association. Medical position statement: nausea and vomiting. *Gastroenterology*. 2001;120:261–263.

Gastrointestinal motility. Barrett KE, Barman SM, Boitano S, Brooks HL, eds. *Ganong's Review of Medical Physiology*. 25th ed New York: McGraw-Hill; 2016.

Horn CC. Why is the neurobiology of nausea and vomiting so important? *Appetite*. 2008;50(2–3):430–434.

Maule WF. Nausea and vomiting. In: Walker HK, Hall WD, Hurst JW, Boston, eds. *Clinical Methods: The History, Physical, and Laboratory Examinations*. 3rd ed. Boston: Butterworths; 1990 chap 84, pp. 437–438.

Sadock B, Kaplan H, Sadock V. Substance-related disorders. In: *Kaplan & Sadock's Synopsis of Psychiatry: Behavioral Sciences/Clinical Psychiatry*. 10th ed. Philadelphia: Lippincott Williams & Williams; 2007. chap 12, pp. 381–466.

Scorza K, Williams A, Phillips JD, Shaw J. Evaluation of nausea and vomiting. *Am Fam Physician*. 2007;76(1):76–84.

Williams N, DeBattista C. Psychiatric disorders. In: Papadakis MA, McPhee SJ, Rabow MW, eds. *Current Medical Diagnosis & Treatment 2017*. 56th ed. New York: McGraw-Hill; 2017 chap 25.

Fever

Extreme changes in body temperature in psychiatric inpatients should be a cause for concern. Depending on the working diagnosis and initial treatment, fever can be an early sign of an impending disease process, with accompanying morbidity and mortality. Even temperature elevations that are not extreme, including those to about 100.4°F (38.0°C), warrant timely evaluation. In any patient on antipsychotic medication with an unrevealing fever work-up and without obvious sign of infection, always consider the possibility of neuroleptic malignant syndrome (NMS), serotonin syndrome, or malignant catatonia.

PHONE CALL

Questions

1. How does the patient look (nurse's estimate of the patient's condition)?
2. What is the temperature, and how was it taken (e.g., orally or rectally)?
3. When was the temperature taken?
4. What are the other vital signs, and were these repeated?
5. What are the associated symptoms and signs (if any)?
6. What has been the trend in the patient's temperature over the past 24 to 48 hours?
7. When was the patient admitted?
8. What is the admission diagnosis?
9. What comorbid medical or surgical conditions exist in this patient? Have there been any recent medical or surgical procedures (e.g., blood transfusion or bronchoscopy)?
10. What is the patient's substance use history? Are results available from a urine drug screen done during this admission?
11. Is the patient taking an antipsychotic? If so, for how long?
12. What other medications is the patient taking?
13. Has the patient's intake or output of fluids changed in any way?

Orders

1. If other vital signs were not taken, take them now.
2. If the patient is hypotensive with fever, order an intravenous setup and give a fluid bolus of 500 mL–1000 mL of normal saline solution or lactated Ringer's. If the patient is hemodynamically unstable, call the medical consult immediately.
3. If the patient has symptoms and signs of meningitis (nuchal rigidity, mental status changes, photophobia), consider ordering a lumbar puncture (LP) tray to the ward or enlisting the help of the neurology consult service.
4. Routine laboratory studies drawn during a fever work-up include blood cultures (aerobic and anaerobic bottles), complete blood count, urinalysis with culture and sensitivity, and if focal signs and symptoms indicate, sputum stain and culture and stool culture. A posteroanterior/lateral chest x-ray film should also be considered.

Inform RN

"Will arrive in … minutes."

The possibility of septic shock, meningitis, pulmonary embolism (PE), delirium tremens, alcohol/benzodiazepine/barbiturate withdrawal, NMS, serotonin syndrome, malignant catatonia, or anti-N-methyl-D-aspartate (anti-NMDA) receptor encephalitis demands that you see the patient immediately.

ELEVATOR THOUGHTS

What are causes of fever and change in temperature in psychiatric patients?

1. Infection: bacterial, viral, parasitic, fungal (e.g., urinary tract infection in an elderly patient, right upper or middle lobe pneumonia in a patient with a history of alcohol abuse, aspiration of excess saliva from clozapine therapy, an infectious agent in an immunocompromised patient, or infection or abscess in a patient who has had a recent surgical or dental procedure)
2. Drug-induced fever (e.g., NMS, serotonin syndrome, medication side effect):
    - For NMS, is the patient on an antipsychotic medication? Although rare, clozapine can also cause transient increases in temperature above 100.4°F (38.0°C) that are generally benign and self-limited. Peak incidence of clozapine-associated fever occurs within 3 weeks of initiating therapy and rarely requires discontinuation of treatment.
    - For serotonin syndrome, is the patient taking L-tryptophan, monoamine oxidase inhibitor (MAOI), amphetamine, selective serotonin reuptake inhibitor (SSRI), buspirone,

tricyclic antidepressant (TCA), serotonin-norepinephrine reuptake inhibitor (SNRI), bupropion, or linezolid?

- Is the patient on anticonvulsants? Carbamazepine and phenytoin are common causes of drug-induced fever.
- Drug-induced fever often begins 5 to 6 days after the drug is initiated and is sometimes accompanied by lymphadenopathy mimicking an infectious mononucleosis. After discontinuations of the drug, these symptoms may take 2 to 6 weeks to abate.

3. PE
4. Deep vein thrombosis
5. Substance withdrawal: namely alcohol, benzodiazepine, or barbiturate withdrawal (as these withdrawal syndromes are potentially lethal)
6. Paraneoplastic syndromes
7. Autoimmune or connective tissue disease; note that a normal erythrocyte sedimentation rate may point toward a noninflammatory process, although not always
8. Postoperative/postprocedure fever (atelectasis, urinary tract infection, wound infections, deep venous thrombosis, PE)
9. Malignant catatonia: catatonia plus triad of (1) severe rigidity, (2) autonomic nervous instability, and (3) altered mental status

MAJOR THREAT TO LIFE

PE
Alcohol withdrawal
Alcohol-related delirium tremens
Benzodiazepine withdrawal
Barbiturate withdrawal
Septic shock
Meningitis
Encephalitis (viral, anti-NMDA receptor, etc.)
NMS
Serotonin syndrome
Malignant catatonia

BEDSIDE

Quick Look Test

Is the patient resting comfortably, sick, distressed, agitated, apprehensive, lethargic, stuporous, catatonic, or comatose?

Airway, Breathing, Circulation, and Vital Signs

1. Airway: Can the patient maintain his or her airway? Are accessory muscles of respiration in use? Is there stridor?

2. Breathing: What are the respiratory rate and quality? Is there evidence of hypoxia (e.g., cyanosis, increased respiratory rate)? If you have evidence of cardiopulmonary arrest or suspect that one is imminent, have the nurse call a cardiac arrest code and get the arrest cart to the bedside. Initiate advanced cardiac life-support protocols.
3. Heart rate: Often the febrile patient is tachycardic; expect a rise in the pulse rate of 10 beats/min with each degree Fahrenheit (or 16 beats for each degree Celsius) increase in temperature.
4. Blood pressure: Hypotension and fever (or a decrease in body temperature) can be indicative of septic shock. Assess the patient's volume status and initiate intravenous fluid challenge (e.g., 500 mL bolus of lactated Ringer's or normal saline solution) via a large-bore peripheral intravenous catheter. Call for a medical consultation, because this probably warrants transfer to a medical ward.
5. Circulation: In addition to assessing the pulse rate and blood pressure, one can determine circulatory status by assessing the skin color, capillary refill, and sensorium.

There are two stages in the development of septic shock. Warm shock occurs first. Increased cardiac output and peripheral vasodilation cause the skin to be warm, dry, and flushed. The second stage is the development of cold shock, in which the patient becomes hypotensive and peripheral vasoconstriction occurs, leaving the skin cool and clammy. Changes in sensorium ranging from lethargy to agitation can occur with fever, particularly in the elderly. If a specific cause for fever is not obvious, consider an LP to rule out meningitis.

Selective Physical Examination I

Keep in mind volume status, signs and symptoms of septic shock, and signs and symptoms of meningitis.

1. Vital signs: Repeat. Check skin for turgor, temperature, color, and moisture.
   - Look for signs of the autonomic hyperactivity associated with substance withdrawal (increase in pulse rate, blood pressure, and temperature, and sweating, tremors, and tongue fasciculations).
   - Look for signs of autonomic instability associated with NMS (blood pressure fluctuations, irregular respiration, cardiac arrhythmia) or serotonin syndrome (tachycardia, diaphoresis with normal skin color) or malignant catatonia.
2. Head, eyes, ears, nose, and throat: Evaluate the tongue, oral mucous membranes, and conjunctivae for moisture.
   - Look for photophobia and neck stiffness associated with meningitis.

- Examine pupils: Dilated pupils, ocular clonus (slow lateral eye movements), can be associated with serotonin syndrome.
3. Respiratory function: Note the rate and quality. Is there any respiratory distress? Assess lung fields for crackles, wheezes, or decreased breath sounds.
4. Cardiac function: Note the pulse rate. Assess the pulse volume, and check the distal capillary refill.
5. Abdomen: Note any tenderness.
6. Neurologic: Assess for acute changes in mental status (agitation, lethargy, catatonia).
   - Look for rigidity associated with NMS or malignant catatonia. Assess for hyperreflexia, inducible clonus, myoclonus, spontaneous clonus, and increased muscle tone (lower limbs > upper limbs) associated with serotonin syndrome.
7. Special maneuvers: Assess the patient for Brudzinski sign and Kernig sign (each is suggestive of meningeal irritation).

MANAGEMENT

Initial Management

Major life-threatening situations include the following:
1. PE: Depending on the size and location of the embolus, the patient's outcome can range from a mild cough with fever to immediate death. You should have a suspicion of PE in patients who are restrained for prolonged periods of time, are bedridden for medical or surgical reasons, or have a history of deep venous thrombosis or hypercoagulable states. Localizing signs and symptoms include shortness of breath, cough, chest pain, hemoptysis, crackles or a friction rub on auscultation, dullness to percussion, egophony and bronchophony, whispered pectoriloquy, Westermark's sign on chest x-ray, and characteristic changes on electrocardiogram. A medical consultation should be called, because the patient will probably require anticoagulation medication (unless contraindications exist) and further radiologic tests.
2. Alcohol/benzodiazepine/barbiturate withdrawal: Please see Chapter 20.
3. Delirium tremens: Please see Chapter 20.
4. Septic shock: Volume-resuscitate aggressively but use caution with patients who have a history of heart failure. While resuscitation is in progress, measure prothrombin and partial thromboplastin times, fibrinogen, fibrin split products, electrolytes, blood urea nitrogen, creatinine, glucose, serum alanine transaminase, serum aspartate transaminase, gamma-glutamyltransferase, alkaline phosphatase, amylase, total and direct bilirubin, lactate

dehydrogenase, creatine phosphokinase (CPK), and procalcitonin. Order a complete blood count with differential count (T-cell profiles in immunocompromised patients). Obtain aerobic and anaerobic blood culture specimens from two separate sites. Obtain urine for urinalysis with microscopic urinalysis, and urine for Gram stain and culture. Obtain sputum for Gram stain and culture, including tests for acid-fast bacilli. Measure arterial blood gas to determine the base deficit. (The greater the deficit, the more profound or prolonged the shock.) A patient in septic shock will most likely be transferred to a medical intensive care unit or a surgical intensive care unit if this has occurred after a surgical procedure. The patient will need broad-spectrum antibiotics and will require intensive monitoring. Other intensive care unit supportive measures may be needed, including intubation and ventilatory support.

5. Meningitis: Perform an ophthalmic examination to rule out papilledema (increased intracranial pressure) and a complete neurologic examination. If meningitis is suspected, a neurologic consultation should be requested. An LP with measurement of cerebrospinal fluid pressures and collection of cerebrospinal fluid for appropriate studies (glucose, protein, cell count with differential, Gram stain, culture) should be performed as quickly as possible. A computed tomography (CT) scan of the head is usually necessary before LP is done to help rule out a mass lesion with increased intracranial pressure and possible herniation. Discuss with neurology or medicine whether IV antibiotics can be deferred until head CT and LP are done. They may need to be started urgently. In addition, blood cultures and laboratory tests, as outlined for septic shock, should be obtained. Fever, headache, seizure, stiff neck, or changes in sensorium should be considered evidence of meningitis until proven otherwise. The appropriate neurologic or medical consultant should be contacted to evaluate the patient. Collection of cerebrospinal fluid should be done as rapidly as possible, unless the patient has a coagulopathy, papilledema is present, or focal neurologic signs exist, which are highly suspicious for the presence of a mass lesion. Inform the consultant of these facts. Again, you may elect to begin intravenous antibiotics empirically and obtain an immediate noncontrast head CT (if available) to rule out any space-occupying lesions.

6. Neuroleptic malignant syndrome/serotonin syndrome/malignant catatonia: CPK level, blood urea nitrogen (BUN) and creatinine levels, basic electrolytes, lactate (to evaluate for metabolic acidosis), complete blood count (CBC), urine, or serum drug screen.

7. Encephalitis or meningitis: If there is a clinical suspicion (comorbid viral infection, sudden change in functioning),

we recommend a thorough neurologic work-up—which may include serum cerebrospinal fluid (CSF) cell count, Gram stain, culture, MRI/non-contrast head computed tomography (NCHCT), and appropriate antibody serologies—and a neurology consult. Of note, anti-NMDA receptor encephalitis, while rare, has appeared in the medical literature as an encephalitic process often associated with children and young adults; this can be especially important, as primary psychiatric disorders often occur at the same age.

Selective Chart Review

If the patient does not have one of the previously discussed causes for fever, do a selective chart review, looking for localizing clues from the following:

Admission history and physical examination

Process of medical clearance to psychiatry (e.g., what was done, what was recommended, what is pending, consultations, tests)

Current medications (e.g., steroids, antipyretics, antibiotics, antipsychotics)

Allergies

Substance use history (when the patient last used a substance)

Recent laboratory values

Temperature trends during hospitalization

Evidence of immunodeficiency (e.g., human immunodeficiency virus infection, acquired immunodeficiency syndrome, cancer chemotherapy, malignancy)

Other reasons for fever (e.g., autoimmune disease, neoplasm, drug fever, substance withdrawal, infections acquired in recent travel)

Selective Physical Examination II

Search to confirm localizing symptoms and signs that may exist as suggested by the chart review:

1. Vital signs: repeat now (rectal temperature, if possible)
2. Head, eyes, ears, nose, and throat:
   Fundi: papilledema (intracranial abscess), Roth's spots (infective endocarditis)
   Conjunctiva: scleral petechiae (infective endocarditis)
   Ears: erythematous tympanic membrane (otitis media)
   Sinuses: tenderness, inability to transilluminate (sinusitis)
   Oral cavity: dental caries and abscess
   Pharynx: erythema, exudate (pharyngitis, thrush, tonsillar abscess)
   Neck: meningeal signs, lymphadenopathy
3. Chest: crackles, friction rub, egophony, bronchophony, other signs of consolidation (pneumonia, PE)
4. Cor: new murmurs (infective endocarditis), pericardial friction rub (pericarditis)

5. Abdomen and back: localized tenderness, guarding, rebound costovertebral angle tenderness (pyelonephritis)
6. Rectal: tenderness or mass (perirectal abscess)
7. Pelvic: tenderness or mass (pelvic inflammatory disease, cervicitis)
8. Extremities: calf swelling and tenderness, Homan's sign (deep venous thrombosis), joint tenderness, swelling, erythema, effusion (septic joint)
9. Skin: Examine thoroughly, including IV sites and any surgical wound, for possible tenderness or rash. Look for rubor, dolor, calor, tumor, pressure sores (infection and abscess), petechiae, Osler's nodes, Janeway lesions (bacterial endocarditis).

Subsequent Management

Any patient with an unexplained rectal temperature of 100.4°F (38.0°C) or greater needs the following:

1. Aerobic and anaerobic blood cultures from two separate sites
2. Urinalysis (with microscopy) and urine culture
3. White blood count and differential
4. Other more selective tests, depending on localizing clues elicited from your chart review, history, and physical examination, such as the following:
   a. Throat swabs for Gram stain and culture
   b. Sputum for Gram stain, acid-fast bacilli stain, and cultures
   c. Chest x-ray
   d. LP
   e. Special-protocol blood cultures (e.g., acid-fast bacilli, fungal)
   f. Swabs for Gram stain and aerobic and anaerobic cultures from all sites that appear infected or are drawing fluid
   g. Studies for parasites and other infectious agents
   h. Obtain CPK level (will be elevated in NMS, serotonin syndrome, or malignant catatonia but also can be elevated in other conditions)

Once the data acquisition and initial fever work-up have begun, appropriate consultation with the medical, neurologic, or surgical services should be obtained to determine the appropriate antibiotic therapy and management of the patient. Although the majority of fevers are self-limited, they do increase oxygen demand and can exacerbate cardiopulmonary illness or cause mental status changes. Unless the patient has a contraindication to specific treatment, symptomatic treatment is generally recommended.

Although aspirin and nonsteroidal antiinflammatory drugs are effective antipyretics, acetaminophen is commonly preferred because it has limited gastrointestinal side effects and should be considered first line in children to avoid any increased risk of

Reye's syndrome. For severe hyperthermia, consider additional use of cooling blankets or tepid sponge baths.

Keep in mind which patients will need broad-spectrum antibiotics immediately:

1. The patient with fever and hypotension
2. The patient with fever and neutropenia ($<1000/mm^3$) or other signs and symptoms or history of immunocompromise
3. The patient who is febrile and appears acutely ill or toxic

The following types of patients need specific antibiotics immediately:

1. The patient with fever and meningeal signs and symptoms
2. The patient with fever and clear localizing signs and symptoms

NMS: discontinue all antipsychotics; supportive care (intravenous fluids); external cooling (ice packs); antipyretics; consider prophylactic intubation in patients with swallowing dysfunction, excessive salivation, coma, acidosis, hyperthermia with severe rigidity

Serotonin syndrome: discontinue all offending medications; supportive care (intravenous fluids); hyperthermia should be aggressively managed with IV hydration, external cooling (ice packs), and benzodiazepines; if temperature is $>41°C$ patient should be intubated with induced neuromuscular paralysis

- Of note, there is limited utility in administering traditional antipyretics since the mechanism of serotonin syndrome is related to muscle tone rather than central thermoregulation.
- If possible, physical restraints should be avoided as they can increase hyperthermia, lactic acidosis, and rhabdomyolysis.
- Dantrolene is generally not recommended.

Malignant catatonia: high-dose benzodiazepines are typically first line, but if no improvement, electroconvulsive therapy (ECT) should be strongly considered (prior to the accepted use of ECT, most patients with malignant catatonia died)

- Antipsychotics (particularly first-generation/typical antipsychotics) should be avoided, as they can worsen catatonia and precipitate NMS.
- Interestingly, NMS and serotonin syndrome are often considered to be iatrogenic subtypes of malignant catatonia secondary to the use of psychiatric medications.

REMEMBER

With any serious change in the status of a patient, inform the patient's attending physician and never hesitate to ask for help from the appropriate attending or consulting service.

Seizures

Seizures are clinical manifestations of an excessive, abnormal electrical discharge of neurons. A seizure can be an isolated event or part of a group of disorders ("the epilepsies") characterized by chronic, recurrent seizures. In the latter case, there may be either an absence of apparent provoking factors or evidence of remote neurologic injury that predisposes recurrence. In the United States an estimated 10% of people experience a seizure in their lifetime, whereas there is a 3% incidence of epilepsy. The physician on call should be able to correctly identify, manage, and give an accurate account of the observed seizure phenomena to the primary clinician or neurologic consultant.

PHONE CALL

Questions

1. Has the seizure stopped? If not, how long has the seizure lasted?

   The patient is in status epilepticus (SE) if the seizure lasts longer than 30 minutes or if the patient has multiple seizures without regaining consciousness. Assume a patient is in status until the history is clarified. Once a seizure lasts greater than 5 minutes, it is unlikely to stop spontaneously without medical intervention. Approximately 50% of patients in status will not have a history of seizures.

2. What is the patient's current level of consciousness?

   Assess if the patient is still actively seizing, postictal, or in any respiratory distress. This includes determining if the patient can maintain an adequate airway.

3. Did someone witness the seizure? If so, ask for a specific description.

   Specifically, ask about the moments prior to the seizure, symmetry of movements, which limbs were involved, was the head turned a specific direction, did either arm become dystonic, was the face involved, did the eyes deviate to one side or the face twitch, was there a gaze preference or blank staring, and were there automatisms? Was there a tongue bite during seizure? Did the patient lose bowel or bladder control? Finally, what was the duration of the seizure?

4. What are the patient's age, sex, diagnosis, and medication profile?

If the patient was on antiepileptic medication, was the medication lowered or changed? Get a stat level and try to maintain it at the upper limit of therapeutic range. Although a level may be checked on any antiepileptic medication, most institutions are only able to check older medications (i.e., phenytoin, carbamazepine, valproate, phenobarbital) without sending it out to a specialized laboratory.

5. What are the patient's vital signs? Does the patient have a fever? Is the blood pressure elevated?

Elevated heart rate (sinus rhythm), dilated pupils, and elevated blood pressure are commonly seen with tonic-clonic seizures because of initial sympathetic discharge.

6. If the patient is female, is she pregnant?

If so, how many weeks? Although more than 90% of pregnant women with seizures have normal vaginal delivery, there is an increased risk of fetal hypoxia, preeclampsia, bleeding, preterm birth, placental abruption, and miscarriage. Furthermore, organogenesis occurs at 5 to 12 weeks' gestation. Mothers who take antiepileptic drugs (see Tables 26.1 and 26.2) during this time have an increased incidence of major and minor malformations and growth retardation. Fear of medication effects on the fetus is often a source of noncompliance in pregnant women.

7. Does the patient have a history of seizures?

If so, when was the last seizure and what medications did the patient respond to? Did the patient ever have an allergic reaction to any prior antiepileptics?

8. Are there any obvious injuries?

Be prepared to do a thorough physical examination to look for signs of any musculoskeletal injury. Shoulder dislocations, head trauma, and lacerations are relatively common complications of tonic-clonic seizures.

9. Are there are any allergies?

Orders

1. Move the patient into the lateral decubitus position to avoid aspiration. Have suction available at the bedside. Lower the bed to the lowest level and put the side rails up with padding. Take special care with head and neck injuries.

2. Have available the following:
   An airway setup
   Intravenous (IV) setup: two large-bore IV lines and 0.9% normal saline

TABLE 26.1		Antiepileptic Drugs: Indications According to Seizure Type, Food and Drug Administration Monotherapy Approval, and Selected Comments		
Medication	**Brand Name**	**Indication**	**FDA Monotherapy Approval**	**Comments**
Carbamazepine	Tegretol	P, G	Yes	For partial seizures: many Rx interactions, P-450, black box warnings for blood dyscrasias and serious dermatologic reaction, increased risk with HLA-B*1502 (Asian descent). Hyponatremia.
Ethosuximide	Zarontin	G	Yes	For absence seizures; may worsen mixed absence.
Gabapentin	Neurontin	P		Renal excretion, minimal Rx interactions, taper slowly (1 week).
Lamotrigine	Lamictal	P, G		Stevens-Johnson syndrome (SJS) <0.4% of adults.
Levetiracetam	Keppra	P		Renal excretion, minimal Rx interactions.
Oxcarbazepine	Trileptil	P	Yes	Minimal Rx interactions, hyponatremia.
Phenobarbital	Barbital	P, G	Yes	Blood dyscrasias, gum swelling, SJS.
Topiramate	Topamax	P, G		At >400 mg/day, cognitive deficits; weight loss, kidney stones.
Valproic Acid	Depakote	P, G	Yes	For GTC, ME, JME; weight gain, hair loss.
Zonisamide	Zonegran	P		Weight loss, hyponatremia, contraindicated in sulfonamide allergies.

FDA, Food and Drug Administration; G, generalized; GTC, generalized tonic-clonic seizures; JME, juvenile myoclonic epilepsy; MC, myoclonic seizures; ME, myoclonic epilepsy; P, partial.

TABLE 26.2 Antiepileptic Drugs: Dosages, Therapeutic Levels, and Additional Comments

Medication	Brand Name	Starting Dose	Titration	Maintenance Dose	Do Not Exceed	Therapeutic Level (mcg/mL)	Labs to Monitor
Carbamazepine	Tegretol	400 mg/day either bid (tablets, extended-release) or qid (liquid)	Increase by up to 200 mg/day at weekly intervals	800 to 1200 mg/day	1600 mg/day	4–12	CBC w/diff, BMP, Fe, Lipids, LFTs, TFTs, UA, b-HCG
Ethosuximide	Zarontin	500 mg/day	Increase by ≤250 mg every 4–7 days, as needed	Individualized	1500 mg/day	40–100	CBC, LFTs
Gabapentin	Neurontin	300 mg tid	Increase based on response and tolerability	900–1800 mg/day given tid	2400 mg/day	4–20	Monitor levels of other AEDs. If adding gabapentin to AED, do so slowly
Lamotrigine	Lamictal	Depends: if added to other AEDs, start at 50 mg daily for 2 weeks, if no other AEDs 25 mg daily. If VPA on board then 25 mg every other day.		Individualized		2–20	LFTs, renal function
Levetiracetam	Keppra	500 mg q12	May increase by 500 mg/dose every 2 weeks	Individualized	1500 mg q12	12–46	Adjust for renal insufficiency

Continued

TABLE 26.2   Antiepileptic Drugs: Dosages, Therapeutic Levels, and Additional Comments—cont'd

Medication	Brand Name	Starting Dose	Titration	Maintenance Dose	Do Not Exceed	Therapeutic Level (mcg/mL)	Labs to Monitor
Oxcarbazepine	Trileptil	300 mg bid	Increase dose by 300 mg daily every 3rd day	600–1200 mg bid	2400 mg/day	8–35	Serum Na in first 3 months especially
Phenobarbital	Barbital	1–3 mg/kg/day or 30–60 mg/day	Give maintenance dose 12 hours after loading	1–2.5 mg/kg/day (s. conc 15–40 mg/L)		20–40	CBC w/diff, LFTs, renal function
Phenytoin	Dilantin	5–7 mg/kg/day or 200–400 mg/day	Give maintenance dose 24 hours after loading	6–8 mg/kg/day based on s. conc of 10–20 mg/L (free phenytoin levels 1–2 mg/L)		10–20	CBC, LFTs, plasma phenytoin
Topiramate	Topamax	25 mg/day	Increase 25–50 mg/day every week	400 mg/day	800 mg/day	20–50	Monitor HCO_3 levels at baseline and periodically
Valproic Acid	Depakote	10–15 mg/kg per day given bid or tid	Increase 5–10 mg/kg per day every week	1000 mg q12	60 mg/kg per day	50–100	CBC, LFTs, serum ammonia with somnolence
Zonisamide	Zonegran	100 mg/day	Increase by 200 mg/day after 2 weeks	300–400 mg/day given bid or tid	400 mg/day	20–40	BUN, Cr, HCO_3

bid, Twice a day; *IV,* intravenous; *PO,* orally; *qd,* daily; *tid,* three times a day.

Lorazepam: 4 mg IV at 2 mg/min should be administered initially, and the dose should be repeated if patient continues to seize after 2 minutes. Patient should be loaded with a nonbenzodiazepine antiseizure medication after this step to maintain seizure control. If unable to get IV access, IM midazolam 10 mg is an alternative until further access is established.

Apparatus for blood collection. Routine labs including basic metabolic panel (BMP), liver function tests (LFTs), magnesium (Mg), and ionized calcium should be sent.

3. If the patient is postictal, remove any dentures and suction the oropharynx.
4. Do a bedside glucose test.
5. Ask someone to stay with the patient.
6. Advise nursing personnel not to restrain the patient. Restraining postictal patients increases agitation and the risk of violence.

Inform RN

"I will arrive in ... minutes."

Note: A patient who is experiencing a seizure must be seen immediately.

ELEVATOR THOUGHTS

Was the attack truly a seizure?

Any paroxysmal event that transiently alters neurologic function can be mistaken for an epileptic seizure. The differential diagnosis includes the following:

1. Cardiac arrhythmias, vasovagal syncope, and postural hypotension can produce loss of consciousness and result in brief generalized tonic or clonic movements if cerebral hypoxia is prolonged. A syncopal loss of consciousness tends to be briefer and recovery tends to be quicker without prolonged confusion and disorientation. Syncope often presents with a loss of consciousness after a patient is frightened suddenly, has a Valsalva maneuver such as a laugh or cough, or is exposed to an extremely hot, crowded environment.
2. Complicated migraine can present as an acute confusional state resembling complex partial SE.
3. Transient ischemic attacks may be manifested as brief, repetitive, stereotyped sensory or motor deficits, amnesia, or aphasia. However, most seizures present as "positive" phenomena as opposed to deficits.
4. Transient global amnesia can produce sudden confusion and acute loss of newly formed memory. Cognitive functions and language remain intact, and these attacks occur rarely and tend not to recur. They are more common in elderly patients.

5. Sleep disorders include narcolepsy, cataplexy (may mimic an atonic seizure), and parasomnias (sleepwalking, night terrors).

6. Movement disorders include tics, Tourette's syndrome, myoclonus, and choreoathetosis.

7. Nonepileptic or psychogenic seizure (hysterical seizures or pseudoseizures) is suggested by concurrent emotional outbursts (e.g., crying), body posturing, opisthotonus, pelvic thrusting, and completely asynchronous thrashing of limbs. However, many of these symptoms may also be seen with frontal lobe seizures. Lack of facial involvement is a sensitive sign for nonepileptic seizures. Nonepileptic seizures are most common in patients with a history of sexual, physical, or substance abuse; personality disorder; or other psychiatric illness. Approximately 10% to 40% of patients may also have coexisting epilepsy, and video electroencephalogram monitoring may be required to make the diagnosis.

Urgent Issues to Consider

Be aware that a minority of seizures may result in sudden death. About 30% to 60% of status patients will have residual cerebral injury as a result of excitotoxicity and hypoxia. Patients may also develop aspiration pneumonia from depressed mental status due to ongoing seizures and sedative effects of medications. Renal failure may occur as a result of rhabdomyolysis. Direct injury from the clonic phase of seizures may result in compression fractures, especially of the thoracic spine, rib fractures, and shoulder dislocation. The rapid response team should be alerted if there is a concern of SE or hemodynamic instability.

What Kind of Seizure Was It?

From The International League against Epilepsy 2010 Revised Classification of Epileptic Seizures:

I. Focal (partial) seizures
   A. Focal seizures with awareness (replaces the term "simple partial seizures")
      1. With motor symptoms
      2. With somatosensory or special sensory symptoms (simple hallucinations, tingling, light flashing, buzzing)
      3. With autonomic symptoms or signs (e.g., epigastric sensation, pallor, sweating, flushing, piloerection, pupillary dilation)
      4. With psychic symptoms (disturbances of higher cerebral function—e.g., déjà vu, jamais vu, fear, distortion of time perception)
      Note: Auras, sensations such as epigastric rising or fear, are a type of simple partial seizure that may immediately precede complex partial and some generalized seizures.

B. Focal seizures without awareness (replaces the term "Complex partial seizures")

C. Focal seizures evolving in to bilaterally convulsive seizures
   1. Tonic
   2. Clonic
   3. Tonic-clonic
   Note: Focal seizures can be localized by the symptoms patients experience. Auditory hallucinations are likely to be associated with a temporal lobe focus, olfactory hallucinations with the orbitofrontal region, visual auras with occipital lobe area, and somatosensory sensations of sinking or choking with parietal lobe regions. Frontal lobe seizures may result in complex motor automatisms involving boxinglike movements of the arms, bicycling of the legs, and speech arrest.

II. Generalized seizures (convulsive or nonconvulsive)
   A. Absence seizures (petit mal): impairment of consciousness alone or with mild clonic, atonic, or tonic components and automatisms
      1. Absence
      2. Atypical absence
      Note: Absence seizures, in contrast to complex partial seizures, tend to last seconds (often patients pause in the middle of a sentence during an absence seizure and complete the sentence when they regain consciousness), do not have a postictal phase, and are not preceded by auras.
   B. Myoclonic
   C. Clonic
   D. Tonic
   E. Tonic-clonic
   F. Atonic seizures

What Caused the Seizure? (Useful Mnemonic—VITAMINNS)

V. VASCULAR

Stroke (ischemic or hemorrhagic), vasculitis, arteriovenous malformation, hypertensive encephalopathy, preeclampsia.

I. INFECTIOUS

Meningitis, encephalitis, central nervous system (CNS) abscess, CNS granuloma, HIV.

T. TRAUMA

Subdural/epidural hematoma, subarachnoid hemorrhage, intraparenchymal contusion.

A. AUTOIMMUNE

Systemic lupus erythematosus (SLE), CNS vasculitis, multiple sclerosis, serum sickness.

M. METABOLIC/TOXIC

Hypo/hyperglycemia, hypo/hypernatremia, hypocalcemia, hypomagnesemia, hypoxia, hypercapnia, azotemia, uremia, carbon monoxide (CO) intox, etoh, intoxication/withdrawal, benzodiazepine (BDZ), barbiturate and baclofen withdrawal, cocaine, phencyclidine (PCP), amphetamine intoxication, and subtherapeutic anti-epileptic drug (AED) levels.

I. IDIOPATHIC/IATROGENIC

Idiopathic epilepsy, febrile seizures, or medications, as below:
a. Lidocaine
b. Antibiotics, such as fluoroquinolones, isoniazid, metronidazole, penicillins, cephalosporins
c. Tricyclic antidepressants
d. Other antidepressants, such as bupropion, maprotiline, trazodone
e. Antipsychotics, especially clozapine
f. Lithium carbonate
g. Hypoglycemic agents
h. Anticholinergic agents
i. Antihistaminergic agents
j. Nonsteroidal antiinflammatory drugs (NSAIDs)
k. Adrenergic agents

N. NEOPLASTIC

Primary CNS neoplasm versus secondary metastasis to brain.

N. NUTRITIONAL

Vitamin B6 (pyridoxine deficiency).

S. STRUCTURAL/CONGENITAL

Neurofibromatosis, Sturge-Weber syndromes, tuberous sclerosis (rare in adults).

MANAGEMENT

Principles of Seizure Management

1. Stabilize the patient and attend to the ABCs: Airway, Breathing, and Circulation. Place the patient in the left lateral decubitus position to decrease the chances of aspiration. Administer oxygen by nasal cannula or face mask.
2. Assess the patient. Note the type of seizure. Meanwhile, check fingerstick glucose, obtain IV access (avoid antecubital area in

case of clonic flexion), monitor vital signs, and arrange for routine and special laboratory tests.
3. Most seizures resolve on their own. However, if the seizure lasts more than 5 minutes, treat it as SE and treat aggressively. Neurologic dysfunction occurs after 20 minutes of continuous seizure activity despite attention to oxygenation and ventilation.

Status Epilepticus: A Medical Emergency

In patients without epilepsy, the causes of SE may include alcohol withdrawal, acute intracerebral events such as stroke and intracerebral hemorrhage, central nervous system infections, neoplasms, drug intoxication, anoxic encephalopathy, and acute metabolic disturbance. Drugs of abuse can also provoke SE. Continue to search for the underlying cause of seizure.

SE is a medical emergency that requires management in the intensive care unit with close monitoring. Time is critical because the morbidity and mortality rates increase with duration of seizure activity. The Neurocritical Care Society recommends the following treatment:
1. Stabilize the vital physiologic functions: Maintain airway, administer O_2, prevent aspiration, and maintain blood pressure. Watch and observe seizures. Draw blood to check glucose, electrolytes, calcium, and magnesium levels, complete blood count, and toxicology screens.
2. Start an IV line and administer 100 mg of thiamine followed by 50 mL of 50% glucose, and start IV abortive therapy. Start with lorazepam 4 mg at a rate of 2 mg/min. If the seizure does not stop after 5 to 10 minutes, repeat for a maximum total dose of 8 mg.
3. If lorazepam fails to stop the SE, administer fosphenytoin in a loading dose of 20 mg/kg IV at a max rate of 150 mg/min.
4. The initial dose may be augmented with another 10 mg/kg. Hypotension and cardiac arrhythmias may occur in older patients; therefore patients should be on a telemonitor continuously. Sometimes it may be necessary to slow the rate of infusion or consider dopamine or other pressor agents.
5. If SE persists, an endotracheal tube should be inserted for respiratory support and phenobarbital 20 mg/kg started at a rate of 50 to 100 mg/min. For refractory SE, pentobarbital, midazolam, or propofol may be used.

SEIZURE PRECAUTIONS

Place bed in the lowest position.
Have oral airway at the head of the bed.
Put side rails (padded for tonic-clonic seizure) up when the patient is in bed.

Provide firm pillow.

Have suction at the bedside.

Have oxygen at the bedside.

Allow bathroom privileges with supervision only.

Allow bath or shower only with a nurse in attendance.

Measure axillary temperature only.

Allow use of sharp objects (e.g., straight razor, nail scissors) with direct supervision only.

There are three stages to the management of new-onset seizures:

1. Control continuing seizure activity
2. Treat any underlying disease
3. Prevent recurrent seizures

Long-term management of seizure disorders should be provided by a neurologist. A neurology consultation should always be obtained when dealing with new-onset seizures.

Suggested Readings

Brophy GM, Bell R, Claassen J, et al. Guidelines for the evaluation and management of status epilepticus. *Neurocrit Care.* 2012;17(1):3–23. https://doi.org/10.1007/s12028-012-9695-z.

LeRoche S, Helmers S. The new antiepileptic drugs scientific review. *JAMA.* 2004;291:605–614.

Manno EM. Status epilepticus: current treatment strategies. *Neurohospitalist.* 2011;1(1):23–31. https://doi.org/10.1177/1941875210383176.

Martindale JL, Goldstein JN, Pallin DJ. Emergency department seizure epidemiology. *Emerg Med Clin North Am.* 2011;29:15.

Sarma AK, Khandker N, Kurczewski L, Brophy GM. Medical management of epileptic seizures: challenges and solutions. *Neuropsychiatr Dis Treat.* 2016;12:467–485.

Falls

The physician on call is often asked to assess a patient who has fallen. All falls must be assessed rapidly and comprehensively. Falls are the leading cause of fatal and nonfatal injury in the elderly. The health care system is acutely aware of this phenomenon, and fall reduction programs are often emphasized in the inpatient setting. The rate of falling is higher in long-term care facilities than at home, because patients often fall when trying to remove restraints, when going to the bathroom, and when trying to get out of bed in an unfamiliar place. In addition, there is increased difficulty at night because of poor lighting, fewer people to assist with transfers, and confusion. Patients who are prone to fall include those who:

Are elderly

Have a history of falling

Have medical problems

Have had recent intravenous therapy

Have had recent electroconvulsive therapy

Have impaired gait

Have poor vision or proprioception

Are taking hypotensive or sedating medication

Have a history of alcohol use disorders

Have dementia or delirium

PHONE CALL

Questions

1. Was the fall witnessed?
2. Did the patient hit his or her head?
3. Is there an obvious injury?
4. What are the vital signs, including orthostatic changes?
5. Are there any acute changes in mental status or in level of arousal?
6. Is the patient receiving anticoagulants, antiepileptics, or sedating medication?
7. What were the medical and/or psychiatric diagnoses on admission?

8. Does the patient have a history of falling?
9. Does the patient have any localized pain, hematoma, or bleeding?

Orders

Ask the nurse to notify you immediately if there are any changes (particularly in the mental status, level of arousal, or vital signs) before you are able to assess the patient. Give other appropriate orders as necessary (e.g., one-to-one observation, bed rest, frequent neurologic examinations). If there is concern that the patient hit his or her head, the patient must be seen immediately, and a STAT head computed tomography may be indicated to rule out intracranial bleeding.

Priorities

All falls must be evaluated as soon as possible (many hospitals have protocols for an MD assessment after a fall). Severe falls may require comprehensive medical and neurologic evaluation. Be aware that some falls may be described initially as minor, but you may find serious or rapidly progressive injury (e.g., head injury in a patient taking an antiplatelet or blood-thinning agent).

ELEVATOR THOUGHTS

Why does a patient fall?

Think primarily of environmental, cardiac, and neurologic causes and medication effect. Your differential diagnosis should include the following:

Myocardial infarction

Arrhythmias (particularly atrial fibrillation)

Orthostasis (volume depletion, drugs, autonomic changes)

Vasovagal reflex (notably in elderly patients going to the bathroom)

Dementia (associated with Parkinson's disease and other subcortical processes, Alzheimer disease, vascular disease, hydrocephalus/normal-pressure hydrocephalus)

Delirium (especially in patients taking narcotics, sedative-hypnotics, tricyclic antidepressants, cimetidine, antihypertensives, alcohol history [ETOH hx])

Transient ischemic attack (defined as occurring for a period less than 24 hours)

Cerebrovascular accident

Seizure (Obtain a clear history, as partial complex seizures are often overlooked.)

Ataxia, including medication-induced ataxia (e.g., from carbamazepine or lithium toxicity)

Hepatic and renal failure (may also increase exogenous drug levels)

Metabolic disorders

Electrolyte abnormalities (think about Ca, Mg, Na, K)

Untended physical disabilities

Diminished muscle strength

Multiple sensory deficits (e.g., poor vision, impaired proprioception)

Environmental causes (e.g., an unfamiliar environment, a call bell that is not accessible, a wet floor, unassisted transfers out of bed, walking without assistance)

Volitional falls (e.g., by psychotic, manic, or personality-disordered patients or by patients seeking primary or secondary gain)

MEDICAL AND NEUROLOGIC EMERGENCIES

A fall may be the result of an underlying medical emergency (e.g., myocardial infarction, pulmonary embolism). Even environmentally induced falls or slips can result in a serious injury that constitutes an emergency. Head injury usually warrants an immediate complete neurologic examination to rule out an intracranial bleed. Order a head computed tomography scan immediately if a new neurologic deficit is identified or if there is external evidence of head trauma, especially in the elderly. For a patient taking anticoagulation medication, an immediate reversal of coagulation should be discussed with the medical or neurology consultant. Order frequent neurologic examinations and vital sign checks if no neurologic deficits are identified after a fall.

BEDSIDE

Quick Look Test

Does the patient look well, sick, or critical? Is there any evidence of injury or pain?

Airway and Vital Signs

What is the heart rate, and how is the rhythm?
    Rule out arrhythmias.
Is the patient breathing normally?
Does the patient have a fever?
What is the patient's level of arousal (awake, lethargic, obtunded, comatose)?

Orthostasis

Are orthostatic changes noted in heart rate or blood pressure?
Are there any drug-induced orthostatic changes?

Look at the actual medication dosing on the nurse's medication sheets.

Is there any evidence of volume depletion (blood pressure and heart rate both change) or autonomic problems (blood pressure drops but heart rate does not change)?

Selective History

Always obtain the full history from the patient, staff, any observers, and the chart. Remember that people's memories are often biased, and relevant facts must always be verified. In addition, you should assess the patient's insight and judgment into what transpired. However, it is worth mentioning that patients with psychiatric conditions are at risk of having their complaints dismissed due to their illness—that is, staff may approach a patient's self-report with skepticism if the patient is thought-disordered or has other impairments (including coarse personality traits that may interfere with care). A thorough history and exam are always warranted, regardless of the patient's established diagnosis.

1. Was the fall witnessed?
2. How did the patient fall?
3. Where did the patient fall?
4. What was the patient doing?
5. Is there any injury or localizing pain (e.g., is there evidence of head trauma)?
6. Were there any warning symptoms or signs of an impending fall?
7. Is there a history of previous falls? If so, were they similar?
8. Is there a history of hypoglycemia or diabetes?
9. Is there a history of cardiac disease or hypertension?

Selective Physical Examination

1. Vital signs (Changes may indicate orthostatic hypotension, infection, or arrhythmias.)
2. Head, eyes, ears, nose, and throat (Be sure to look for any sensory deficits, "raccoon eyes," blood, cerebrospinal fluid loss, or significant bruising.)
3. Cardiac (Listen for arrhythmias, extra heart sounds, or rubs.)
4. Musculoskeletal, especially pelvis (Always have the patient fully rotate joints, because lack of movement may obscure a complete examination, and press on back, pelvis, and hips to check for pain on palpation.)
5. Skin (Look for hematomas or lacerations.)
6. Neurologic (including testing strength, reflexes, sensory, and especially gait—Is there any evidence of a tia or stroke?)
7. Mental status examination (especially orientation and cognition)

1. Note the reasons for admission for both medical and psychiatric diagnoses.
2. Look for a history of arrhythmia, hypertension (increased stroke risk), seizures, autonomic dysfunction, nocturnal confusion, diabetes, dementia, multiple sensory deficits, or any other potentially causative medical diagnoses.
3. Review all current medications, including all available as needed ("prns"). Look especially for hypotensive agents, including cardiac medication, low-potency neuroleptics, tricyclic antidepressants, and other sedating medications.
4. Review the most recent laboratory tests and any changes (e.g., comprehensive metabolic profile, complete blood count with differential count, acutely elevated liver function tests, elevated prothrombin and partial thromboplastin times and international normalized ratio, drug levels, toxicology screens). Consider repeating laboratory tests that may be significant.

At this point, if you have any questions or concerns, contact the medical or neurologic consultant on call.

MANAGEMENT

Provisional Diagnosis

Establish the reason for the fall. The reasons for a fall may often be multifactorial, and all contributing factors should be taken into account, and documented in the note.

Complications

1. Fractures (hip fractures are the most common and carry a significant risk of morbidity and mortality)
2. Hemorrhage, hematoma (including those in nonobvious areas such as the thoracic cavity, the thigh, the retroperitoneal space, or the subdural space)
3. Lacerations
4. Other injuries

Call medical, neurologic, surgical, or orthopedic consultants immediately as appropriate.

TREAT THE CAUSE

As previously described, a fall may be a symptom of medical or psychiatric illness or may be related to side effects of medication or environmental causes. Identify and treat the illness (e.g., correct fluids and electrolytes, abort a seizure, hydrate) and discontinue or adjust the suspected medication. Warn the patient and provide for safety precautions with a call bell, one-to-one or close observation, and adequate light. Consider lowering the bed to the floor. Discuss the interventions fully with the nursing staff. Correct all reversible factors, including treating occult urinary tract infections and nocturia, and address withdrawal from drugs or alcohol. Be aware that chronic alcoholic patients are prone to Wernicke's encephalopathy from acute thiamine depletion in the presence of a carbohydrate load.

Follow up with any consulting physicians already involved in the case. Take a proactive approach, and obtain pertinent laboratory results with complete blood count, therapeutic drug monitoring, prothrombin and partial thromboplastin times, comprehensive metabolic profile, chemical strips for glucose, urinalysis, and urine toxicology.

Finally, ensure that your full evaluation, consultation notes, tests obtained, and actions taken are fully documented in the chart. If this is not done, then other members of the health care team may not be aware of what has happened. If there are any significant changes, be sure to speak directly to the patient's primary physician. Many institutions have a specific form that must be completed in the case of a fall, but it does not supplant good medical notes in the chart.

Suggested Readings

Papadakis MA, McPhee SJ, Rabow MW. *Current Medical Diagnosis and Treatment.* 55th ed. New York: McGraw-Hill Medical; 2016.

Blood Pressure Changes

The on-call resident will sometimes be contacted because a patient's blood pressure (BP) is either high or low. This chapter focuses on BP changes pertinent to psychiatric patients.

PHONE CALL

Questions

1. What are the patient's BP and other vital signs? Are they outside of the usual range for that patient?
2. Does the patient have any other symptoms (e.g., altered mental status, syncope, headache, rigidity, dizziness, confusion, tremor, chest pain or discomfort, shortness of breath)?
3. Does the patient have a history of hypertension or hypotension? Is he or she taking an antihypertensive medication?
4. Does the patient have a history of alcohol or other substance use? When was the last use?
5. What medications is the patient taking? When was the last dose? Has the patient had previous reactions to medications?

Orders

The patient should be evaluated before any medications are ordered. However, the physician may want to ask the nurse to do the following:

1. Repeat the vitals.
2. Hold any medication that could further elevate or lower BP until the patient can be assessed.

Inform RN

"Will arrive in … minutes."

If the patient is in any distress, the person on call should see him or her as soon as possible. If the patient has other acute findings (such as altered mental status, focal neurological findings, chest pain, low oxygen saturation, etc.), the psychiatrist should consider concurrently calling the appropriate acute hospital team, if available (such as a "rapid response team," a stroke team, etc.).

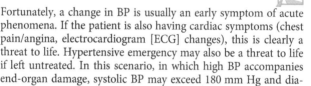

ELEVATOR THOUGHTS

What are common causes of BP changes in patients on psychiatric wards?

Normal physiology

Essential hypertension

Medication side effects (including neuroleptic malignant syndrome [NMS])

Substance use or withdrawal

Drug withdrawal (e.g., abrupt withdrawal of some antihypertensives may cause rebound hypertension)

Drug interactions (monoamine oxidase inhibitors are particularly dangerous)

Drug noncompliance (during admission or outside of the hospital)

MAJOR THREAT TO LIFE

Fortunately, a change in BP is usually an early symptom of acute phenomena. If the patient is also having cardiac symptoms (chest pain/angina, electrocardiogram [ECG] changes), this is clearly a threat to life. Hypertensive emergency may also be a threat to life if left untreated. In this scenario, in which high BP accompanies end-organ damage, systolic BP may exceed 180 mm Hg and diastolic pressure may exceed 120 mm Hg, though an acute rise in BP beyond the patient's normal range that does not meet these values may still be considered a hypertensive emergency. Also, potentially lethal cerebrovascular problems must be considered, including neurologic emergencies such as intracranial bleeding.

NMS is another condition that may present a serious threat to life. Although the hallmark of NMS is rigidity (specifically "lead-pipe" rigidity), many symptoms may be more prominent in its early stages, such as hypotension, hypertension, tachycardia, and hyperthermia. This is a dangerous side effect of antipsychotic medications that must be considered in any patient taking these medications. The patient may require transfer to a medical ward where he or she can be watched more closely. If NMS is on the differential, the medical consultant should be involved early on.

Serotonin syndrome may also be life-threatening. Symptoms may include mental status changes, autonomic instability (tachycardia, hypertension), and musculoskeletal findings such as hyperreflexia and myoclonus. The medical service should also be involved early in the care of a patient for whom serotonin syndrome is being considered.

BEDSIDE

Quick Look Test

How does the patient look (comfortable, ill, in acute distress)?

This will give you a quick clue to the urgency of the situation (though a complete assessment should be done even if the patient appears well).

Airway and Vital Signs

1. What is the BP?

    Retake the BP yourself in both arms using a sphygmomanometer (BP gauge). Certain medical conditions produce unilateral differences in BP in their stable state. Improperly fitting BP cuffs may produce false results. Orthostatic vital signs may also be useful—a decrease in systolic BP of 20 mm Hg or a decrease of diastolic BP of 10 mm Hg within 3 minutes of standing from a sitting or supine position suggests orthostasis.

2. What are the heart rate and temperature?

    These may help refine the diagnosis, especially in the case of substance-related problems or an underlying medical process such as fever or sepsis.

3. How is the patient breathing?

    Patients in cardiac distress may complain of difficulty breathing.

Chart Review

In addition, the following information should be obtained:

1. Look for pertinent underlying medical conditions—that is, renal failure, infection, etc.
2. Look for a baseline ECG.
3. Has the patient been started on any medication recently?
4. What has the patient's BP been? Has there been a particular trend?
5. Was a urine toxicology screen or a blood alcohol test performed on admission? Alternatively, is there concern the patient obtained access to contraband on the unit and that a urine toxicology should be repeated?
6. Is the patient on a special diet (e.g., low sodium)?

Selective History

Although some of the answers may be in the chart or obtained by talking to the nurse, the patient should also be interviewed directly. It is not uncommon for patients to forget to tell the doctor important information during the initial assessment.

Selective Physical Examination

1. Vital signs: If these have not already been reassessed, take the vital signs now.
2. General: Is the patient in any distress or diaphoretic? What is the skin appearance?
3. Lungs: Are there crackles or wheezes? Absent lung sounds?
4. Cardiovascular: Are there abnormal heart sounds? Is the rhythm regular?
5. Neurologic: What is the level of consciousness? Is the patient confused or tremulous? Are there any focal neurologic signs?
6. Musculoskeletal: Does the patient have cogwheeling or rigidity? What is the patient's muscle tone?

MANAGEMENT

If the patient is in acute medical danger, alert the medical consultant immediately. Fortunately, most BP changes will be relatively simple to handle, and at times are transient. If the BP has not returned to normal by the time the clinician performs a full assessment, however, the following are some management suggestions.

Neuroleptic Malignant Syndrome and Serotonin Syndrome

Both syndromes may present very subtly. Signs of autonomic instability, including hypotension or hypertension, may be the initial clues to the diagnosis. If NMS or serotonin syndrome is suspected:

Stop the patient's antipsychotic and/or serotonergic medication.
Draw the patient's blood for creatine kinase determination, complete blood count, blood chemistry, and hepatic function panel.
Obtain an ECG.
Contact the medical consultant, because transfer to a medical ward or intensive care unit may be indicated; the medical consultant should also be involved in the provision of supportive care (possibly fluids, cooling blankets, etc.).
Retake the patient's temperature and other vital signs.

Hypertension

One of the most common causes of hypertension, especially in newly admitted psychiatric patients, is alcohol withdrawal. Early signs include increased BP, tachycardia, hyperthermia, and tremor. Even if the patient denies or minimizes alcohol use, if the clinician suspects withdrawal, it should be treated to prevent progression. First-line treatment is the administration of benzodiazepines, in which a chlordiazepoxide protocol is commonly used.

However, in the case of patients with liver disease or impaired hepatic function, lorazepam, oxazepam, or temazepam may be the benzodiazepine of choice. Lorazepam and oxazepam are preferred agents because they only undergo glucuronidation in the liver (bypassing oxidation) and have no active metabolites. It is important to remember that oxazepam is only available orally, while lorazepam is available orally, intramuscularly, and intravenously.

Commonly used psychiatric medications can also cause BP fluctuations (e.g., monoamine oxidase inhibitors in patients who are noncompliant with the special tyramine diet) or the use of venlafaxine, which can cause dose-dependent increases in diastolic BP in some patients. If hypertension is a suspected medication side effect, that medication should be withheld until the primary team can make a decision on treatment options.

If the patient has a history of high BP and is taking an antihypertensive medication, ask the nurses when the last dose was given and when the next dose is expected. Find out the usual range for this patient. It may be warranted for the patient to receive the next dose early. If the hypertension is mild and has been persistent, the clinician should recommend to the treating team that the dose be evaluated, a new medication tried, or a medical consultant called.

If the patient has no history of high BP and this is an isolated finding (no previous high readings and not now acute), have the patient's vital signs monitored regularly to watch for an impending problem. If there seems to be a pattern suggesting a new diagnosis of hypertension and the patient's condition is not acute, the patient should undergo regular vital sign monitoring and evaluation by an internist who may choose an appropriate medication; though chronic mild hypertension carries long-term risks, acutely, the patient could be at greater risk from overly aggressive pharmacologic treatment. This option allows the treatment team to choose an appropriate antihypertensive. It is seldom necessary to start antihypertensive therapy immediately. Unless there are signs of target organ damage, it is often preferable to try nonpharmacologic modification for 4 to 6 weeks. Nonpharmacologic interventions may include diet modification, regular exercise, smoking cessation, and weight loss.

Hypotension

The most common cause of hypotension in psychiatric patients (other than normal variations) is medication side effect. Orthostatic hypotension is a common side effect of antipsychotic medications (such as clozapine and olanzapine) that often occurs on the initiation of new medication or an increase in dose, but can also occur in a patient who has been taking a stable dose. Generally, patients will adapt to mild hypotension in time. If the patient is asymptomatic and tolerating the lowered BP, monitoring the vital signs for changes may be sufficient.

If the patient is experiencing hypotension with mild symptoms (e.g., dizziness, light-headedness), withhold the next dose of the medications that might be causative and inform the primary treatment team of this change.

Another common cause of hypotension is dehydration. This may occur in depressed patients with decreased appetite, patients with eating disorders, or catatonic or psychotic patients. If dehydration is suspected, assess for sources of fluid loss (vomiting/diarrhea), check orthostatics and other vital signs to make sure that the patient is stable, and order laboratory tests such as blood chemistries to check for any electrolyte imbalances or kidney injury. Staff should also be included in redirecting the patient to take more fluids. Also, consider fall precautions if appropriate, especially in elderly patients. If the patient is clinically unstable, contact the medical consultant and consider transfer to a ward where the patient can receive any necessary interventions not available on the psychiatry unit (e.g., some psychiatric units cannot safely manage patients with intravenous access or are otherwise unequipped to administer medications or fluids intravenously). Consider also that if the patient has any other unstable vital signs, such an arrhythmia, the patient may need telemetry or other monitoring.

REMEMBER

Always leave a note. Events that happened during the night often do not get reported during the morning rounds. If the patient needed to be seen, it is probably important enough for the treatment team to know about. The best course of action is to contact the treatment team directly. Also, many hospitals have phlebotomy services or nurses to draw blood samples; however, the clinician should always be prepared to obtain his or her own labs.

Suggested Readings

Boyer EW. Serotonin syndrome (serotonin toxicity). Uptodate; 2016, In: Post TW, ed. UpToDate. MA: Waltham; 2016. Accessed December 6, *www.uptodate.com.*

Elliott WJ, Varon J. Evaluation and treatment of hypertensive emergencies in adults. In: Post TW, ed. *UpToDate.* Waltham, MA: Uptodate; 2016 *www.uptodate.com.* Accessed November 30, 2016.

Grossman A, Messerli FH, Grossman E. Drug induced hypertension—an unappreciated cause of secondary hypertension. *Eur J Pharmacol.* 2015;763:15–22.

Kosten T, O'Connor P. Management of drug and alcohol withdrawal. *N Engl J Med.* 2003;349:1786–1795.

Lanier JB, Mote MB, Clay EC. Evaluation and management of orthostatic hypotension. *Am Fam Physician.* 2011;84(5):527–536. http://www.aafp.org/afp/2011/0901/p527.html.

Perry EC. Inpatient management of acute alcohol withdrawal syndrome. *CNS Drugs.* 2014;28(5):401–410.

Telepsychiatry

The on-call psychiatrist is increasingly expected to utilize telepsychiatry as a means of expanding access to psychiatric care. Telepsychiatry initially was conceptualized as a care delivery system primarily for the most rural and remote populations; however, current trends in psychiatric care show a growing nationwide demand for services that far exceeds the supply of mental health professionals (both in number and geographical distribution) needed to deliver these services. Telepsychiatry continues to show significant promise as one of the solutions to the national shortage of psychiatric providers.

The vast majority of the literature to date has found telepsychiatry to be as effective as in-person psychiatry, and specifically with respect to safety assessment, disposition recommendations, diagnostic reliability, response to treatment, patient satisfaction, and ability to establish rapport and a therapeutic alliance from the perspective of the patient *and* the provider.

The term "telepsychiatry" has evolved over time (as the definition previously included phone, fax, email, the Internet), but is now understood to be the use of videoteleconferencing (VTC), meaning live interactive two-way audio-video communication over high-capacity (high-bandwidth) networks, to provide clinical psychiatric care from a distance.

As the on-call psychiatrist, telepsychiatry is most likely to be used for emergency psychiatric evaluations, urgent psychiatric consultations for medical/surgical services, and possibly for brief medication consultations regarding the management of an acutely agitated patient.

BEFORE THE PHONE CALL

It is imperative for the on-call telepsychiatrist to be properly educated and trained in the specifics of your telepsychiatry service with regard to administrative issues.

Questions

(Questions you should be able to answer prior to being on call.)

1. What specific telepsychiatry equipment is available and working currently? Is the on-call telepsychiatrist able to control the camera in the remote location (i.e., zoom in and zoom out on patient, adjust the camera to the left or to the right)?
2. Where is the telepsychiatry equipment located (i.e., close to the emergency room [ER] or tucked away in a corner of the hospital)? Is the equipment in a quiet and private area?
3. Who is responsible for familiarizing the patient with the equipment and introducing the patient to the psychiatrist? Who will be available to the patient, should there be any technical or medical issues, and where is this individual(s) located?
4. What is the policy or protocol for abrupt VTC connection loss in the middle of an interview with a patient? One example might include having the patient speak with the on-call telepsychiatrist over the phone until the VTC connection is fixed.
5. What mental health resources (inpatient and outpatient) and law enforcement resources are available in the community (where the patient is currently located)?
6. What is the written protocol for addressing psychiatric emergencies that includes a list of key team members, with their respective roles and responsibilities?
7. Is the remote staff comfortable handling emergency psychiatric assessments? Do the staff members have the designation of psychiatric training (i.e., are they psychiatric registered nurses [RNs], psychiatric NPs, psychiatric PAs)? What is the level of experience/expertise of the staff in managing acutely agitated or dangerous patients? Are there written policies in place that stipulate the extent of responsibility for the on-call telepsychiatrist versus the responsibilities for the staff on site in managing acute dangerousness?
8. What is the role of the on-call telepsychiatrist in terms of the particular clinical setting (e.g., the emergency room)?
9. What are the documentation requirements? If the electronic medical system is unavailable, how should the on-call psychiatrist document the encounter? Who should the on-call psychiatrist contact in order to obtain the patient's chart to review (in a timely manner)?
10. Will you be responsible for seeing child and adolescent cases?

ELEVATOR THOUGHTS

1. If there are safety concerns during an interview, it is appropriate to interrupt your interview and follow clinic emergency psychiatric policy or protocol, which may include contacting local staff, a local mental health crisis team, or law enforcement.

2. Depending on the level of concern for safety, it may become imperative to involve local law enforcement for assistance in deescalating the situation. Providing law enforcement with information regarding the situation, possible diagnosis, and how that may manifest when confronting the patient, as well as a phone number to assuage their concerns real-time, all contribute to patient, staff, and officer safety and comfort.

3. Given the cultural differences in the meaning and prevalence of firearm ownership between urban and rural environments, it is important to be sensitive to the implications of firearm disposition in this patient population. Though the initial steps in removing firearms from patients involves addressing the various layers of safety measures (i.e., unloading gun and separating bullets), in cases with high suspicion of danger, law enforcement may be called to remove guns from the home.

4. Be familiar with state-specific "duty to warn" laws to appropriately warn potential targets in the event that the patient voices violent or homicidal ideation with a specific threat in mind.

PHONE CALL

Questions

1. Is this an urgent situation? Are you concerned about any immediate danger to the patient, staff, or others? Is the patient suicidal or homicidal?

2. How would you like safety concerns to be communicated with you in the event that a dangerous patient terminates the videoconference interview prematurely? Are there emergency protocols in place?

3. What is your initial diagnostic impression? Are you concerned for your own safety?

4. Are you concerned that the patient demonstrates dangerousness to self in the form of suicidal ideation or grossly disorganized behavior?

5. Are you concerned that the patient demonstrates dangerousness to others in the form of homicidal ideation or violent thoughts?

6. Does the patient have access to firearms? Type of firearms? Locked versus unlocked? Loaded versus unloaded?

7. Do you suspect that the patient is using substances?

8. Does the patient have any acute or chronic medical conditions that could be causing or contributing to psychiatric symptoms?

9. Have you told the patient that the psychiatrist is located remotely and will conduct the interview and exam via VTC and **not** in-person? Did the patient express any feelings or

concerns about this? Did the patient have any specific questions about the process?

10. Has the patient been oriented to the VTC equipment? Is the patient aware of what to do and where to go at the conclusion of the psychiatric evaluation?

Prior to Videoteleconferencing Interview and Exam

- If available, collect data via chart review; review labs, studies, imaging, and physical exam as you normally would in any emergency psychiatric evaluation.

Videoteleconferencing With Patient

- Given that the on-call psychiatrist will not be in the same physical space as the patient, rapport building and therapeutic alliance are essential.
- Make the patient feel as comfortable in the room as possible; ask if the volume is sufficient and ask if the patient is able to see you well enough.
- Ideally you should be able to see the patient's entire body (and not just the patient's face); the patient can be seated in a chair in front of the camera with you adjusting the zoom settings accordingly.
- Patients often have concerns about privacy with telepsychiatry; thus with every patient you should:
    - explicitly verbalize that the interview is not being recorded
    - emphasize confidentiality
    - if it is possible to manipulate the camera that is transmitting video of you to the patient, you can pan the camera around the room you are in so that the patient can actually see that there is no one else in the room with you
- You also should take a few minutes to manage the patient's expectations and explain your role as the on-call psychiatrist.
- For example, you should always explain the protocol and specifically what the patient should do if the VTC connection is lost during the interview.
- State that if necessary you may ask the patient to come closer to the camera—for example, in order to evaluate for possible tardive dyskinesia—if you do not have an adequate view where the patient is sitting during the interview.
- Ask if the patient has any questions, concerns, or feelings specifically concerning VTC.
- If appropriate, you can empathize (and even use humor) with the patient by acknowledging that at first the interview may feel uncomfortable or awkward, but is necessary.
- You can occasionally check-in with the patient to see if there are any technical issues on the patient's end.

AFTER VIDEOTELECONFERENCING INTERVIEW AND EXAM

Communicate with the clinical staff (ideally interdisciplinary team) at the remote site (MD, PA, RN, social worker):

- As soon as the interview is completed, explicitly verbalize if there are any acute safety concerns (harm to self or others, medical concerns) and whether or not the patient warrants constant (1 to 1) monitoring by clinical staff.
- Explain what the next steps will be—for example, collateral gathering and waiting for lab results.
- You should essentially be making the same recommendations you would make if you were seeing this patient in person in that clinical setting.
- Both verbally communicate your recommendations to the clinical staff and document your recommendations.
- Ensure that your recommendations are clear and specific.
- If necessary, you can have the clinical staff bring the patient back to the VTC area in order to personally discuss your recommendations with the patient.
- If time permits, you can debrief with the clinical staff regarding what went well and what could be improved upon.

REMEMBER

Given that telepsychiatry is still relatively new to most patients and clinical staff, there will undoubtedly be a learning curve. As the on-call psychiatrist who potentially may need to utilize telepsychiatry, you want to do everything you can to be knowledgeable about site-specific procedures and policies. Feeling comfortable with the logistics and equipment will allow you to focus on providing the best psychiatric care for the patient, regardless of the system through which the care is delivered.

Suggested Readings

Hilty DM, Ferrer DC, Parish MB, et al. The effectiveness of telemental health: a 2013 review. *Telemed J E Health.* 2013;19:444–454.

Narasimhan M, Druss BG, Hockenberry JM, et al. Quality, utilization, and economic impact of a statewide emergency department telepsychiatry program. *Psychiat Serv.* 2015;66(11):1167–1172. http://doi.org/10.1176/appi.ps.201400122.

Shore JH, Hilty DM, Yellowlees P. Emergency management guidelines for telepsychiatry. *Gen Hosp Psychiatry.* 2007;29:199–206.

Sorvaniemi M, Ojanen E, Santamaki O. Telepsychiatry in emergency consultations: a follow-up study of sixty patients. *Telemed J E Health.* 2005;11:439–441.

Williams M, Pfeffer M, Boyle J, et al. *Telepsychiatry in the Emergency Department: Overview and Case Studies.* California HealthCare Foundation: Oakland; 2009.

Yellowlees P, Burke MM, Marks SL, et al. Emergency telepsychiatry. *J Telemed Telecare*. 2008;14:277–281.

Cross-Cultural Issues

Cultural diversity presents unique challenges to mental health care. According to the DSM-5:

> *Culture refers to systems of knowledge, concepts, rules, and practices that are learned and transmitted across generations. Culture includes language, religion and spirituality, family structures, life-cycle stages, ceremonial rituals, and customs, as well as moral and legal systems. Cultures are open, dynamic systems that undergo continuous change over time; in the contemporary world, most individuals and groups are exposed to multiple cultures, which they use to fashion their own identities and make sense of experience. These features of culture make it crucial not to overgeneralize cultural information or stereotype groups in terms of fixed cultural traits.[a]*
>
> **(Lewis-Fernández et al.)**

Psychiatric illness is affected by culture in numerous ways. Culture influences the development and manifestation of psychiatric illness, the individual's experience of and response to the illness, and the ways in which psychiatric illness can be effectively treated. As the United States grows more diverse, psychiatrists must become practiced at addressing the complexities presented by the culturally diverse individuals they treat. Cultural sensitivity is an essential skill for a psychiatrist to establish a therapeutic working alliance, conduct an accurate diagnostic evaluation, and create an appropriate treatment plan. The goal of this chapter is to characterize these tasks and outline approaches to assessment and management in an on-call setting. For the on-call psychiatrist, understanding the impact of culture enables him or her to assess and respond to any individual encountered over the course of the shift.

---

[a]Reprinted with permission from the Diagnostic and Statistical Manual of Mental Disorders, Fifth Edition, (Copyright © 2013). American Psychiatric Association. All Rights Reserved.

The first goal of the psychiatrist is to understand the psychiatric illness presented. In order to accomplish this, he or she must understand the patient's conceptualization of the illness, which is often influenced by others in the individual's cultural network. The psychiatrist may need to incorporate multiple sources of information to formulate this cultural conceptualization. With an accurate understanding of the individual's background, the on-call psychiatrist can then recommend an effective and sustainable treatment plan.

The following guide is based on the DSM-5 Cultural Formulation Interview and has been adapted for an on-call setting.

PHONE CALL

Questions

1. Does the individual speak English fluently?
   a. If not, what is the individual's preferred language of communication?
   b. Is an in-person interpreter needed and available? As an alternative, is a telephone interpreter available?
2. Does the individual identify with any specific ethnicity, race, gender, sexual orientation, or religion?
   a. Was the individual's identification self-reported or interpreted from secondary sources?
3. Does the individual have any family members or friends who are involved in the individual's care?
   a. Are these family members or friends potential sources of collateral information, support, or stress?
   b. Do they speak English fluently? Is an interpreter needed?
   c. How do the family members or friends understand the individual's illness?
4. What is the individual's history with psychiatric care?
   a. Have there been notable challenges or barriers to care that may be related to the individual's cultural background?

ELEVATOR THOUGHTS

1. How does the individual's cultural identification factor into his or her psychiatric illness and treatment?
   a. How might the individual interpret and communicate his or her psychiatric symptoms?
   b. Would the individual be more open about physical/somatic symptoms versus psychological ones?
   c. How might the individual expect to be treated by a psychiatrist?
   d. How might the individual expect to be helped?
   e. What aspects of the individual's culture may present barriers or opportunities for psychiatric treatment?

2. Religion and spirituality are often beneficial for mental wellness. Incorporating an individual's religious/spiritual beliefs may strengthen alliance and treatment adherence.

BEDSIDE

1. Use the language the individual uses, with the assistance of an interpreter if needed (although an in-person interpreter is preferred, a telephone interpreter is an alternative).
2. Focus on the individual's own way of understanding the problem and ask how he or she would describe his or her problem to his or her social networks.
   a. *People often understand their problems in their own way, which may be similar to or different from how doctors describe the problem. How would you describe your problem?*
   b. *Sometimes people have different ways of describing their problem to their family, friends, or others in their community. How would you describe your problem to them?*
   c. *What do you think are the causes of your [problem]*[b]*? Why do you think this is happening to you? What do your family, friends, or others in your community think is causing your [problem]?*
3. Focus on aspects of the problem that matter most to the individual.
   a. *What troubles you most about your [problem]?*
4. Elicit information about the individual's supports and stressors.
   a. *Are there any kinds of support that make your [problem] better?*
   b. *Are there any kinds of stresses that make your [problem] worse?*
5. Focus on the most salient elements of the individual's cultural identity. Elicit aspects of the identity that make the problem better or worse.
   a. *For you, what are the most important aspects of your cultural identity? Are there any aspects of your background or identity, such as race, religion, gender, sexual orientation, or religion, that make a difference to your [problem]?*
   b. *What gender pronoun do you prefer?*
   c. *Do you consider yourself a religious person? Does spirituality play an important role in dealing with your [problem]?*
6. Elicit information about how the individual self-copes and his or her various sources of help.
   a. *Sometimes people have various ways of dealing with problems like your [problem]. What have you tried on your own to cope with your [problem]? What has been beneficial, and what has not been beneficial?*

---

[b]Use the patient's own description of his or her psychiatric problem.

b. *Often people seek help from many different sources, including doctors, helpers, healers, religious leaders, family, or friends. What kinds of help or healing have you sought for your [problem]? What was most useful? Not useful?*

7. Clarify the barriers to seeking help, accessing care, and engaging in previous treatment. Money, work, family commitments, stigma, discrimination, or language barriers are some examples.
   a. *Has anything prevented you from getting the help you need?*

8. Clarify the individual's current perceived needs and expectations.
   a. *What kinds of help do you think would be most useful to you at this time? Are there other kinds of help your family/friends have suggested that you think would be helpful for you now?*

9. Elicit the individual's concerns about the current provider or treatment, including perceived racism, language barriers, or cultural differences.
   a. *Sometimes doctors and patients misunderstand each other because they come from different backgrounds. Have you been concerned about this? Is there anything we can do to provide you with the care you need?*

MANAGEMENT

1. Just as in the assessment portion of your evaluation, focus on presenting your professional assessments and recommendations in a culturally sensitive manner to facilitate understanding in the individual and family.
   a. Focus on communicating with the individual in a manner that he or she can understand. Consider using the individual's own terms used to describe his or her illness to present your diagnosis and treatment.
   b. Focus on making culturally sensitive recommendations, taking into consideration issues such as access to care, stigma, health literacy, and psychosocial support.
   c. Elicit support, if available, from the individual's family and friends to facilitate the individual's understanding of his or her illness and access to the recommended treatment.

Long-term, consider referring the individual to a provider who will be able to provide culturally sensitive care. Consider factors such as the individual's preferred language and provider factors such as gender, ethnicity, and religion (would involving a chaplain or pastor be beneficial?) to facilitate the patient-provider alliance.

FURTHER THOUGHTS

Culture plays a critical role in an individual's experience of psychiatric illness, treatment, and health care providers. It is critical to assess the individual and family members directly for an accurate assessment of how an individual's beliefs and behaviors inform psychiatric presentation and management. Equipped with a culturally attuned psychiatric formulation, the on-call psychiatrist can provide meaningful support to the individual, family, and other providers.

Suggested Readings

Lewis-Fernández R, Aggarwal NK, Hinton L, Hinton DE, Kirmayer LJ. *DSM-5 Handbook on the Cultural Formulation Interview.* Arlington, VA: American Psychiatric Association; 2015.

MoCA

The Montreal Cognitive Assessment (MoCA) is a structured, 30-item assessment of cognitive ability. It is intended to be used as a screening tool to detect mild cognitive impairment (MCI) by testing a number of cognitive domains (including visuospatial, working memory, attention, and abstraction, as well as orientation). Sensitivity and specificity for MCI (score ≤25) are 90% and 87%, respectively, according to a 2005 validation study (Nasreddine et al., 2005). This exam takes approximately 10 minutes to administer. A full-length English language form of the exam is reprinted later. To ensure validity and consistency, one should administer the test using the script provided in the instructions online at www.mocatest.org.

It is important to keep in mind that the MoCA is not a diagnostic test. A 2015 Cochrane review found existing data "insufficient to make recommendations on the clinical utility of MoCA for detecting dementia in different settings" (Davis et al., 2015). Therefore a score of less than or equal to 25, although strongly suggestive of MCI, warrants additional testing.

Some clinicians may be familiar with another cognitive screener, the Mini-Mental State Examination, or Folstein test. Advantages of the MoCA include the fact that the test is available in more than 50 languages and dialects, has a basic version for subjects who are illiterate, and has a version for subjects with visual impairment. For access to these expanded resources, clinicians may register at www.mocatest.org.

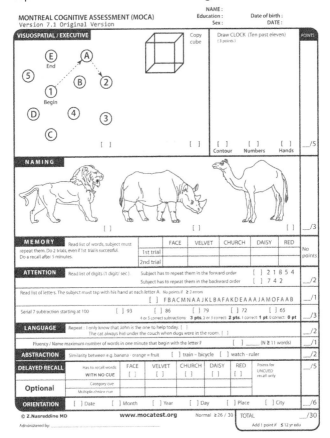

Suggested Readings

Davis DHJ, Creavin ST, Yip JLY, Noel-Storr AH, Brayne C, Cullum S. Montreal Cognitive Assessment for the diagnosis of Alzheimer's disease and other dementias. *Cochrane Database Syst Rev.* 10: 2015. https://doi.org/10.1002/14651858.CD010775.pub2.

Nasreddine ZS, Phillips NA, Bédirian V, et al. The Montreal Cognitive Assessment, MoCA: a brief screening tool for mild cognitive impairment. *J Am Geriatr Soc.* 2005;53(4):695–699.

Mental Status Exam

The mental status examination (MSE) is the psychiatric equivalent of a physical examination. Like the physical exam, the MSE is a "snapshot" of the patient's status at the time of the examination. The standardized structure and vocabulary of the MSE outlined next assist the examiner to organize and present the most clinically relevant aspects of the patient's mental status in the most objective way possible.

1. Appearance
   - Notable physical characteristics (e.g., age, appearance related to stated age, race, dress)
   - Grooming/hygiene
   - Posture
   - Facial expressions
   - Emotional appearance (e.g., anxious, tense, panicky, sad, unhappy, angry)
   - Presence of significant objects/environmental factors (e.g., wheelchair, stuffed animal)
2. Behavior
   - Level of cooperation with exam (e.g., cooperative, hostile, superficially cooperative)
   - Eye contact
   - Relatedness: the patient's style of connecting with you (e.g., odd, distant, overattached, intense)
   - Level of activity (e.g., psychomotor agitation or retardation)
   - Tics or tremors
   - Automatisms: involuntarily performed movements
   - Mannerisms, grimacing, gestures
   - Stereotypy: constant repetition of a meaningless gesture
   - Apraxia: inability to voluntarily perform a specific purposeful movement or use a known object
   - Gait
   - Akathisia: inability to remain seated due to motor restlessness
   - Dyskinesia: insuppressible, stereotyped, awake-state involuntary movements

3. Speech
   - Primary language and accent
   - Aphasia or impaired communication by speech, writing, or signs resulting from dysfunction of the brain centers in dominant hemisphere
   - Prosody or rhythmic quality, a nondominant hemisphere–mediated ability (e.g., normal, impaired, atonal)
   - Rate (e.g., slow, fast, pressured, uninterruptable)
   - Volume
   - Spontaneity
   - Enunciation/phonation (e.g., hoarse, slurred; may test k, t, and m sounds for localizing weak musculature)
   - Pitch
   - Paraphasia: word interposition and substitution causing unintelligible speech
   - Neologism: use of a new word often made up by the patient in a novel or incorrect manner
   - Clang associations: use of words similar in sound but not in meaning
   - Echolalia: involuntary repetition of a phrase spoken by another person
   - Muteness: lack of speech
4. Attitude: the way of thinking, feeling, or acting toward a situation (e.g., cooperative, irritable, aggressive, seductive, guarded, defensive, indifferent, sarcastic)
5. Mood: the patient's subjective experience of his or her emotional state
   - Should be quoted directly whenever possible (e.g., gloomy, sad, angry, tense, happy)
6. Affect: the evaluator's observations of the patient's emotional state. Affect should be named (e.g., dysphoric, euthymic, euphoric) and can be described using the following:
   - Range: full, constricted, restricted
   - Intensity and amplitude: flat (nearly complete absence of affective expression), blunted (decreased amplitude), expansive (increased amplitude)
   - Mood congruity: does the stated mood align with the observed affect?
   - Appropriateness of affect to the situation or interview
   - Stability (e.g., stable or labile)
7. Thought process: the means by which ideas are formed and connected
   - Logical versus illogical
   - Linear and goal directed
   - Circumstantial: taking detours but arriving at a point, or returning to the original topic

- Tangential: taking detours but never returning to the original topic (e.g., if a question is asked it is not answered)
- Flight of ideas: rapidly moving between topics with some connection or logical progression
- Loosening of associations: moving between topics without logical progression
- Word salad: lack of connections even within a single sentence
- Thought blocking: train of thought is abruptly lost
- Perseveration: inability to move thought away from a topic; a response appropriately given to one question is repeated to different questions.

8. Thought content
- Suicidal and homicidal ideation: include specifics about degree of intent and any planning
- Delusions: fixed false beliefs that are not shared by members of the patient's culture. Note details including quality (paranoid, grandiose, religious, somatic) and how well formed and salient they appear
- Thought broadcasting, insertion, or withdrawal: the specific delusion that ideas are taken from, put into, or removed from a patient's mind
- Ideas of reference: delusion that occurrences carry special meaning relating to oneself
- Phobias: objectively unfounded fears that result in avoidance, despite potential awareness of the irrational nature of the fear
- Obsessions: recurring thoughts, urges, or images that are experienced as intrusive and/or unwanted
- Compulsions: repetitive behaviors or mental acts that the individual feels driven to perform, usually in response to an obsession (and usually to relieve distress)
- Depersonalization: feeling of detachment or disconnection from one's self or body
- Derealization: feeling of the external environment being false or unreal
- Magical thinking

9. Perception
- Hallucinations: subjective experiences without basis in reality (e.g., olfactory, auditory, tactile, gustatory, visual)
- Illusions: misperceptions of real sensory experiences
- Feelings of unreality
- Déjà vu: mental impression that a new experience has happened before
- Jamais vu: false feeling of unfamiliarity with a familiar experience
- Time loss and amnesia

10. Cognition. If indicated, perform complete standardized cognitive assay (e.g., MoCA, SLUMS; see appendix). Domains that may be relevant include the following:
    - Sensorium and level of arousal (e.g., alert, lethargic, obtunded, stuporous, comatose)
    - Orientation to person, place, time, and situation
    - Concentration (ask to give days of week or months of year backwards)
    - Immediate recall (give three words and ask patient to repeat)
    - Short-term recall (ask for the three words in 5 to 10 minutes)
    - Long-term recall/fund of knowledge (ask about former presidents/cultural figures, keeping in mind the patient's cultural or national background)
    - Calculation (serial 7's or how many quarters in $1.75)
    - Abstraction (ask patient to explain idiomatic phrases, such as "What does it mean that people living in glass houses should not throw stones?")
    - Language (including speaking, reading, writing, naming, and repetition)
11. Impulse control (e.g., strained, intact, or impaired)
12. Insight: understanding of one's psychological and psychiatric condition, as well as understanding of the situation occurring at the time of interview (e.g., poor, limited, fair, good)
13. Judgment: the ability to make decisions that benefit the patient's health and well-being (e.g., poor, limited, fair, good)

Medical Conditions Manifesting as Psychiatric Disorders

The following Table C.1 lists medical disorders that are commonly associated with psychiatric symptoms, with an emphasis on those disorders that are most often considered in the psychiatric differential diagnosis.

TABLE C.1 Medical Disorders and Commonly Associated Psychiatric Symptoms

	Common Medical Presentation	Psychiatric Complaints	Diagnostic Tests	Comments
Acute intermittent porphyria	Abdominal pain, nausea, vomiting, peripheral neuropathy, constipation, tachycardia, hypertension	Anxiety, insomnia, depression psychosis, delirium	Urine porphyrins, Watson-Schwartz or Hoesch test, seizures	Autosomal dominant, attacks may be induced by medications or diet
Adrenal cortical	Hyperpigmentation, orthostatic hypotension, dizziness	Depression, anorexia	Serum and urine cortisol, serum renin, potassium, urine sodium, abdominal CT	Multiple causes (e.g., Addison disease)
Anemia	Dyspnea on exertion, anxiety,	Mood changes, poor concentration, worsening of dementia	CBC, blood smear	
Any cancer	Various	Depression, anxiety	Tests depend on etiology	May be reactive
Arsenic poisoning	Abdominal pain, GI symptoms, headache, exposure: hyperpigmentation, hepatic disease, weakness, alopecia	Delirium, psychosis	Urine heavy metal screen	Occupational exposure
Chronic hypoxia	Possible evidence of congestive heart failure	Confusion, fatigue, anxiety	Arterial blood gas, pulmonary function tests, chest x-ray	Multiple causes
Renal insufficiency	Peripheral neuropathy, signs of multisystem failure, seizure	Fatigue, mood changes, irritability, bizarre hallucinations, cognitive slowing	Serum electrolytes, CBC, urinalysis, renal imaging	Diabetes mellitus and hypertension most common causes

Continued

TABLE C.1   Medical Disorders and Commonly Associated Psychiatric Symptoms—cont'd

	Common Medical Presentation	Psychiatric Complaints	Diagnostic Tests	Comments
Cryptococcal meningitis	Headache, nausea, vomiting, ataxia, ocular changes	Personality change, confusion, lethargy, dementia	Head MRI or CT, CSF and serum cryptococcal antigen	Occurs in 5%–10% of HIV-infected patients; insidious onset
Giant cell arteritis/polyarteritis nodosa	Headache, joint and muscle pain, fever, vision loss, jaw claudication, polymyalgia	Depression, confusion, psychosis	Temporal artery biopsy	Rapid diagnosis and treatment may prevent blindness
Hepatic encephalopathy	Ataxia, asterixis, seizure, jaundice, fector hepaticus, confusion	Mood and sleep changes, agitation, confusion	Liver function tests, ammonia level	Avoid alcohol and hepatotoxic medications (Tylenol)
Hepatolenticular degeneration	Abdominal pain, hepatitis, Kayser-Fleischer rings	Mood and personality changes, psychosis, dementia	Serum and urinary copper, ceruloplasmin, slit-lamp examination	Autosomal dominant, hemolytic anemia
Herpes simplex virus	Seizure, anosmia	Gustatory and olfactory hallucinations, personality change, psychosis, Kluver-Bucy syndrome	CSF analysis, CT or MRI, EEG	Predilection for temporal and inferomedial frontal lobes
HIV infection	Fever, weight loss, lymphadenopathy, neurologic changes	Anxiety, depression, dementia	HIV serology and neurologic changes, CD4 count, Western blot, consider head imaging and CSF studies	CD4 < 600 associated with increased likelihood of psychiatric symptoms
Huntington disease	Dystonic posturing, rigidity, choreiform movements	Depression, euphoria, psychosis, personality changes	Test for Huntington gene	Autosomal dominant disease

Continued

Hyperadrenalism/ Cushing hypertension	Central obesity moon facies, striae, weakness, acne, diabetes, osteoporosis	Depression, mood liability, psychosis	Serum and urine cortisol, dexamethasone suppression test, imaging studies	Most common cause is iatrogenic syndrome
Hypercalcemia	Weakness, fatigue, constipation, anorexia, QT interval shortening, polyuria, renal stones, nausea, dyspepsia, soft tissue calcification	Depression, confusion	Serum calcium and parathyroid hormone	Multiple causes
Hyperglycemia	Polyuria, polydipsia, dehydration, weight loss	Agitation, delirium	Blood glucose	
Hypernatremia	Respiratory paralysis, seizures, coma	Somnolence, confusion	Serum sodium and urine osmolality	
Hyperdyspepsia	Hypercalcemia, weight loss, confusion, muscle weakness, bone pain, constipation	Depression, anxiety, irritability, psychosis	Serum calcium, phosphorus and parathyroid hormone	
Hyperthyroidism (thyrotoxicosis)	Tremor, weight loss, palpitations, warm moist skin, malaise	Anxiety, depression, irritability, insomnia, psychosis	Thyroid hormones, thyroid stimulation test, imaging studies	Rapid onset resembles anxiety; slow onset resembles depression
Hypoglycemia	Sweating, tachycardia, tremor, seizure	Anxiety, agitation, confusion	Blood glucose, serum and urine ketones	
Hypoparathyroidism	Hypocalcemia, dry skin, diarrhea congestive heart failure, numbness, tingling, tetany	Irritability, paranoia, depression, psychosis	Serum calcium, phosphorus and parathyroid hormone	Most common cause iatrogenic (postsurgical)

TABLE C.1 Medical Disorders and Commonly Associated Psychiatric Symptoms—cont'd

	Common Medical Presentation	Psychiatric Complaints	Diagnostic Tests	Comments
Hypothyroidism (myxedema)	Dry skin, coarse hair, cold intolerance, weight gain, anorexia	Fatigue, depression, anxiety, psychosis, personality change	Thyroid function tests (TSH, free T4, T3RIA), thyroid stimulation test, imaging studies	Slow onset resembles depression or sleep apnea
Intracranial tumor	Headache, vomiting, dementia, papilledema	Personality change, psychosis	Head CT or MRI, LP (after head imaging)	
Ischemic heart	Chest pain, heart failure, myocardial infarction	Anxiety panic, depression	Chest x-ray, electrocardiogram, stress test, coronary arteriography	Must differentiate from anxiety without cardiac disease
Lead poisoning	Abdominal pain, headache, seizures, focal neurologic signs	Irritability, delirium, GI symptoms, dementia	Serum and urine lead, blood smear for basophilic stippling	Children and persons with patient and industrial exposure most commonly affected
Limbic encephalitis	Agitation, possible fever, stereotyped movements in later stages, seizurelike behaviors, tachycardia	Confusion, disinhibition, maniclike symptoms, psychosis	Anti-NMDA antibodies in spinal fluid, abdominal CT for ovarian teratoma, MRI, EEG	Onset can mimic manic/psychotic episode
Lyme disease	Flulike symptoms, erythema migrans, encephalitis	Fatigue, irritability, confusion, labile mood, sleep disturbance, cognitive impairment	ELISA, Lyme Western blot, PCR assay or culture	Borrelia burgdorferi is the tick-borne spirochete
Mercury poisoning	Tremor, GI distress, dermatitis, sensorimotor impairments	Fatigue, anxiety, depression, irritability	Serum and urine mercury levels	

Continued

Mitral valve prolapse	Usually asymptomatic, arrhythmias, chest pain		Electrocardiogram	More common in women
Multiple sclerosis	Waxing and waning focal neurologic deficits, parenthesis, optic neuritis	Anxiety, panic, mood changes Chronic fatigue, memory impairment	White matter lesions on MRI, CSF assay for gamma globulins and oligoclonal bands	May be mistaken for somatization
Neurosyphilis	Headache, vertigo, Robertson Argyll pupils, stroke, dementia, ataxia, bladder disturbances, hyperreflexia	Insomnia, mood and personality changes, psychosis	CSF serology	
Niacin deficiency/ Pellagra	Diarrhea, peripheral neuropathy, angular stomatitis, glossitis, rash in sun-exposed skin, chronic wasting, encephalopathy, dementia	Insomnia, fatigue, irritability, anxiety and depressed mood	Urine N-methylnicotinamine or erythrocyte NAD/ NADP ratio	More common in alcoholics, refugee populations, vegetarians in less developed countries
Normal pressure hydrocephalus	Abnormal gait, urinary incontinence, dementia, psychomotor retardation, apathy	Dementia	Head CT or MRI	A treatable cause of dementia
Pancreatic carcinoma	Abdominal pain, weight loss, anorexia, nausea, vomiting	Depression, lethargy	Abdominal imaging, ERCP	Insidious onset
Pheochromocytoma	Paroxysmal hypertension, paroxysmal headache, sweating, palpitations, tachycardia	Anxiety, panic	24-hour urine assay for catecholamines, metanephrines, and vanillylmandelic acid	May have family history of the disorder

TABLE C.1   Medical Disorders and Commonly Associated Psychiatric Symptoms—cont'd

	Common Medical Presentation	Psychiatric Complaints	Diagnostic Tests	Comments
Prion disease	Myoclonic jerks, ataxia, seizures, intellectual decline	Mood lability, cognitive impairment, perceptual disturbances. Psychiatric symptoms are more prominent early	CT, MRI, EEG, CSF	Very rare, rapidly progressive fatal condition
Rabies	Parasthesias, fasiculations, confusion, encephalitis, coma	Psychosis, combativeness, hydrophobia	RT-PCR from saliva and skin biopsy, rabies antibody titers in CSF and serum	Transmitted via bite from an infected animal (often raccoons, foxes, skunks, bats)
Seizure disorder	Episodic staring, tonic-clonic jerking, automatisms, aura	Memory problems, personality changes, illusions and sensory hallucinations	Electroencephalogram	
SIADH	Lethargy, seizures, increased thirst, increased urination	Confusion, personality changes	Serum electrolytes (Na), serum and urine osmolarities	Can be secondary to psychiatric disorders or many medical disorders including CHF, CNS trauma/infection
Subdural hematoma	Headache, focal weakness	Irritability, confusion, hypersomnolence, dementia	Head CT or MRI	Precipitating trauma may be minor or not
Systemic lupus erythematosus	Arthritis, malar rash, lymphadenopathy, oral ulcers, photosensitivity	Depression, fatigue, psychosis, mania	ESR, ANA, serum complement levels	Female predominance 10:1; corticosteroid treatment may complicate psychiatric features

Condition	Physical signs	Psychiatric signs	Tests	Notes
Thiamine deficiency/Wernicke-Korsakoff syndrome	Neuropathy, ophthalmoplegia, confusion	Amnesia, confabulation	Thiamine level	Common in alcoholics, s/p bariatric surgery, prolonged malignancy, hyperemesis gravidarum
Tuberculosis	Fever, weight loss, headache, obtundation, meningeal signs	Lethargy, confusion	CSF assay for meningitis; CSF cultures; acid-fast bacteria	SIADH
Vitamin B12 deficiency	Ataxia, peripheral neuropathy, GI symptoms	Mood changes, anxiety, psychosis, dementia, fatigue	Serum B12 and folate, red cell indices	Pernicious anemia and bariatric surgery are common causes
Wilson disease	Liver disease, Kayser-Fleischer corneal rings, choreoathetosis, clumsiness	Behavior changes, decline in school performance	Low serum ceruloplasmin, increased copper in urine, liver function tests	Autosomal recessive disorder of copper metabolism; usually in adolescents

ANA, Antinuclear antibody; CBC, complete blood count; CHF, congestive heart failure; CNS, central nervous system; CT, computed tomography; CSF, cerebrospinal fluid; ERCP, endoscopic retrograde cholangiopancreatography; ESR, erythrocyte sedimentation rate; GI, gastrointestinal; HIV, human immunodeficiency virus; LP, lumbar puncture; MRI, magnetic resonance imaging; TSH, thyroid-stimulating hormone.

Data from Beck BJ. Mental disorders due to a general medical condition. In: Stern TA, Rosenbaum JF, Fava M, Biederman J, Rauch SL, eds. Comprehensive Clinical. 1st ed. Philadelphia, PA: Elsevier; 2008:257–281. Goldman L, Bennett JC, eds. Cecil Textbook of Medicine. 21st ed. Philadelphia, PA: WB Saunders; 2000; Fauci AS, Braunwald EB, Isselbacher KJ, et al., eds. Harrison's Principles of Internal Medicine. 14th ed. New York: McGraw-Hill; 1998; Sadock B, Sadock V, eds. Kaplan and Sadock's Synopsis of Psychiatry. 9th ed. Philadelphia, PA: Lippincott Williams & Wilkins; 2003; Wyszynski AA, Wyszynski B. A Case Approach to Medical-Psychiatric Practice. Washington, DC: American Psychiatric Press; 1996; Jenkins SC, Hansen MR. A Pocket Reference for Psychiatrists. 2nd ed. Washington, DC: American Psychiatric Press; 1995:76–88.

Neurologic Examination

The neurologic examination provides focused information regarding how a patient's nervous system is working and where problems may lie. A directed neurologic examination is indispensable for certain on-call situations and as a screen for patients to be admitted to an inpatient service. It can be done swiftly and does not always need to cover all the details listed here. It should be guided by the patient's history.

The neurologic examination consists of the following:

- Mental status
- Cranial nerves
- Motor
- Sensory
- Coordination
- Gait
- Reflexes

The *italicized* terms in parentheses indicate the most likely localizations for the deficits elicited by the tested function.

Mental Status

The mental status examination must be conducted in a systematic fashion. The neurologic exam portion of the mental status will focus on six hierarchical domains.

1. Level of Consciousness (*ascending reticular activating system in upper pons and midbrain, septal nuclei, hypothalamus, thalamus, cerebral cortex*):

    The level of consciousness of a patient can be described as states on the continuum from full alertness to deep coma:

    - **Alert** (self-awareness to external and internal stimuli, in other words, ability to interact in a meaningful manner with the examiner).
    - **Lethargy** (impaired awareness such that patient slowly drifts to drowsiness if not externally stimulated).
    - **Stupor** (vigorous or painful stimulus required for arousal).

- **Coma** (unresponsive drowsiness to any sort of external or internal painful stimulus).

  In addition to the aforementioned, you should also describe how the patient responds to various intensities of external stimulation and what the patient does upon the cessation of stimulus, because each of the previous states are qualitative and can encompass variable points on the continuum of consciousness.

  You may use the **Glasgow Coma Scale (GCS) in certain situations (e.g., traumatic brain injury [TBI])**, which measures three parameters and assigns points to each:

- Eye opening (spontaneous, 4; to voice, 3; to pain, 2; none, 1)
- Best motor response (obeys commands, 6; localizes to pain, 5; withdraws to pain, 4; flexor posturing, 3; extensor posturing, 2; none, 1)
- Best verbal response (conversant and oriented, 5; conversant and disoriented, 4; uses inappropriate words, 3; makes incomprehensible sounds, 2; none, 1)

  The final score is obtained by adding the points assigned to each parameter. This will help to determine the severity and prognosis from the injury. In general, a score ≥13 indicates mild TBI, 9 to 12 a moderate TBI, and ≤8 suggest severe TBI and worst prognosis. A score of 3 to 5 on the GCS correlates well with coma, a score of 7 to 8 with stupor, 12 to 14 with lethargy, and 15 with full alertness on the grade of levels of consciousness described previously.

2. Attention/Concentration *(frontal lobes):*

   This should be tested by having the patient perform a task that requires working memory, such as recite numbers by serially subtracting 7 from 100 (also tests for calculation), spell *WORLD* forward then backward, or recite a string of numbers backward and forward (6 to 7 forward and 4 to 5 backward is normal). For patients with low educational attainment, naming the months in a year or days in a week forward and backward is an equivalent test.

3. Orientation *(frontal, temporal lobes): Assessment of orientation is a test of attention and recent memory:*
   - Situation (related to insight)
   - Time: year, season, month, date, day of week
   - Place: type (hospital), name, city, floor, county
   - Person: governor, mayor, president, spouse, not self
   - General current events

4. Language *(dominant frontal and temporal lobes):*

   Specific deficits in language function can inform localization of brain pathology. These include aphasias in which there is a defect in higher-order integrative language function leading to errors of grammar and word choice secondary to brain pathology and should be differentiated from dysarthria (speech articulation dysfunction), apraxia, alexia, and other speech problems seen in dementia and schizophrenia.

- Fluency: Is the patient speaking swiftly with normal volume and flow of words, or is there a paucity of words and delay in producing speech?
- Comprehension: Can the patient follow commands and understand what is said?
- Repetition: Can the patient repeat short phrases or sentences ("no ifs, ands, or buts"; "today is a sunny day"; or "the spy fled to Greece")?
- Naming: Ask the patient to name both high-frequency (watch, table, pen, door) and low-frequency (watchband, watch face/crystal, clasp, lapel, cuff) words.

Other areas of language: During conversation, note the use of paraphasic errors—these may be phonemic, wherein one syllable is substituted for another (e.g., "pair" for "chair"), or semantic, wherein one word is replaced with a semantically related one (e.g., "car" for "bus")—clang associations, neologisms or inappropriate syntax, diction, prosody (the patterns of stress and intonation in a language), rate of speech, and volume of speech. The prosody of patients with a lesion to the nondominant parietal lobe is abnormal and may mimic the flat affect of patients with depression. In addition, the fluent, yet nonsensical, speech of a patient with a Wernicke aphasia may be confused with the disorganized speech patterns seen in some patients with schizophrenia (see the following table).

Classification of Aphasias

	Fluency	Comprehension	Naming	Repetition
Broca aphasia (motor)	0	+	0	0
Wernicke aphasia (sensory)	+	0	0	0
Transcortical motor aphasia	0	+	0	+
Transcortical sensory aphasia	+	0	0	+
Global aphasia	0	0	0	0

Conduction aphasia	+	+	+	0
Anomic aphasia	+	+	0	+
Mixed transcortical aphasia	0	0	0	+

0, abnormal; +, normal.

5. Memory *(mesial temporal, hippocampus):*
   Name three objects (an emotion, an object, and a place) and have the patient repeat them out loud 1 or 2 times. After 5 minutes, ask the patient to repeat the three objects; if the patient is unsuccessful, you may give multiple choice or other cues. Normally, a person should not need any cues.
6. Higher Cognitive Functions:
   Thought content/process, abstraction, insight, judgment, mood, and affect are all discussed earlier.
   - Praxis: the ability to execute learned/commanded behavior—such as "brush teeth" or "comb hair" *(dominant parietal)*
   - Visuospatial orientation: drawing pentagons/clock, cardinal directions *(nondominant parietal)*
   - Left-right confusion/crossing midline: "touch left ear with right thumb" *(dominant parietotemporal)*
   - Follow multistep commands: "point to the ceiling after touching your nose."

Differential Diagnosis of a Disorganized, Fluent, Rambling and Neologistic Speech

	Schizophrenia (Word Salad)	Dementia (Circumlocutory Speech)	Wernicke Speech (Fluent Jargon)
Age	Young	Older	Elderly
Vascular risk factors	Absent	May be present	Present
Onset	Chronic	Gradual onset	Acute
Paranoid delusions	Common and complex	Less common and simple (e.g., delusions of someone stealing personal items or spouse cheating with somebody)	Rare

Neologisms	Consistent and symbolic	Only seen in setting of word finding difficulties and associated with circumlocutory and paraphasic speech	Random and nonsymbolic
Comprehension	Intact	Intact	Impaired
Repetition	Intact	Intact	Impaired
Word naming	Intact but associated with disordered thought process	Impaired but less severe than aphasics and less bizarre than schizophrenics	Impaired with significant paraphasic errors

Cranial Nerves

I Olfactory: Test smell with nonnoxious agents (coffee, vanilla, or peppermint), especially for head trauma. Bilateral loss of smell sensation is seen in rhinitis, smoking, and aging, whereas unilateral loss is seen in peripheral lesions such as deviated nasal septum and meningioma *(frontal)*.

II Optic: Test for visual acuity (with Snellen chart), color vision *(optic nerve, occipital cortex, lens, retina)*, and visual fields *(retina, optic nerve, optic chiasm, optic tracts, lateral geniculate bodies, optic radiations, occipital lobes)* test in each eye separately. For visual fields, be sure to assess all regions—nasal, temporal, superior, and inferior—by confrontation (have the patient count fingers or identify a moving finger from the periphery).

- Also test for accommodation, direct and consensual pupillary response. Abnormalities include red color desaturation and afferent pupillary defect (tested on swinging flashlight test) seen in severe dysfunction of optic nerve.

III (Oculomotor), IV (Trochlear), and VI (Abducens) nerves: These nerves are tested together by having the patient look in all directions without moving their head (smooth pursuit). Saccades are fast conjugate movements of eyes in either direction *(contralateral frontal lobes)*. The III nerve is responsible for all extraocular movements except abduction and depression while the eye is adducted.

- Third nerve palsy is characterized by ptosis (drooping of an eyelid). Mydriasis (a fixed, dilated pupil) and depressed and abducted eye (due to unopposed action of IV and VI nerves) *(midbrain or third cranial nerve)*.

- The fourth cranial nerve intorts and depresses the eye in adduction. A IV nerve palsy would cause an inability to look down and in. Patients often try to compensate by tilting the head in contralateral side *(midbrain)*.

VI Cranial nerve is tested by abduction of the eyes. In VI nerve palsy, the affected eye appears adducted *(pontomedullary junction)*.

V Trigeminal: The trigeminal nerve is sensory in three divisions (V1, V2, V3) to the face. Use the pin/light touch test to assess the sensory function, evaluate bilateral motor function (muscles of mastication, masseters/pterygoid), and test reflexes (corneal and jaw jerk) (pons).

VII Facial: This nerve innervates the muscles of facial expression. Ask the patient to smile and raise eyebrows and look for asymmetries. The facial nerve also supplies the anterior two thirds of the tongue with taste sensation.
- If the forehead is involved (absence of forehead creases and inability of close eye), the lesion is peripheral or Bell palsy.
- If only the lower face is involved (flattening of the affected nasolabial fold and drooping of the lower face, inability to puff the cheek), the lesion is in central pathways *(contralateral frontal lobe)* (ipsilateral cerebellopontine angle, VII nerve).

VIII Vestibulocochlear: This nerve is responsible for hearing and vestibuloocular reflexes. Whisper multisyllabic words in each ear or rub the fingers by each ear with the patient's eyes closed *(cerebellopontine angle, VIII nerve)*.
- The Rinne and Weber tests (in which a tuning fork is struck and held directly on the frontal bone or in front of the auditory canal) can be used to differentiate hearing loss resulting from conduction abnormalities from hearing loss resulting from damage to the nerve itself.

IX Glossopharyngeal: This nerve raises the palate and is responsible for the gag reflex. Have the patient open the mouth wide and say "aah." Look for symmetric palatal rise and midline uvula. This nerve also supplies taste sensation to the posterior one third of the tongue.
- The uvula points to the side of the lesion *(medulla)*.

X Vagus: This nerve is responsible and testable for the same functions as cranial nerve IX and also for autonomic functions *(medulla)*.

XI Spinal accessory: Have the patient shrug the shoulder and turn the head, and look for weakness or asymmetry *(medulla)*.

XII Hypoglossal: This nerve is responsible for motor function of the tongue. Have the patient stick the tongue out and move it from side to side. The tongue tends to point to the side of the lesion and is slower or weaker in movements on the ipsilateral side of the lesion (*medulla*).

Motor

- Test for motor function by:
  1. Observing for posture and abnormal movements (tics, tremors, chorea, athetosis, myoclonus, dystonias, and dyskinesias) as well as for any slowness of movement.
  2. Inspection of muscles for any overt atrophy, hypertrophy, or fasciculations.
  3. Palpating for any tenderness and for assessing tone (normal vs. hypo/hypertonia).
  4. Functional testing of each group of muscles. Confrontational testing involves checking strength by providing resistance to active contraction and then comparing each muscle to the other side to note the difference.
     - **Graded system:** 5/5, normal full strength; 4/5, against resistance but not fully (may be 4+ or 4−); 3/5, against gravity but not resistance; 2/5, not against gravity but can move in plane perpendicular to vector of gravity; 1/5, flicker of contraction but no movement; 0/5, no contraction. Always compare one side with the other for each muscle at the time it is tested.
     - **Confrontational testing:** deltoids, biceps, triceps, wrist flexors/extensors, intrinsic hand muscles, iliopsoas (hip flexion), gluteus maximus (hip extension), quadriceps, hamstrings, thigh abductors/adductors, tibialis anterior (dorsiflexion/inversion of foot), gastrocnemius/soleus (plantarflexion of foot/toes), peronei (eversion of foot).
     - **Subtle testing for weakness:** pronator drift of outstretched arms with palms up (even a slight curl of the extended fingers is abnormal), fine finger movements, heel and toe walking, hopping on one foot (*peripheral nerve, plexus, nerve root, spinal cord, brainstem, internal capsule, corona, frontal*).
       - In functional weakness as seen in conversion disorder and malingering, patients often have "collapsing weakness" wherein the limb collapses with light touch, and variable effort on strength testing is seen with improvement on further encouragement.
- Tone can be checked by passive movement of limbs at joints (especially at wrist). It can be decreased in lower motor neuron lesions (e.g., spinal cord or peripheral nerve injuries) when it is called hypotonia or increased as in hypertonia. Hypertonia can be classified into spasticity (velocity dependent resistance to

motion) that is seen in upper motor neuron lesions of cortico-spinal tracts (as in strokes) and rigidity (resistance throughout the passive range of motion) seen in upper motor neuron lesions of extrapyramidal system (commonly seen in Parkinson disease). Patients with advanced dementia or catatonic patients have difficulty in relaxation and tend to exert more resistance against a passive movement despite normal tone. This phenomenon is called "paratonia" or "gegenhalten."

Sensory

The sensory exam is the most difficult part of a neurologic exam. It is subjective in nature and requires cooperation and attention on the part of the patient. Testing should be done by comparing dermatomes on both sides of the body and different areas on the same side of the body. For assessment, you should ask "Does it feel the same on both sides?" rather than "Which one feels sharper?"

There are four modalities: pain/temperature (pinprick) (contralateral spinothalamic system/tract), light touch, proprioception (joint position)/vibration (the posterior columns), and cortical (double simultaneous extinction [tactile/visual/auditory], stereognosis, graphesthesia) *(peripheral nerve, plexus, nerve root, spinal cord, brainstem, thalamus, parietal lobe)*.

- Patterns of sensory disturbances seen in disease state include hemisensory loss (cortical lesions), stocking glove sensory loss (neuropathy), spinal level and Brown Séquard syndrome (spinal cord lesions), dermatomal sensory loss (nerve root lesions), peripheral nerve sensory loss (mononeuropathy), and saddle anesthesia (lesion in cauda equina or conus medullaris).
- In functional sensory loss, patients can present with inconsistent sensory loss that does not obey dermatomal distribution and occasionally have midline splitting to pinprick and vibration.

Coordination

Test finger-nose-finger, rapid alternating movements, and heel-knee-shin for dysmetria. Test Romberg sign (by asking the patient to stand straight with feet together and eyes closed—be sure to take precautions that the patient does not fall), and look for nystagmus *(spinocerebellar tracts in spinal cord, cerebellum, thalamus, basal ganglia)*.

Gait

Test stance and walk, noting foot excursion off the ground, length and sureness of stride, ataxia, initiation, turning, and tandem (tightrope walking). *(May be multifactorial with contributors from nearly any of the previous systems.)*

- Certain gait disturbances are characteristic and diagnostic of neurologic disorders, for example the hemiplegic gait (dragging or circumduction of the affected leg with ipsilateral arm flexion) seen in stroke, and the short, shuffling gait with reduced arm swing in Parkinson disease. Patients with functional gait disorders tend to have slow initiation with cautious and decreased length stride, often falling towards or away from the examiner (the astasia abasia gait pattern).

Reflexes

- Testing for reflexes helps in localization of the pathology on the neuraxis.
  - **Graded system:** 0, no reflex; 1+, hyporeflexia; 2+, normal; 3+, hyperreflexia possibly with unsustained clonus; 4+, marked hyperreflexia with sustained clonus. Always compare both sides before moving to the next reflex.
  - **Deep tendon reflexes:** biceps (C5, C6), triceps (**C7**, C8), brachioradialis (C5, C6), patellar (L3, **L4**), Achilles (S1).
  - **Superficial reflexes:** abdominal (stroke lightly on the abdomen), cremasteric, plantar (Babinski: big toe goes up and rest of toes fan out).
  - **Other:** finger flexors (hyperreflexia if fingers have exaggerated flexion when tapped lightly on the palmar surface), Hoffman (hyperreflexia if thumb and forefinger flex when flicking the nail of the middle finger), jaw jerk (if exaggerated, will place lesion at the level of cranial nerve V in the brainstem or above).
    - For upper motor neuron signs (hyperreflexia, Babinski, spastic weakness), place the lesion above the conus medullaris of the spinal cord and in the CNS. For lower motor neuron signs (hyporeflexia, fasciculations, flaccid weakness), place the lesion distal to the conus or cord in the case of root or plexus lesions.
  - **Frontal release signs:** primitive reflexes are often seen if the frontal lobe is involved; glabellar (with tapping on forehead, patient cannot stop blinking even if asked); palmomental (stroking palm produces flexion of ipsilateral mentalis muscle); forced grasp (placing fingers between thumb and first finger, patient will grasp); root (patient will move lips to stimulus at corner of mouth); snout (tapping slightly on lips produces puckering).
- Of note, impaired pursuit eye movements are often seen in schizophrenia, which may indicate frontal lobe dysfunction. Tracking dysfunctions commonly occur in affective psychoses. High rates of catch-up saccades during eye tracking may be specific to schizophrenia.

Suggested Readings

Blumenfeld H. *Neuroanatomy Through Clinical Cases.* Sunderland, MA: Sinauer Associates; 2010.

Boks MP, Russo S, Knegtering R, van den Bosch RJ. The specificity of neurological signs in schizophrenia: a review. *Schizophr Res.* 2000; 43:109–116.

Flyckt L, Sydow O, Bjerkenstedt L, et al. Neurological signs and psychomotor performance in patients with schizophrenia, their relatives and healthy controls. *Psychiatry Res.* 1999;86:113–129.

Ismail BT, Cantor-Graae E, Cardenal S, McNeil TF. Neurological abnormalities in schizophrenia: clinical, etiological and demographic correlates. *Schizophr Res.* 1998;30:229–238.

Sharpe M, Stone J, Hibberd C, et al. Neurology out-patients with symptoms unexplained by disease: illness beliefs and financial benefits predict 1-year outcome. *Psychol Med.* 2010;40(4):689–698.

Strub RL, Black FW. *The Mental Status Examination in Neurology.* Philadelphia: FA Davis Co; 2000.

Urine Toxicology

TABLE E.1   Urine Toxicology Screen

Drug	Screening Cutoff Concentration (ng/mL)	Urine Detection Time[a]	Potential False Positives	Potential False Negatives
Alcohol	300,000	7–12 h	Short-chain alcohols	
Amphetamine and methamphetamine	1000	48 h	Many[b], notably: amantadine, bupropion, chlorpromazine, desipramine, ephedrine, labetalol, methylphenidate, phenylephrine, pseudoephedrine, ranitidine, selegiline, trazodone	3,4-Methylenedioxymethamphetamine (MDMA) (~50% lower sensitivity for MDMA)
Barbiturates	200			
Short acting		24 h		
Long acting		3 weeks		
Benzodiazepines	200		Oxaprozin, sertaline	Midazolam, chlordiazepoxide, flunitrazepam. Tends to be manufacturer specific[c].
Short acting		3 days		
Long acting		30 days		
Cocaine	300	1–3 days	Cross-reactivity is nearly nonexistent	Addition of eye drops to urine sample (benzalkonium chloride can act as a buffer)
Marijuana	50	Single use, 1–3 days	Dronabinol, efavirenz, hemp-containing foods, nonsteroidal antiinflammatory drugs (NSAIDs), proton pump inhibitors	
		Chronic use, >30 days		

Continued

TABLE E.1	Urine Toxicology Screen—cont'd			
Drug	Screening Cutoff Concentration (ng/mL)	Urine Detection Time[a]	Potential False Positives	Potential False Negatives
Opioids	2000		Dextromethorphan, diphenhydramine, poppy seeds, quinine, quinolones, rifampin, verapamil	Fentanyl, oxycodone[d]
Codeine		2 days		
Heroin		2 days		
Hydromorphone		2–4 days		
Morphine		2–3 days		
Oxycodone	300	2–4 days		
Methadone		3 days		
Phencyclidine	25	8 days	Dextromethorphan, diphenhydramine, doxylamine, ibuprofen, imipramine, ketamine, meperidine, mesoridazine, thioridazine, tramadol, venlafaxine	

[a]May vary widely depending on amount ingested, compound, physical state of subject, and other factors.

[b]Amphetamine urine drug screen is prone to false positives. In addition to those listed above, known potential false-positive results also includes: benzphetamine, clobenzorex, l-deprenyl, dextroamphetamine, fenproporex, isometheptene, isoxsuprine, methamphetamine, l-methamphetamine (Vicks inhaler), phentermine, phenylpropanolamine, promethazine, ritodrine, thioridazine, trimethobenzamide, trimipramine.

[c]Benzodiazepine detection varies with manufacturer. Primarily, commercial assays are based on detection of urinary metabolites oxazepam and nordiazepam; neither lorazepam nor clonazepam have these as urinary metabolites. This test does not detect newer hypnotics known as "z-drugs": zolpidem, zaleplon, and eszopiclone.

[d]To avoid false-positives from poppy seed ingestion, the urine screening detection limit was increased from 300 to 2000 ng/mL of morphine. Due to this, detection of opiate use is less sensitive. However, many clinical laboratories continue to use the lower cutoff.

Although ingestion of some foods and medications may result in positive preliminary tests, most medical centers use alternative methods to confirm positive screening results. Gas chromatography–mass spectrometry (GC-MS) is the most reliable, most definitive procedure for drug identification.

From Moeller KE, Lee KC, Kissack JC. Urine drug screening: practical guide for clinicians. *Mayo Clin Proc.* 2008;83(1):66–76.

Substance Detoxification Regimens

Alcohol Detoxification Regimens

Reminders:

- Early withdrawal signs/symptoms include headache, anxiety, sleep disturbance, anorexia, nausea, vivid dreams, tachycardia, elevated blood pressure, hyperactive reflexes, sweating, tremor, perceptual distortions.
- In more severe withdrawal, hallucinations (visual most common) may occur, with or without other symptoms.
    - In 90% of patients, withdrawal is mild or moderate and peaks between 24 and 36 hours.
    - In 10% of patients, withdrawal symptoms progress to a life-threatening delirium with an autonomic storm (delirium tremens [DTs]).
- Provide thiamine by oral supplementation (e.g., 100 to 250 mg daily) for several weeks to prevent Wernicke disease and Korsakoff psychosis, both with and without glucose loading as needed.
- Be alert for needing a higher level of care in patients with high daily use or history of severe withdrawal.
- Patients with seizures or DTs should be in a monitored or intensive care unit (ICU)–level setting.

REGIMEN 1: SYMPTOM-TRIGGERED THERAPY

- Is as effective as fixed-dose therapy (later) but leads to less medication use overall, reduces overtreatment, and significantly shortens treatment duration.
- Monitor the patient every 4 to 8 hours using CIWA-Ar (Clinical Instrument Withdrawal Assessment for Alcohol—revised version) until score has been less than 8 to 10 for 24 hours

(CIWA-Ar, a score of <9 is mild, 10 to 18 is moderate, and >18 severe withdrawal).
- Administer one of the following medications when CIWA-Ar is greater than 8 to 10:
  - Chlordiazepoxide 25 to 100 mg PO; these doses may be repeated hourly
  - Diazepam 5 to 10 mg IV every 5 to 10 minutes (presence of active metabolites ensure long-acting benzodiazepine (BZD) coverage; be on lookout for oversedation and respiratory depression)
  - Lorazepam 2 to 4 mg IV every 15 to 20 minutes (preferable if hepatic insufficiency)
  - Other benzodiazepine at equivalent substitution
- Repeat CIWA-Ar at appropriate intervals for chosen medication to assess need for further medication. Increasing CIWA-Ar scores are an indication to reevaluate your treatment plan and consider transferring the patient to a higher level of care.

REGIMEN 2: FIXED-DOSE THERAPY

- Useful if:
  - Ward where staff are not trained in CIWA-Ar or other scales.
  - Patients with known history of withdrawal seizures or other symptoms with high morbidity as fewer symptoms manifest.
  - Patient with acute medical or surgical complications to avoid the stress of symptomatic detox.
- Sample protocols:
  - Chlordiazepoxide 50 mg PO every 6 hours for four doses and then 25 mg q 6 hours for eight doses.
  - Diazepam 10 mg IV every 6 hours for four doses and then 5 mg IV q 6 hours for eight doses.
  - Lorazepam 2 mg IV every 6 hours for four doses and 1 mg IV q 6 hours for eight doses.
- More severe withdrawal may require starting doses at 50% to 100% higher than listed previously, with more gradual taper. Provide additional medication as needed (PRN) for breakthrough symptoms.

Sedative-Hypnotic Detoxification Regimens

Reminders:
- Time and severity of sedative-hypnotic (i.e., benzodiazepines, barbiturates, and nonbenzo/barbiturate agents) withdrawal syndrome are influenced by dose, duration of use, and duration

of drug action (i.e., half-life). Clinical syndromes and time of onset are highly variable.

- Longer periods of higher daily use predict more likelihood of severe withdrawal; however, even short periods of use cause habituation.
- Similar symptoms to alcohol withdrawal but can progress quickly to delirium and confusion without tremor or seizure and can present with psychosis.
- Evidence of delirium should prompt treating patient in a monitored setting such as ICU.
- The Clinical Instrument Withdrawal Assessment for Benzodiazepines (CIWA-B) is a 22-item scale based on the CIWA-Ar and is currently undergoing validation. It, along with the Benzodiazepine Withdrawal Symptom Questionnaire (BWSQ), can be useful aids in tracking symptom response to treatment.

REGIMEN 1: SLOW TAPER (OUTPATIENT)

- Taper existing total daily dose in a fixed schedule, decreasing dose by 10% per week.
- Last ¼ of taper should be slower as anxiety will increase.
- Difficult to do with short half-life agents such as alprazolam.

REGIMEN 2: SUBSTITUTION AND TAPER

- Use cross-tolerant long-acting benzodiazepine at equivalent daily dose and taper similar to alcohol protocols.
- Examples: chlordiazepoxide or clonazepam. The selected drugs have consistent serum levels at steady state, therefore reducing emergence of withdrawal symptoms.
- Phenobarbital may be preferable in patients with multiple drugs of dependence and high dose-dependence but should be used with caution.

Opioid Detoxification Regimen

Reminders:
- Opioid withdrawal progresses through two phases: acute withdrawal and protracted abstinence syndrome.
  - Acute withdrawal generally begins within 4 to 6 hours of the last dose of heroin (short half-life) and up to 36 hours after the last dose of methadone or continuous release synthetic opiates (longer half-life).
  - Withdrawal signs and symptoms include gastrointestinal distress, insomnia, muscle and joint pain, anxiety, dysphoria, poor thermoregulation, and piloerection.
  - Unless comorbid medical problems or comorbid benzodiazepine/alcohol abuse is present, opiate withdrawal is not

usually life-threatening. Protracted and severe vomiting or diarrhea could potentially cause metabolic derangement.

- For accurate characterization of withdrawal symptoms, perform a brief physical exam and use a standardized symptom measurement tool, such as the COWS (Clinical Opiate Withdrawal Scale).
- Symptomatic treatments including antinausea agents, ibuprofen, and clonidine can augment withdrawal treatment.
- Long-standing methadone maintenance patients will require much longer taper.

REGIMEN 1: METHADONE TAPER

- WARNING: Methadone should NOT be used in patients with a QTc > 500.
- Overdose of methadone can be lethal and should be reversed by using 0.4 to 0.8 mg naloxone with repeated doses as necessary and transfer to an MICU.
- Because of methadone's long half-life, it should be dosed cautiously over the first 24 hours as it will accumulate faster than it is eliminated.
- After physical signs of withdrawal begin to appear as assessed by a standardized measure (such as the Clinical Opiate Withdrawal Scale, COWS), may give up to 20 mg methadone in initial dose and reassess after 2 hours, dose again and repeat until symptoms controlled. Do not exceed 40 mg over the first 24 hours.
- Find the dose at which the patient's symptoms are stabilized. Then after day 2 taper methadone by 20% per day for inpatients (for outpatients, may taper by 5% per day, or even 3% per week for very gradual detoxification).

REGIMEN 2: CLONIDINE DETOXIFICATION

- Clonidine is an alpha-2 adrenergic agonist that is helpful for reducing autonomic symptoms, such as rhinorrhea, anxiety, sweating, and gastrointestinal (GI) distress. It is less helpful for myalgias, insomnia, and cravings.
- Benefits include lack of potential for physical dependence and shorter detoxification period; negatives include more likely relapse.
- To initiate, abruptly stop opioids and check blood pressure to make sure it is at or above 90/60, pulse is greater than 60, and there is no orthostatic hypotension.
- Dose clonidine 0.1 mg × 1 dose, then check Clinical Opiate Withdrawal Scale (COWS) and blood pressure parameters,

and if symptoms remain prominent (COWS > 8), can administer additional 0.1 mg dose and repeat every 45 to 60 min up to 4 doses. After this, dose 0.1 mg to 0.3 mg every 6 hours based on COWS score. Total daily dose should not exceed 0.8 mg/day (or 1.2 mg/day if patient is 200 lbs or more). Monitor blood pressure closely as hypotension is a prominent side effect.

- For day 2 through day 4, the total daily dose from day 1 is divided into 3 or 4 doses per day.
- By day 5 to 7, if symptoms are minimal, taper may begin by decreasing the dose by 0.1 to 0.2 mg daily to avoid rebound hypertension, headache, and reemergence of withdrawal symptoms.

Suggested Readings

Dickinson W, Eickelberg S. Management of sedative-hypnotic intoxication and withdrawal. In: Ries R, ed. *The ASAM Principles of Addiction Medicine*. 5th ed. New York, NY: Wolters Kluwer; 2014:652–667.

Tetrault J, O'Connor P. Management of opioid intoxication and withdrawal. In: Ries R, ed. *The ASAM Principles of Addiction Medicine*. 5th ed. New York, NY: Wolters Kluwer; 2014:668–684.

Wartenberg A. Management of alcohol intoxication and withdrawal. In: Ries R, ed. *The ASAM Principles of Addiction Medicine*. 5th ed. New York, NY: Wolters Kluwer; 2014:635–651.

Wilkins J, Danovitch I, Gorelick D. Management of stimulant, hallucinogen, marijuana, phencyclidine, and club drug intoxication and withdrawal. In: Ries R, ed. *The ASAM Principles of Addiction Medicine*. 5th ed. New York, NY: Wolters Kluwer; 2014:685–704.

Wright T, Cluver J, Myrick H. Management of intoxication and withdrawal: general principles. In: Ries R, ed. *The ASAM Principles of Addiction Medicine*. 5th ed. New York, NY: Wolters Kluwer; 2014:625–634.

Abuse and Neglect of Children and Elders

Child Abuse and Neglect

Child abuse, as defined by the Child Abuse Prevention and Treatment Act (CAPTA), is "any recent act or failure to act resulting in death, serious physical or emotional harm, sexual abuse, or exploitation involving a child, by a parent or caretaker (including any staff providing out-of-home care) who is responsible for the child's welfare." In the United States in 2014, 700,000 incidents of child abuse were substantiated out of a total of 3.6 million referrals involving 6.6 million children and resulted in 1500 fatalities. Diagnostic evaluation of a suspected victim of child abuse must include a determination of whether the index of suspicion is high enough to report to Child Protective Services (CPS). Although serious consequences can result from an unsubstantiated report of abuse, the risks associated with failure to report are far more grave. An abused child is at a 50% risk of being abused again. Parental risk factors for child abuse include young age, low educational attainment, single status, and substance abuse. Child risk factors include minority status, former prematurity, congenital anomalies, mental retardation, hyperactivity, adoption, stepchild status, and age younger than 3 years. Parents are the perpetrators in greater than 75% of cases of abuse, and greater than half (54% in 2014) of perpetrators are female.

Child abuse is rarely the chief complaint to the on-call psychiatrist during a child's presentation. The pediatrician providing medical care may discover physical injuries inconsistent with the presenting complaint or history provided by the parents or other adults. A detailed history and a careful examination inform initial suspicion of abuse. All available collaterals should be questioned. A vague and changing history provided by a caretaker or one inconsistent with the developmental stage of the child should raise concern.

Obtaining a verbal history directly from the child may be difficult. If the child is old enough to speak, the on-call psychiatrist should begin with open-ended questions, aimed at the child initially, with the parents present. Interaction between parent and child should be observed; verbal or physical hostility or the absence of touching and eye contact may raise suspicion of parental abuse of the child. If abuse is suspected, a request to interview the child alone should be made because the child may resist providing information in the presence of the caretaker secondary to fear of retribution by the abuser. Most parents will consent to a child being interviewed alone. Refusal should be documented in the chart and may raise suspicion. The use of dolls or drawing during the interview is often helpful.

Physical examination of the child should include an observation of his or her attire for cleanliness and appropriateness for size, season, and situation. A complete examination should follow after removing all the child's clothes, which can be done sequentially. The torso can be exposed while the extremities are still covered. One common physical clue is a bathing-suit pattern of bruises, so-called because of a distribution that is not apparent to a casual observer.

A complete laboratory evaluation should be performed, including a complete blood count (anemia may reflect neglect and nutritional deprivation), basic chemistries, and coagulation studies (if bleeding is present). Elevated liver and pancreatic enzymes may reflect damage to these organs. In addition, toxicology screening and a thorough radiologic evaluation geared toward the presenting symptoms may be necessary.

Child abuse will not always be the result of violence or neglect. Some parents or caretakers cause medical illnesses in children (i.e., Munchausen syndrome by proxy, or factitious disorder imposed on another [*Diagnostic and Statistical Manual of Mental Disorders*, 5th Edition (DSM-5)]).

All states require physicians to report suspicion of child neglect or abuse to the CPS, but definitions of child abuse and reporting procedures vary. Most hospitals have a child abuse team that should be contacted if there is a suspicion of child abuse and can assist with the decision to report to the CPS. If no such team is available, each state has a "hotline" phone number run by the agencies designated to receive and investigate reports of child abuse and neglect; this information can be found at the website https://www.nccafv.org/child-abuse-reporting-numbers. Hospitalization is indicated for a child if it is deemed unsafe for him or her to return to the care of the guardian or if further information must be collected.

The National Clearinghouse on Child Abuse and Neglect (https://www.childwelfare.gov/) can provide additional resources and information, including state-specific abuse definitions, reporting procedures, and services.

Elder Abuse and Neglect

Elder abuse and neglect has several definitions which continue to evolve; the Centers for Disease Control and Prevention (CDC), along with a group of elder abuse experts, have released guidelines defining elder abuse as the "intentional act or failure to act by a caregiver or another person in a relationship involving an expectation of trust that causes or creates a serious risk of harm to an older adult." Abuse can be approximately divided into categories of physical, sexual, and psychological abuse or neglect; financial exploitation; self-abuse or self-neglect; and abandonment. Each of these categories, including signs and symptoms, will be discussed.

Elder abuse been estimated to occur in 10% of people older than 65 years. According to one study, up to 550,000 older Americans are abused each year, but only one-fifth of those cases are documented and reported. Patients with cognitive and functional disability are most vulnerable to abuse and neglect; a 2009 study found that nearly 50% of patients with dementia experience some form of elder abuse. Physicians on call or in the emergency room are the most likely to encounter patients suffering from abuse and neglect, so their ability to recognize the condition and provide resources is significant.

Abuse or neglect is rarely the chief complaint to the on-call psychiatrist at presentation. Pay attention to the interaction between the patient and the caregiver. Be alert to inconsistencies between the history given by the patient and the caregiver, and be wary of caregivers who do not allow a patient to be examined or interviewed out of their presence. Suspicion should be raised in a patient with a history of missed appointments, poor medication compliance, or poor activities of daily living, even though such signs are not specific for abuse. Elders at high risk for abuse and neglect include those with a functional, medical, or cognitive disability and those whose disability is worsening, leading to increased caregiver stress. Other risk factors include female gender, low socioeconomic status, past traumatic experience, and living with a large number of household members other than a spouse. The highest proportion of elder abusers are adult children of elderly parents. Spouses, grandchildren, paid caregivers, staff, and visitors to other patients in a hospital or institutional setting should also be considered when abuse is suspected. Caregivers with emotional, psychiatric, financial, legal, or substance abuse problems are at higher risk to commit elder abuse or neglect, especially when the caregiver is an adult child who is dependent on the elderly parent.

The on-call physician is most likely to encounter the following signs and symptoms of abuse and neglect, either at the bedside or in the emergency room. Importantly for the on-call psychiatrist, these forms of abuse may manifest themselves as depression or anxiety in the patient. In addition, assertions by the patient of any type of abuse or neglect should be taken seriously and investigated. Patients with dementia may be capable of expressing signs or reporting symptoms of abuse or neglect; elderly patients' reports should not be discounted—nor should patients not be questioned—due to cognitive impairment.

Physical Abuse

Physical abuse involves force leading to bodily injury, pain, or physical impairment, including acts of violence, physical punishment, inappropriate use of physical or chemical restraints, inappropriate use or withholding of medications, and force feeding or withholding of nutrients or fluids.

Signs and symptoms include the following:

- Bruises at different stages of healing
- Burns
- Lacerations
- Bone fractures
- Untreated injuries
- Evidence of use of restraints
- Laboratory findings consistent with dehydration
- Excessive or inappropriately low use of medication
- Sudden change in behavior
- Delirium
- Report by the patient of being mistreated
- Refusal by the caregiver to allow access to the patient

Sexual Abuse

Sexual abuse involves any nonconsensual sexual contact, including contact involving an individual who is not competent to provide consent to such contact. Physicians sometimes wrongly discount an elderly patient's report that they are being sexually abused, attributing this to delusions in a patient with dementia.

Signs and symptoms include the following:

- Bruising, abrasions, or bite marks on the breasts, genitals, or buttocks
- Unexplained vaginal/anal bleeding or lacerations
- Unexplained or newly acquired sexually transmitted infections
- Urinary tract infections
- Report by the patient of being sexually assaulted

Emotional Abuse

Emotional abuse involves infliction of emotional pain or distress via verbal or nonverbal acts. This can include verbal abuse, intimidation or humiliation, harassment, and isolating the patient via enforced social isolation or verbal withdrawal.

Signs and symptoms include the following:
- Emotional lability or agitation
- Flat, withdrawn affect
- Regressive behaviors, such as rocking and sucking
- Hypervigilance or excessive fearfulness
- Subtle signs of intimidation, such as deferring questions to a caregiver

Neglect

Neglect involves either intentional or inadvertent failure to provide necessary care for an elder, including failing to provide food, clothing, shelter, medication, a clean body and clothing, and an appropriate living environment. This may involve either a service provider such as a home attendant or a family member.

Signs and symptoms include the following:
- Dehydration or malnutrition
- Poor personal hygiene
- Untreated health problems such as decubitus ulcers
- Nonadherence to medication regimen
- Urine, feces, and/or dirt on patient and/or patient's clothing
- Attire that is inappropriate for the season
- Evidence or a patient's report of inadequate living conditions, including lack of heat, air conditioning, and running water

Financial Exploitation

Financial exploitation refers to the misuse of an elder person's assets or property. Although matters relating to financial exploitation may not be likely to come up while on call, you should be alert to warning signs of financial exploitation by a caretaker or relative of an elderly patient.

Signs include the following:
- An elder patient's allegation of financial exploitation
- Evidence of poor financial decision making or changes in financial patterns
- Forged or altered patient signature
- Provision of unneeded services
- Unexplained disappearance of valuables
- Inability to pay for medicine, medical care, food, rent, or other necessities
- Nonadherence to medical treatment

Self-Neglect and Self-Abuse

Self-neglect and self-abuse refer to the inability of an elderly person to maintain adequate self-care, jeopardizing his or her health or safety. The signs and symptoms parallel those for neglect or abuse by someone other than the elder. In this situation, homelessness or a severely inadequate or dangerous living arrangement may also be considered an indicator of self-neglect or self-abuse.

However, as with other situations involving assessment of danger to self, the person being evaluated must be deemed mentally incompetent to be legally regarded as self-neglecting or self-abusive. This is different from a capacity evaluation, which is in response to specific treatment decisions. Nonetheless, if you are concerned about a patient, you should strongly consider encouraging the patient to accept additional consultations (e.g., from a social worker or substance abuse counselor).

Abandonment

An elderly person is considered abandoned if he or she has been deserted by someone—either a family member or other caregiver—who was previously providing essential care. Frequent sites for abandonment include emergency rooms, public areas such as parks or stores, hospitals, and nursing facilities.

If You Suspect Elder Abuse or Neglect

Criteria for elder abuse are currently defined by state laws, and these laws can vary widely. Nonetheless, most states have mandatory laws regarding reporting even suspected abuse. All 50 states and the District of Columbia have some type of adult protective services (APS) to facilitate the reporting, investigating, and reduction of elder abuse. Because APS service provisions are voluntary (unless the patient is determined to lack capacity), patients must provide consent for treatment and should be included in decision making as much as possible. In addition, the least restrictive option should be chosen. Patients also are allowed to withdraw from the program.

In a hospital setting, if abuse is suspected, the social work department can usually provide assistance in reporting potential abuse and in determining what, if anything, must be done to ensure safety for those at risk. As with child abuse, when elder abuse is suspected, the safety of the patient is primary.

For a referral to a state agency if abuse and/or neglect is suspected: Call National Eldercare Locator at 1-800-677-1116 (Monday to Friday 9 a.m. to 8 p.m. Eastern time), run by the US Department of Health and Human Services (HHS).

To locate an adult protection service (for domestic abuse/neglect) or an ombudsperson (for nursing home and other institutional abuse) in any state, log on to www.eldercare.gov.

Suggested Readings

Acierno R, Hernandez MA, Amstadter AB, et al. Prevalence and correlates of emotional, physical, sexual, and financial abuse and potential neglect in the United States: the National Elder Mistreatment Study. *Am J Public Health.* 2010;100(2):292–297. https://doi.org/10.2105/AJPH.2009.163089.

American Psychiatric Association. *Diagnostic and Statistical Manual of Mental Disorders.* 5th ed. Arlington, VA: American Psychiatric Publishing; 2013.

Dong X, Chen R, Simon MA. Elder abuse and dementia: a review of the research and health policy. *Health Aff (Millwood).* 2014;33:642–649.

Friedman B, Santos EJ, Liebel DV, Russ AJ, Conwell Y. Longitudinal prevalence and correlates of elder mistreatment among older adults receiving home visiting nursing. *J Elder Abuse Negl.* 2015;27(1):34–64. https://doi.org/10.1080/08946566.2014.946193.

Hall JE, Karch DL, Crosby AE. *Elder abuse surveillance: uniform definitions and recommended core data elements for use in elder abuse surveillance, version 1.0.* Atlanta, GA: National Center for Injury Prevention and Control, Centers for Disease Control and Prevention; 2016.

Harrell R, Toronjo CH, McLaughlin J, et al. How geriatricians identify elder abuse and neglect. *Am J Med Sci.* 2002;323:34–38.

Lachs M, Pillemer K. Elder abuse. *N Engl J Med.* 2015;373:1947–1956. https://doi.org/10.1056/NEJMra1404688.

Laumann E, Leitsch S, Waite L. Elder mistreatment in the United States: prevalence estimates from a nationally representative study. *J Gerontol B Psychol Sci Soc Sci.* 2008;63(4):S248–S254.

Peterson J, Burnes D, Caccamise P, et al. Financial exploitation of older adults: a population-based prevalence study. *J Gen Intern Med.* 2014;29(12):1615–1623. https://doi.org/10.1007/s11606-014-2946-2.

Quinn K, Benson W. The states' elder abuse victim services: a system in search of support. *Generations.* 2012;36(3):66–71.

U.S. Department of Health & Human Services, Administration for Children and Families, Administration on Children, Youth and Families, Children's Bureau. Child Maltreatment 2014. 2016. Available from http://www.acf.hhs.gov/programs/cb/research-data-technology/statistics-research/child-maltreatment.

Index

Note: Page numbers followed by *t* refer to tables; *b*, boxes.